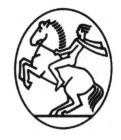

Wolfgang Seeger

Microsurgery of the Cranial Base

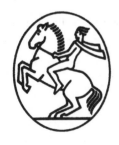

Springer-Verlag Wien New York

Prof. Dr. med. WOLFGANG SEEGER
Medical Director of the Department of General Neurosurgery
and Chairman of Neurosurgery of the Neurosurgical Clinic,
University of Freiburg i. Br., Federal Republic of Germany

With 200 Figures

© 1983 by Springer-Verlag/Wien
Softcover reprint of the hardcover 1st edition 1983

Design: Hans Joachim Böning, Wien

Library of Congress Cataloging in Publication Data. Seeger, Wolfgang, 1929–   . Microsurgery of the cranial base. 1. Basicranium-Surgery. 2. Microsurgery. I. Title. RD529.S44. 1983. 617'.514. 83-14652.

ISBN 978-3-7091-3090-2   ISBN 978-3-7091-3088-9 (eBook)
DOI 10.1007/978-3-7091-3088-9

Preface

The preceding volumes having considered micro-surgery of the brain as well as microsurgery of the Medulla spine, with its surrounding structures, it then seemed logical to cover microsurgery of the areas near the brain. In addition to daily work at the operation table, the increasing experience of the University of Freiburg Neurosurgical Hospital in the bordering areas of ophthalmology and ENT was stimulating. Of significance was the work with Prof. Dr. Renate Unsöld, Freiburg University Ophthalmological Hospital (Director: Prof. Dr. G. Mackensen) whose experience, published together with C. B. Ostertag, J. DeGroot, and T. H. Newton in "Computer Reformations of the Brain and Skull Base" offered valuable diagnostic ideas. Some of the findings attributed to Prof. Dr. R. Unsöld and Doz. Dr. C. B. Ostertag are again covered here. I thank Prof. Dr. Chl. Beck, Director of University Freiburg ENT-Hospital, for his critical review of the chapter on oro-nasal hypophysis approach. Special appreciations go to my colleagues Doz. Dr. J. M. Gilsbach, Dr. H. R. Eggert, Dr. W. Hassler, and Dr. E. Gröbner for suggestions and assistance in providing literature. Several anatomical preparations were made possible with the help of Prof. Dr. N. Boehm, Deputy Direc-tor of Freiburg University Institute of Pathology and Prof. Dr. J. Staubesand, Director of Freiburg Univer-sity Anatomical Institute I. The translation of the text was undertaken by my colleague, Dr. E. Gröbner, and Mrs. S. Godine, Freiburg. I am grateful to Mrs. E. Hilsenbeck-Hottek for typing the manuscript.
Once again I am especially grateful to Dr. W. Schwabl, and his colleagues, of the Springer-Verlag, Wien and New York, who have published this exten-sive work with their usual speed, generous presenta-tion and precision.

Freiburg, October 1983   Wolfgang Seeger

Contents

Introduction

Operations in the skull base area are performed by neurosurgeons, ear-nose- and throat physicians and ophthalmologists, as well as by facial surgeons, since the skull base is characterized as a transition area of intracranial space, sinuses and orbitae. In this volume the areas of neurosurgical interest to be covered are basically limited to intra- and extradural relations of dura, cranial nerves and brain. Some of these operative procedures may be carried out in cooperation with colleagues in related fields, as when sinuses or orbitae are opened. Other operations, for example those in the area of A. carotis int. path within Os petrosum, are left completely to specialists in other fields, since the neurosurgeon rarely has sufficient experience in the problematic anatomical topographical relations of the skull base.

A few neurosurgical procedures are not dealt with in this volume, since the author has insufficient personal operative experience in these areas; for example, Glomus tumors of Foramen jugulare and aneurysms of A. basilaris or vertebralis are covered neither in the volume "Microsurgery of the Brain" nor in the present volume. Other operations, relating to but not strictly limited to the skull base, were included because of their great clinical importance, such as extra-intracranial bypass operations. It seemed unsuitable to expand this volume to include processes of the skull convexity and/or convexity dura, since a later volume will cover microsurgical operations in the area of cerebral veins, giving special attention to skull and brain convexity. This volume is already in preparation. The present volume is composed along guide-lines similar to previous volumes. Drawings were done by the author this time as well, since it is impossible to find an artist capable of making drawings from the author's extremely detailed operation sketches, even given years' time. The technical quality of the drawings is less important than providing as detailed as possible microsurgical information. In this connection may I mention that, in this volume as well, only the anatomical structures are enlarged to scale; this scale does not apply to the instruments, usually sketched on a smaller scale. In reality (and contrary to the drawings) the instruments cover a large area of the operation site; therefore a realistic presentation such as photography has less didactic value than these sketches. The author's mode of presentation is justified since this book does not seek to document specific operations. Rather, as in previous volumes, it seeks through individual cases to assist the neurosurgeon who is in training and/or especially interested in microsurgery in his understanding of the anatomical structures of the operation site and, together with his already assimilated anatomical knowledge, to improve his operative technique.

FIG. 1 ═══════════════════════════════════════ 2

Chapter 1
Oronasal Hypophysis Operations
(Figs. 1 to 49)

Fig. 1. Special anatomical features and special techniques of hypophysis operations
Vestibulum oris, varying topographical **relations to Apertura piriformis** (broken-lines) in 5 normal individuals of various age groups

a Distance of Apertura piriformis from juncture of Gingiva and Labium sup.

b Distance between first incisor and juncture of Vestibulum oris or between toothless Processus alveolaris sup. and Vestibulum oris (**C**)

Abbreviations:

(api)   Apertura piriformis (projection)

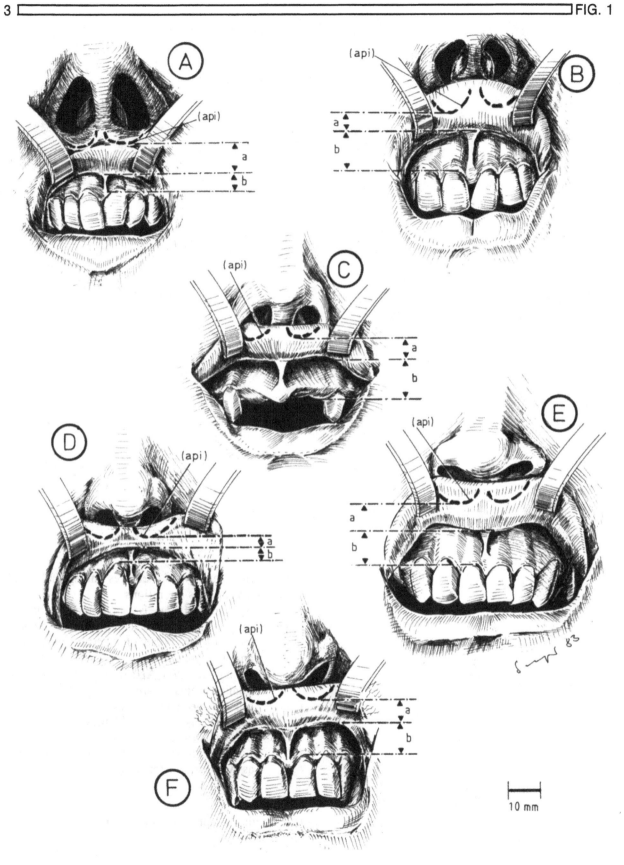

FIG. 2 [=================================] 4

Fig. 2. Special anatomical features and special techniques of hypophysis operations

A – F   **Apertura piriformis,** anatomical variants. Section lines **c** and **d** see Fig. 3, note varying width of lower half of Apertura piriformis and its asymmetries

G + G'   Upper area of Apertura piriformis with Lamina mediana –*lm*–

G   **Lamina mediana** reaches as far as anterior edge of nasal bone and thus to Apertura piriformis (arrow)

G'   Lamina mediana –*lm*– does not reach as far as Apertura piriformis (arrow)

Abbreviations:

(cs)   Cartilago septi nasi (projection)
lm   Lamina mediana

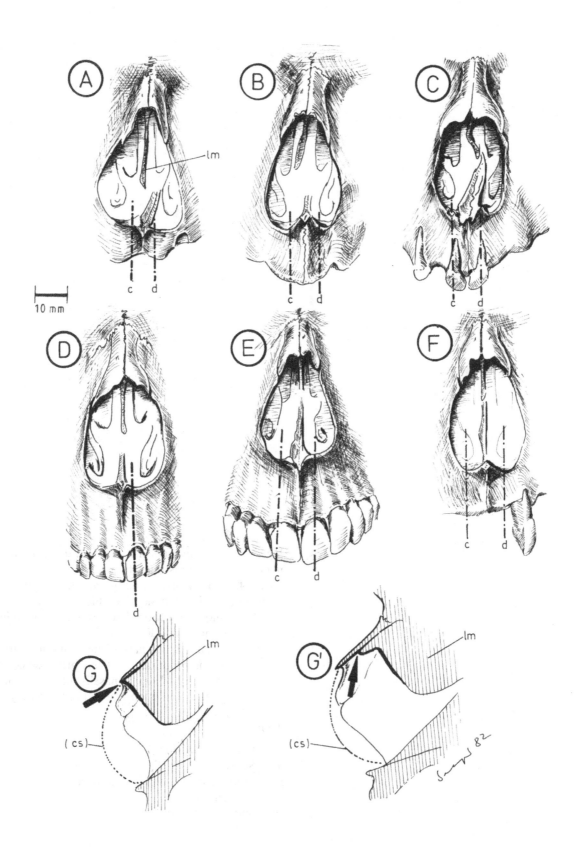

FIG. 3 ⬚ 6

Fig. 3. Special anatomical features and special techniques of hypophysis operations

Floor of nasal cavity. Parasagittal section planes **c** (right side) and **d** (left side) see Fig. 2

A' – F'   Showing section sketches of the anatomical samples **A – F** of Fig. 2

Behind Spina nasalis ant. Palatum durum –*p*– is prominent. At this prominence the mucosa of Meatus nasalis inf. may tear if preparation is not carried out carefully

Abbreviations:

c   Section right, Fig. 2
d   Section left, Fig. 2
p   Prominent area of Palatum durum
pd   Palatum durum
spa   Spina nasalis ant.

FIG. 3

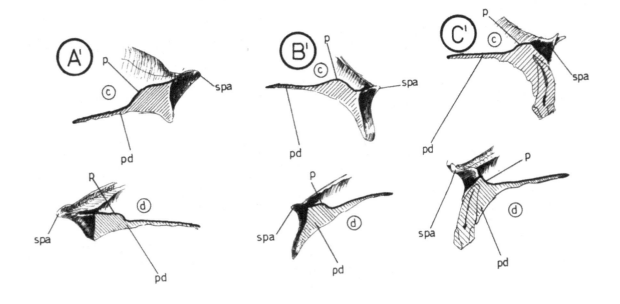

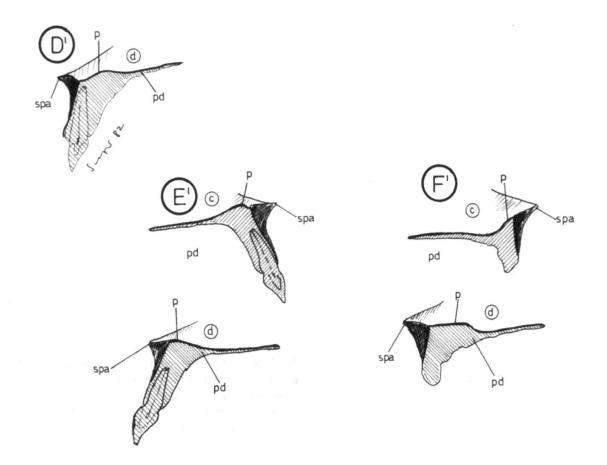

FIG. 4 ⌐━━━━━━━━━━━━━━━━━━━━━━━━⌐ 8

Fig. 4. Special anatomical features and special techniques of hypophysis operations
Spina nasalis ant., variants
Five skeletal samples with varying widths and asymmetries of Spina nasalis ant. and adjoining areas of Vomer

FIG. 4

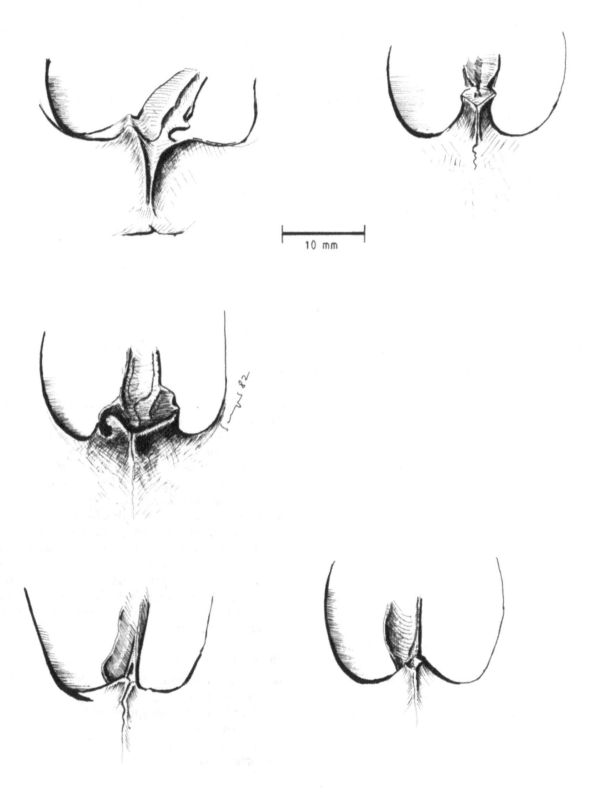

10 mm

FIG. 5 ⊏⊐ 10

Fig. 5. Special anatomical features and special techniques of hypophysis operations

Septum nasi, sample. Slight bony asymmetry, more extensive asymmetry of cartilage *–(cs)–*

A Bone preparation, anterior view

A' Same view, enlarged with Cartilago septi *–(cs)–*. (Transparently sketched)

B Same preparation, anterior-caudal view

B' Same preparation, cartilage not sketched in. This view corresponds to view during operation. Only by slight septum deviation one can see Lamina cribrosa *–lc–* deeper rostrally, still farther rostrally Apertura sphenoidalis *–asp–*, below it Ala vomeris *–av–*. Extensive asymmetry of Spina nasalis ant. *–spa–*

Abbreviations:

asp Apertura sphenoidalis
av Ala vomeris
(cs) Cartilago septi nasi (projection)
lc Lamina cribrosa
lm Lamina mediana
spa Spina nasalis ant.
vo Vomer

FIG. 5

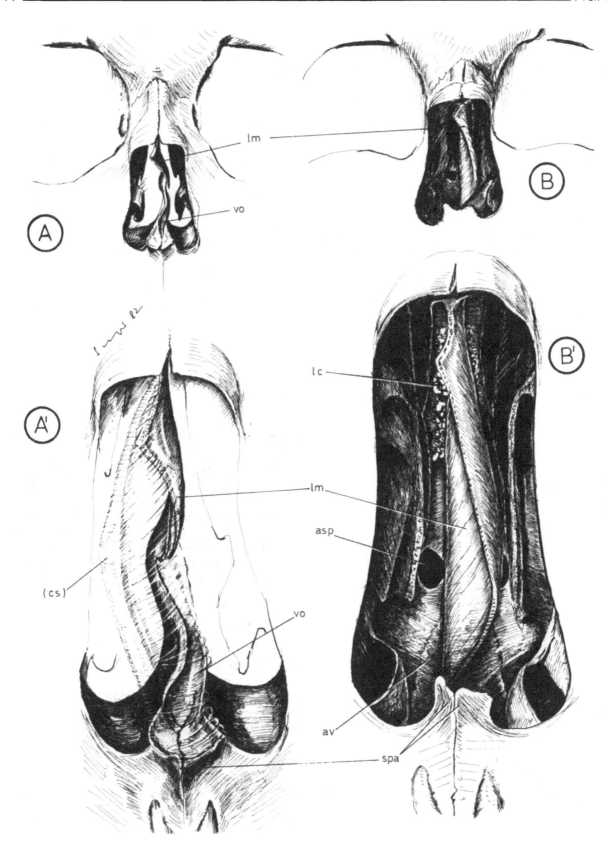

FIG. 6 ⊏════════════════════════════════════⊐ 12

Fig. 6. Special anatomical features and special techniques of hypophysis operations

Topography of **Sinus sphenoidalis,** anatomical overview. Sagittal view of preparation is, however, not as low as the view during operation

A Skull preparation, anterior view with removal of parts of Apertura piriformis and Maxilla on the right side, as well as removal of Maxilla, Os zygomaticum and the major portion of Os ethmoideum on the left side. Vomer resected

B Sectional enlargement of **A**

Abbreviations:

apa	Ala parva
asp	Apertura sphenoidalis
av	Ala vomeris
cet	Cellulae ethmoidales (residuals)
fos	Fissura orbitalis sup.
fosp	Facies orbitalis of Os sphenoidale
lc	Lamina cribrosa
lm	Lamina mediana (resected)
na	Os nasale
op	Canalis opticus
rt	Foramen rotundum
vo	Vomer (resected)

FIG. 6

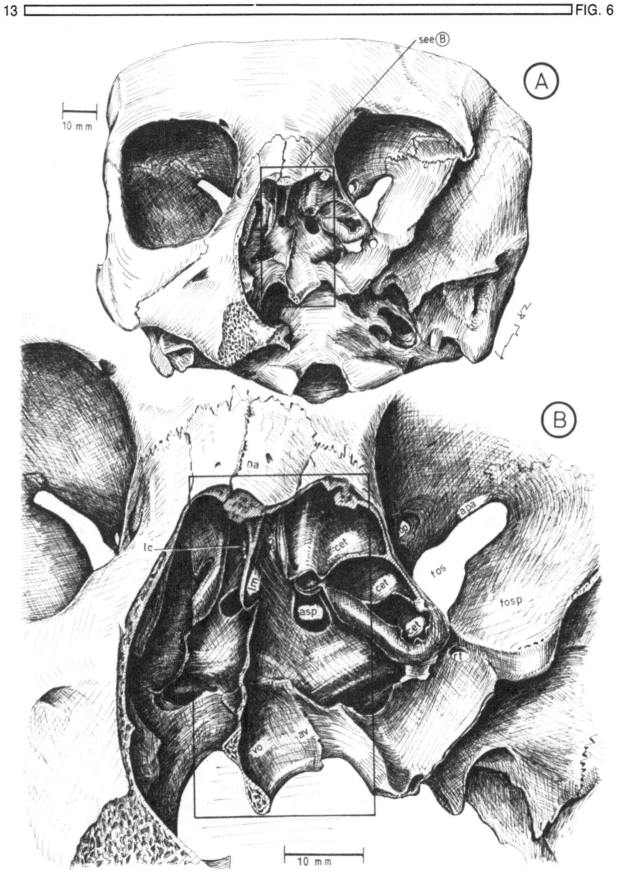

see(B)

(A)

(B)

10 mm

na

lc

vo   av

10 mm

FIG. 7 ⊏⟝⟞ 14

Fig. 7. Special anatomical features and special techniques of hypophysis operations

Topography of **Sinus sphenoidalis,** anatomical overview. View of Preparation is from an inferior direction as during operation, however obliquely lateral (not sagittal as during operation)

A Skull preparation, oblique view from a left inferior direction

B Detail view of **A**

Abbreviations:

apa Ala parva
asp Apertura sphenoidalis
av Ala vomeris
cet Cellulae ethmoidales (residuals)
fos Fissura orbitalis sup.
fosp Facies orbitalis of Os sphenoidale
lc Lamina cribrosa
lm Lamina mediana (resected)
na Os nasale
op Canalis opticus
rt Foramen rotundum
vo Vomer (resected)

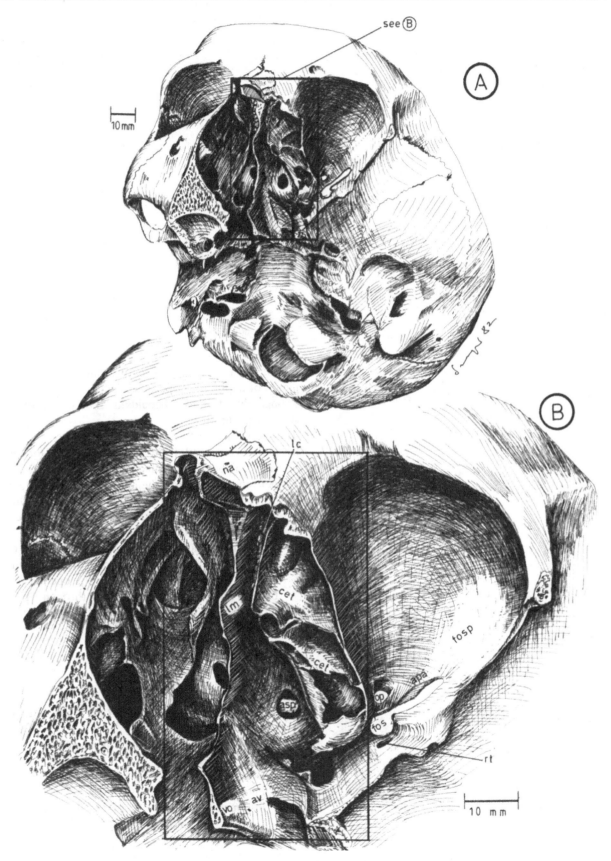

FIG. 8 ☐━━━☐ 16

Fig. 8. Special anatomical features and special techniques of hypophysis operations
Topography of **Sinus sphenoidalis,** skull preparation, superior posterior view

A Overview

B Detail, enlarged from **A**. Sella floor, Dorsum sellae, Tuberculum sellae and adjoining posterior portions of Planum sphenoidale are removed, in order to open view into Sinus sphenoidalis. One sees that Sinus sphenoidalis extends so far laterally, that its medial wall can border medial wall of Foramen rotundum –rt–. Ridges in the floor of Sinus sphenoidalis –pe–; open arrows: Canalis opticus, the medial wall of which is opened up. Beyond Sinus sphenoidalis looking through Apertura sphenoidalis –asp– one sees the medial margin of Concha superior –cs–

Abbreviations:

asp	Apertura sphenoidalis
cs	Concha sup.
(csp)	Juncture of Concha sup. to the floor of right Sinus sphenoidalis
[csp]	Bony cleft at juncture of Concha sup.
op	Canalis opticus
pe	Bony rigdes in the floor of Sinus sphenoidalis
psp	Planum sphenoidale
rt	Foramen rotundum
ssp	Septum sphenoidale

FIG. 8

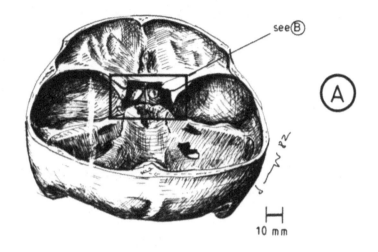

see Ⓑ

Ⓐ

10 mm

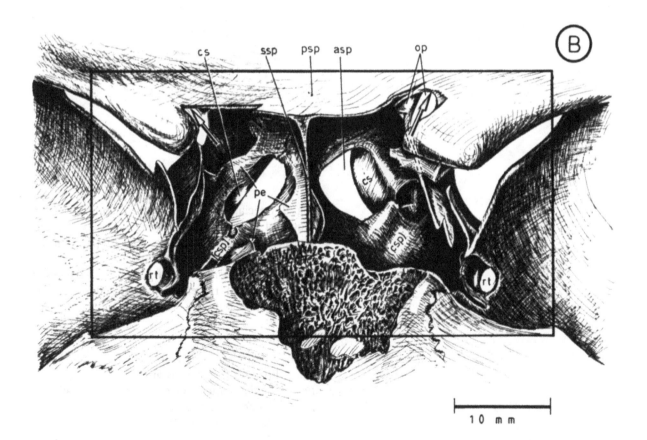

Ⓑ

cs   ssp   psp   asp   op

pe

csp

rt

cs

csp

rt

10 mm

FIG. 9 ▭ 18

Fig. 9. Special anatomical features and special techniques of hypophysis operations

Sinus sphenoidalis, the same skull preparation as in Fig. 8, superior view from above

A – C Progressive enlargements. Irregularily shaped ridges –pe– in the floor of Sinus sphenoidalis

Abbreviations:

asp Apertura sphenoidalis
pca Processus clinoideus ant.
pe Ridges in the floor of Sinus sphenoidalis
psp Planum sphenoidale
ssp Septum sphenoidale
rt Foramen rotundum

FIG. 9

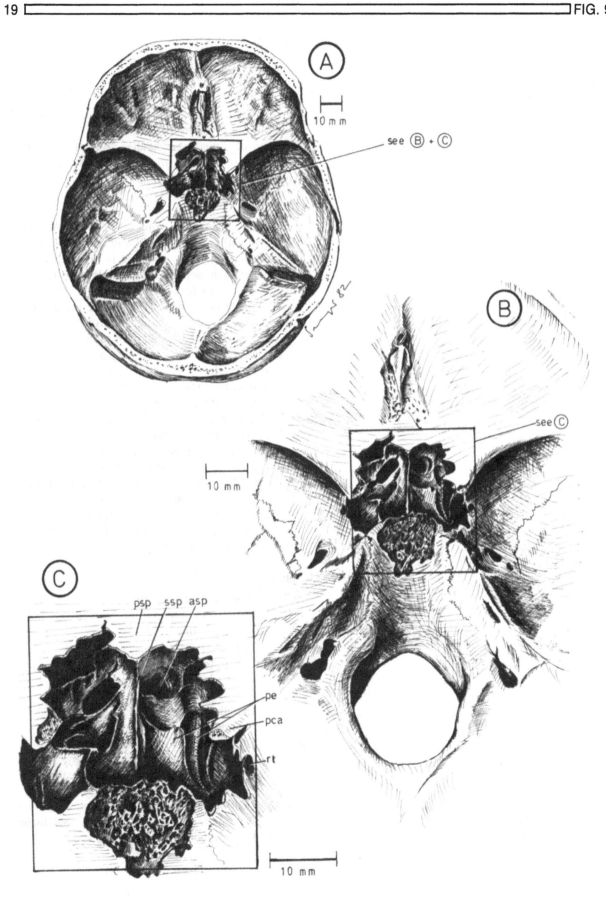

FIG. 10 20

Fig. 10. Special anatomical features and special techniques of hypophysis operations

Anatomy of **Sinus sphenoidalis,** topographical relation to N. opticus, A. carotis int. and N. maxillaris. Asymmetry of Septum sphenoidale

A Position of frontal section planes. View as in Fig. 9 **B**

B Section plane at the level of Apertura sphenoidalis –*asp*–. Medial wall of Canalis opticus –*(wop)*–, which was removed in the preparation, is sketched in. Septum sphenoidale –*ssp*– is nearly at the median (otherwise relation to median is often very asymmetrical). Only the midpoint between Aperturae sphenoidales –*asp*– lies approximately in the median plane of the skull

   a Distance between median plane of skull and medial edge of Apertura sphenoidalis

   a' The same distance contralaterally

C Farther posterior section plane parallel to **B** through Processus clinoideus ant. and through Foramen rotundum with N. maxillaris -N.V2-. Because roof of Sinus sphenoidalis was removed in preparation, contours were sketched in afterwards. A. carotis int. lies in Sulcus caroticus –*(suc)*–. This portion of the dorso-lateral wall of Sinus sphenoidalis may protrude into Sinus sphenoidalis. A. carotis int. –*cl*– is sectioned in the anterior siphon area

Abbreviations:

asp	Apertura sphenoidalis
cet	Cellula ethmoidalis
cl	A. carotis int.
fos	Fissura orbitalis sup.
fptp	Fossa pterygopalatina
(fse)	Floor of Sella (projection)
lm	Lamina mediana nasi
op	Canalis opticus
pca	Processus clinoideus ant.
pe	Ridges in floor of Sinus sphenoidalis
sip	Sinus sphenoidalis divided (by Septum sphenoidale –*ssp*–) in separate cavities
(suc)	Sulcus caroticus (projection)
(wop)	Wall of Canalis opticus (projection)
(wsuc)	Dorso-lateral wall of Sinus sphenoidalis below Sulcus caroticus (projection)

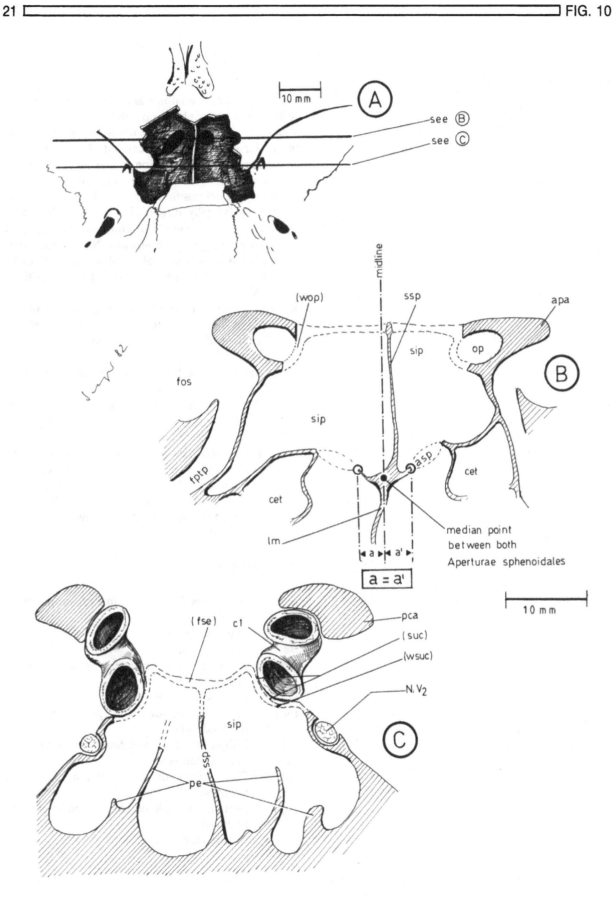

FIG. 11 ⌐━━━━━━━━━━━━━━━━━━━━━━━━━━━━━━━━━━⌐ 22

Fig. 11. Special anatomical features and special techniques of hypophysis operations

Anatomy of **Sinus sphenoidalis** in presence of **intrasellar processus.** Displacement of A. carotis int.

A Schematic frontal section at the level of carotis syphon. Floor of Sella *–fse–* is inferiorly displaced from original position, *–(fse)–*, and A. carotis int. *–cl–* is laterally displaced. Processus clinoideus ant. *–pca–* is thinned out and laterally displaced from original position *–(pca)–*. Note topographical relation of Sinus sphenoidalis *–sip–*, floor of sella *–fse–*, A. carotis int. *–cl–* to N. maxillaris -N.V2-

B The same topographical situation as in **A,** superior view. Here too one sees the lateral displacement of both Aa. carotis intt.

Asymmetries of A. carotis int.:

a short distance between midline and Curvatura ant. of A. carotis int. (variant)

a' short distance of Curvatura post. of A. carotis int. from midline anterior to Dorsum sella *–dos–*

In the presence of intrasellar processus both Aa. carotis intt. are laterally displaced. Displacement of A. carotis int. towards the midline very rarely occurs. Position of A. carotis int. must be ascertained by means of preoperative angiography

Abbreviations:

cl	A. carotis int.
(cl)	A. carotis int. (projection of normal findings)
dos	Dorsum sellae
fse	Floor of Sella
(fse)	Floor of Sella (projection of normal findings)
pca	Processus clinoideus ant.
(pca)	Processus clinoideus ant. (projection of normal findings)
pe	Ridges in the floor of Sinus sphenoidalis
sip	Sinus sphenoidalis
(sip)	Sinus sphenoidalis (projection of normal findings)
(ssp)	Septum sphenoidale (projection of normal findings)
ts	Tuberculum sellae

FIG. 11

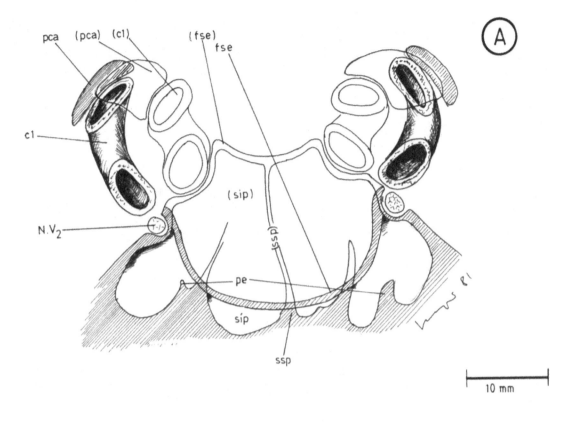

A

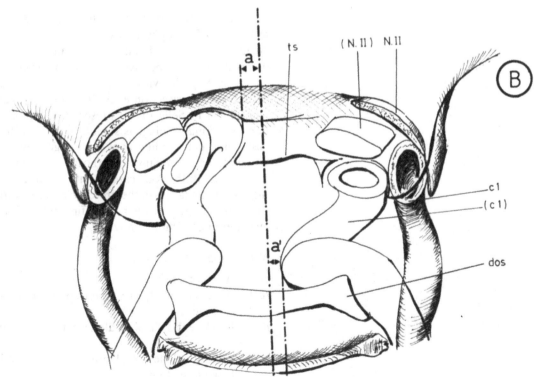

B

FIG. 12 ▭━━━━━━━━━━━━━━━━━━━━━━━━▭ 24

Fig. 12. Special anatomical features and special techniques of hypophysis operations

Anatomical model of inner sella wall according to observations of hypophysis tumors by transcranial approach. Superior view. Cutting plane –s– of Dura corresponds to resection edge of Dura at operation. Dura lining of Sella in the presence of tumors contrary to normal findings is smooth and show numerous round and cleftlike gaps with slight seepage of venous blood (from Sinus cavernosus and Sinus intercavernosi). Both Aa. carotis intt. protrude only slightly into Sella –p– in the presence of large intrasellar tumors contrary to the normal findings. This facilitates thorough tumor removal

Abbreviations:

c1   A. carotis int.

(c1)   A. carotis int. (projection of path within Sinus cavernosus)

p   Prominent sella wall along path of A. carotis int.

s   Cutting plane of Dura after removal of hypophysis tumor

FIG. 12

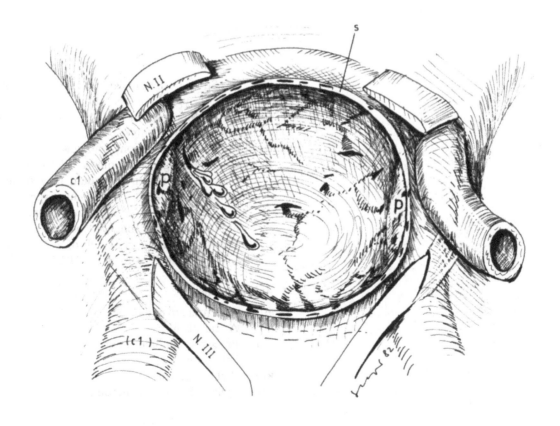

FIG. 13 ⊏───────────────────────────────────────⊐ 26

Fig. 13. Special anatomical features and special techniques of hypophysis operations

Anatomy of **Sinus sphenoidalis,** sagittal section of topographical relationship

A Anatomical preparation, overview

B Sectional enlargement from **A.** Walls of Canalis opticus and Foramen rotundum may stand out prominently against the Sinus sphenoidalis *–wop–* and *–wrt–*. Danger of injury during operations on Sinus sphenoidalis

C Preparation as **B,** with sketch of A. carotis int. *–cl–*. -N.II- and N. maxillaris -N.V2-

Abbreviations:

asp Apertura sphenoidalis
cl A. carotis int.
pca Processus clinoideus ant.
se Sella turcica
wop Wall of Canalis opticus
wrt Wall of Foramen rotundum

FIG. 13

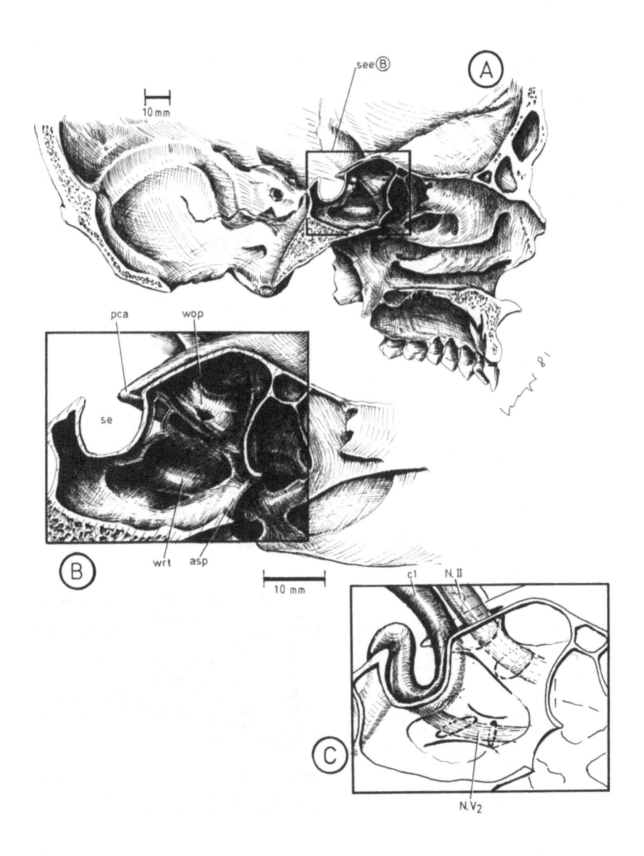

FIG. 14 [──────────────────────────────────] 28

Fig. 14. Special anatomical features and special techniques of hypophysis operations
Continuation of Fig. 13. Topographical relationship of intrasellar processes
A Path of A. carotis int. –cl–, N. opticus -N.II- in the presence of balloon sella
B Path of A. carotis int. –cl–, N. opticus -N.II- and N. maxillaris -(N.V2)- in the presence of flatly enlarged sella
C Normal findings

Abbreviations:

cl A. carotis int.
(N.V2) N. maxillaris (projection)

FIG. 14

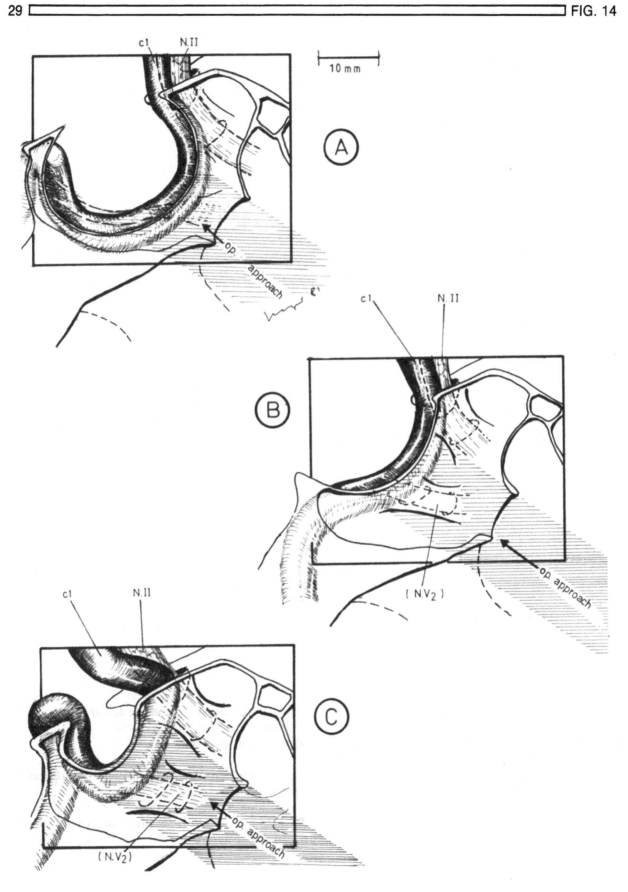

10 mm

A

B

C

FIG. 15 ⊏━━━━━━━━━━━━━━━━━━━━━━━━━━━━━━━━━⊐ 30

Figs. 15–24. Special anatomical features and special techniques of hypophysis operations
Principles of operation

Fig. 15. Position of gingiva incision, and operative approach towards sella
A Position of **gingiva incision**
B Fold-back of upper lip after soft tissue incision, **operative approach** sketched (arrow)

FIG. 15

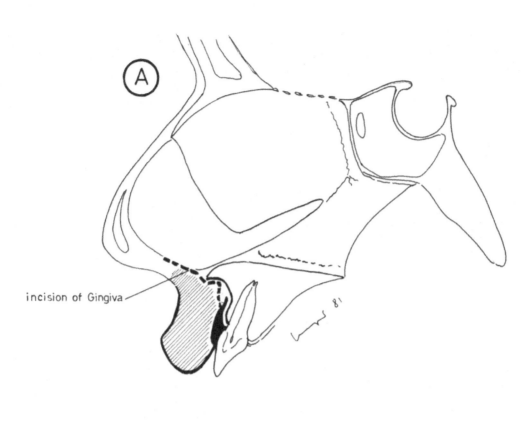

incision of Gingiva

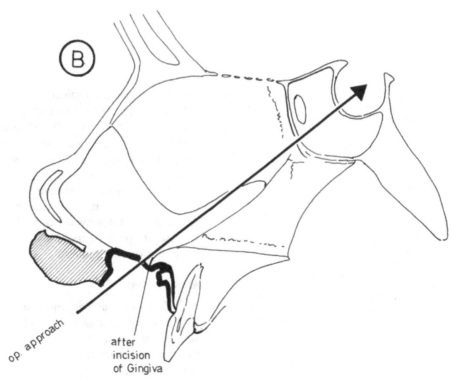

op. approach

after
incision
of Gingiva

FIG. 16 ⬚ 32

Fig. 16. Special anatomical features and special techniques óf hypophysis operations

Principles of operations. **Detachment of nasal mucosa** –*muc*– from the cartilaginious nasal septum –*cs*– and from Spina nasalis ant. –*spa*–, as well as from floor of Meatus nasalis inf. –*fn*–

A Frontal schematic presentation
B Correct detachment of mucosa from floor of nasal cavity with downward-curved instrument
B' Use of upward-curved instrument carries the risk of perforating mucosa

Abbreviations:

cs   Cartilaginious Septum nasi
fn   Floor of Meatus nasalis inf.
muc Mucosa nasi
pd   Palatum durum
spa Spina nasalis ant.

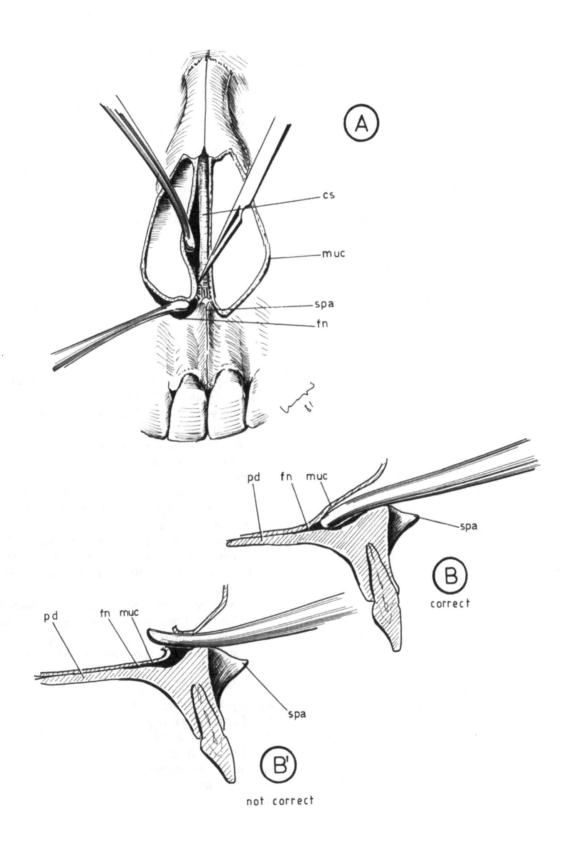

FIG. 17 ⊏▭⊐ 34

Fig. 17. Special anatomical features and special techniques of hypophysis operations
Principles of operation. **Resection of Septum nasi**

A   Resection of Septum nasi, measurements. In the area of Spina nasalis ant. *–spa–*, a part of Septum nasi can be saved, if the approach is only from **one** side

B   Anatomical preparation, overview. Upper edge of speculum, Apertura sphenoidalis and Canalis opticus lie in **one** plane

C   Speculum is at first inserted (see also **A**) only 50 mm deep measured from Spina nasalis ant.
    1   Detachment of mucosa from Vomer residual *–vo–*
    2   Arrows: Farther insertion of speculum into final position after mucosa preparation. Apertura sphenoidalis (s. also **B**) appears at the upper edges of speculum, on both sides

Abbreviations:

asp   Apertura sphenoidalis
cs   Cartilaginious Septum nasi
lm   Lamina mediana
pd   Palatum durum
sip   Sinus sphenoidalis
spa   Spina nasalis ant.
vo   Vomer

FIG. 17

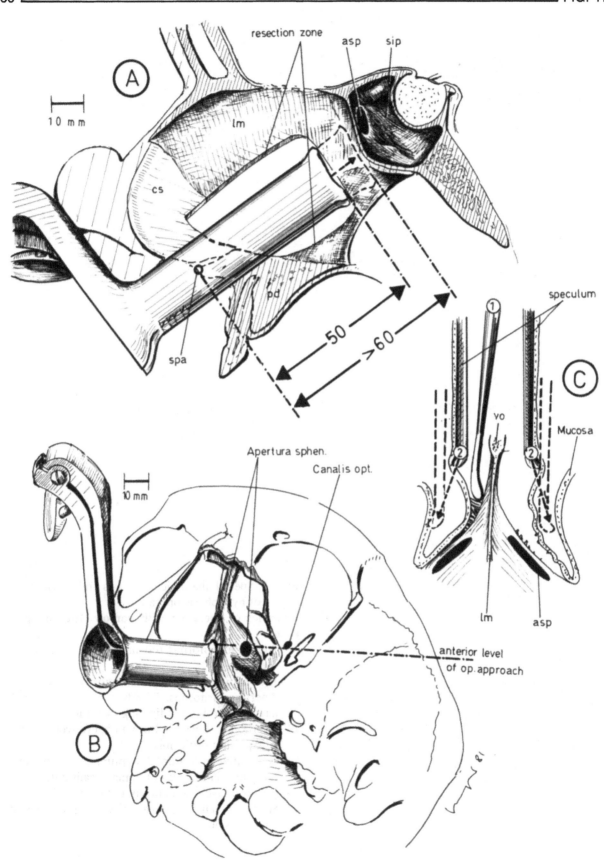

A

resection zone asp sip

10 mm

lm

cs

pd

spa

50

>60

speculum

1

vo

2 2

Mucosa

C

lm asp

Apertura sphen.

Canalis opt.

10 mm

anterior level
of op. approach

B

FIG. 18 ⌷━━━━━━━━━━━━━━━━━━━━━━━⌹ 36

Fig. 18. Special anatomical features and special techniques of hypophysis operations

Principles of **operation with narrow Apertura piriformis**

A Apertura piriformis too narrow for insertion of speculum

B Alternative procedure 1: resection of bony wall of Apertura piriformis. Disadvantage: Sinus maxillaris and teeth are adjoining (see Fig. 19)

B' Insertion of speculum through operatively enlarged Apertura piriformis

C Alternative procedure 2: Septum nasi is cut anteriorly also in the area of Spina nasalis ant. –spa–. Disadvantage: cosmetically unfavourable

C' Speculum can be inserted if cut Septum nasi is pushed aside

FIG. 18

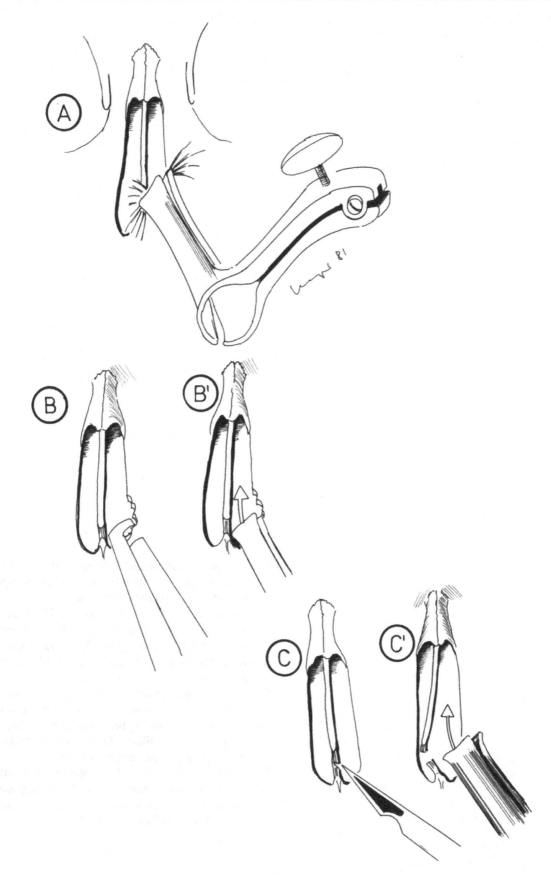

FIG. 19 ⌧ 38

Fig. 19. Special anatomical features and special techniques of hypophysis operations. Dangers in operative widening of **Apertura piriformis**

A   Favourable for operation: Sinus maxillaris is located at a considerable distance from Apertura piriformis (thin bony wall of Apertura piriformis)

A'   Bone resection of lateral margin of Apertura piriformis

B   Unfavourable situation (in younger persons). Sinus maxillaris –(sma)– adjoins Apertura piriformis. The bone quickly broadens laterally because it hugs Sinus maxillaris. Dental roots –(ro)– approach closely Apertura piriformis

B'   If one tries to resect lateral margin of Apertura piriformis, Sinus maxillaris might be opened up and one or several dental roots may be injured.
Preop. X-ray-studies important

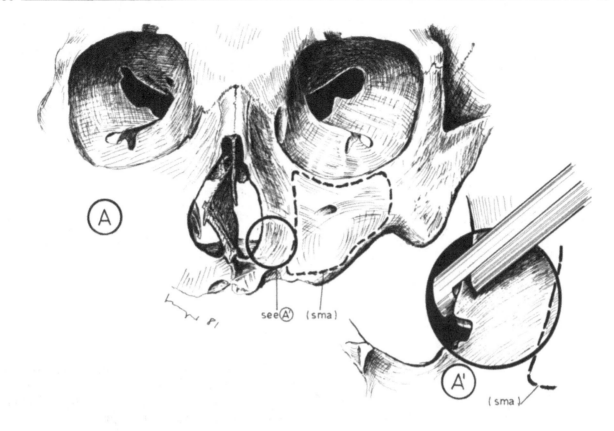

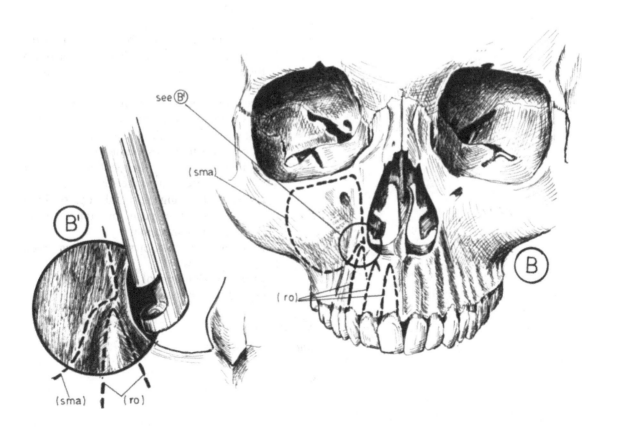

FIG. 20 ⊏━━━━━━━━━━━━━━━━━━━━━━━━━━━━━━━⊐ 40

Fig. 20. Special anatomical features and special techniques of hypophysis operations

Principles of operation. Tear of mucosa of Septum nasi with resulting **obstructed approach**

Corrected position of speculum

A – C	Anatomical sketch
A' – C'	Operation site
A	Speculum –*sp*– pushes back mucosa on the right side only. On the left –*L*– mucosa is torn and is not pushed back by speculum –*muc*–
A'	The torn mucosa overlaps anterior wall of Os sphenoideum on the left side
B	Insertion of two flexible spatulas –*spt*–
B'	Operation site corresponding to **B**
1a + 1b	Removal of speculum –*sp*– after insertion of the spatula –*spt*–
2a + 2b	Bending of spatula tips on both sides of speculum after removal
C	Reinsertion of speculum
1a + 1b	Branches of speculum are eased forward
2a + 2b	Removal of spatulas
C'	Operative site, corresponding to **C**

Abbreviations:

muc torn mucosa
sp Speculum
spt Spatula

FIG. 20

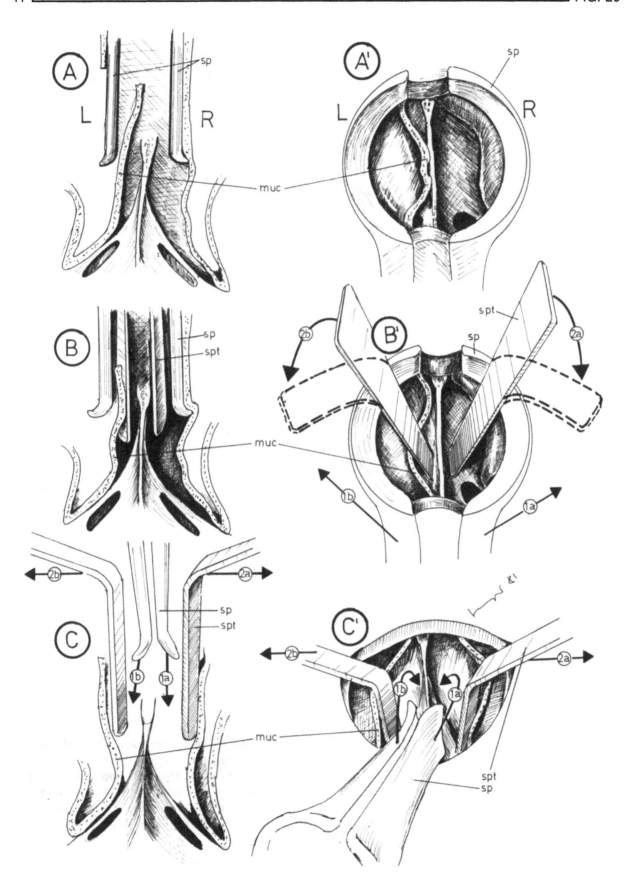

FIG. 21 ⬚══════════════════════════════⬚ 42

Fig. 21. Special anatomical features and special techniques of hypophysis operations
Principles of operation. **Operative approach** into **skull base** sketched in. Basal view after nearly complete resection of facial part of skull, resection planes at Septum nasi (Lamina mediana, Vomer)

FIG. 21

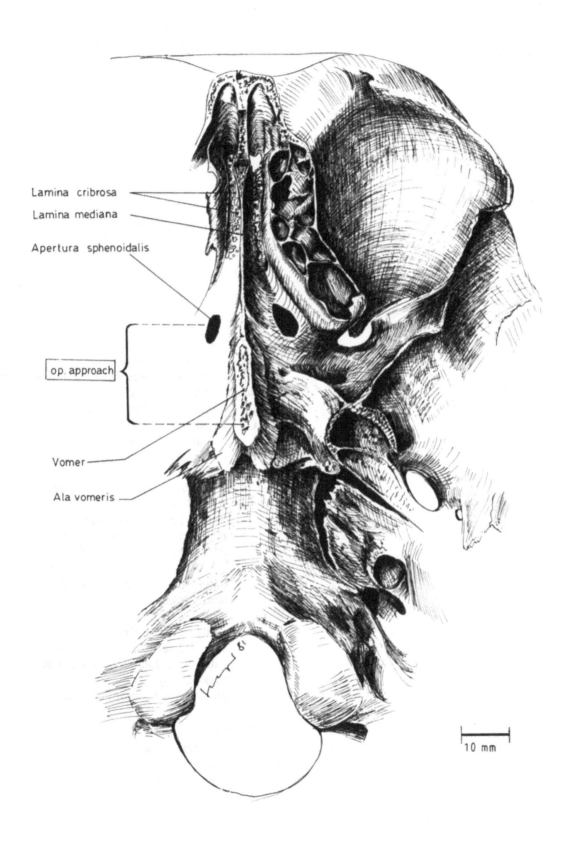

Lamina cribrosa

Lamina mediana

Apertura sphenoidalis

op. approach

Vomer

Ala vomeris

10 mm

FIG. 22 [   ] 44

Fig. 22. Special anatomical features and special techniques of hypophysis operations

Principles of operation. **Determination of midline and resection of Sinus sphenoidalis floor**

A – C	Basal view, detail from Fig. 21
A' – C'	Sagittal view, detail
A	Detail of preparation, sketched according to Fig. 21. Vomer –*vo*– deviates from mid-line
A'	Situation as **A** during Vomer resection, sagittal section
B	After Vomer resection one recognizes that the insertion of Vomer, with juncture to Alae vomerris –*av*–, is in the median position. The midline lies between both Aperturae sphenoidales –*asp*–. Beginning of Sinus sphenoidalis resection
B'	Situation as **B,** sagittal section
C	Sinus sphenoidalis opened up. Septum sphenoidale nearly always has an oblique path; it seldom lies in the midplane or parasagittaly
C'	Situation as **C**, sagittal section

Abbreviations:

asp Apertura sphenoidalis
av Ala vomeris
sip Sinus sphenoidalis
vo Vomer

FIG. 22

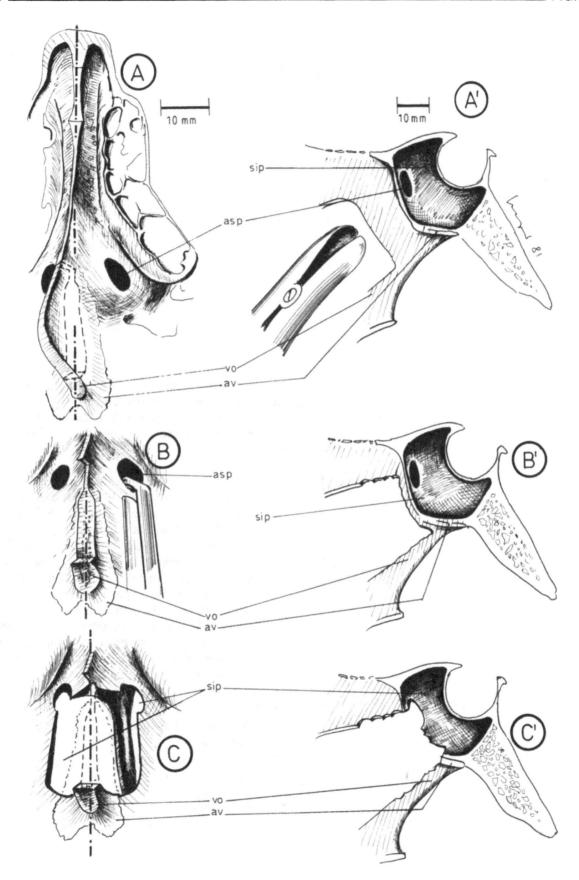

FIG. 23 ⌐━━━━━━━━━━━━━━━━━━━━━━━━━⌐ 46

Fig. 23. Special anatomical features and special techniques of hypophysis operations

Principles of operation. **Os sphenoidale preparation, anterior view, microsurgical operation site** sketched in

A Overview

B Detail enlargement from **A.** Presentation of topographical relation of Vomer and Alae vomeris to Spina sphenoidalis –*spsp*–. Spina sphenoidalis and/or Alae vomeris –*av*–, contrary to Vomer –*vo*–, are of nearly symmetrical configuration. Lamina mediana –*lm*– too is nearly mid-positioned at the juncture of Os sphenoidale. In the area of Aperturae sphenoidales –*asp*– slight asymmetries are to be expected.

Portions of Septum nasi are often very asymmetrical; however, the more nearly they approach Os sphenoidale, the more they tend toward midplane-location

Abbreviations:

asp   Apertura sphenoidalis
av   Ala vomeris
fos   Fissura orbitalis sup.
lm   Lamina mediana
psp   Planum sphenoidale
rt   For. rotundum
spsp Spina sphenoidalis

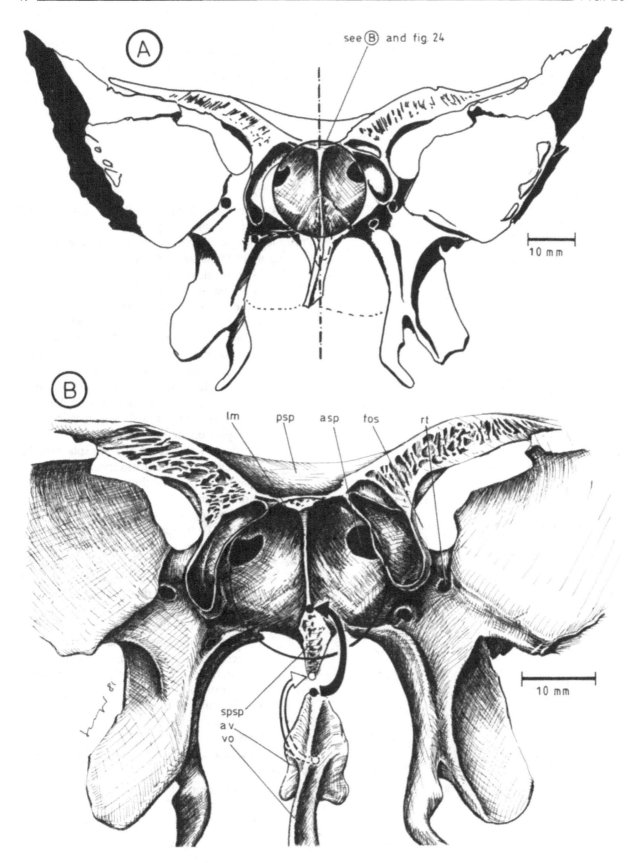

see (B) and fig. 24

10 mm

lm   psp   asp   fos   rt

spsp
a v.
vo

10 mm

FIG. 24 ⬚━━━━━━━━━━━━━━━━━━━━━━━━━━━━━⬚ 48

Fig. 24. Special anatomical features and special techniques of hypophysis operations

Principles of operation. Continuation of Fig. 23.

Opening up of Sinus sphenoidalis

A – C	Microsurgical site
A' – C'	Anatomical sketch, sagittal view
A	Presentation similar to Fig. 23
A'	1 The exposure of Sinus sphenoidalis starts with the resection at the anterior wall, beginning at Apertura sphenoidalis –*asp*–
B	After opening the anterior wall of Sinus sphenoidalis, resection of basal Vomer portions –*vo*–, and resection of Ala vomeris –*av*– one can view grossly asymmetrical Septum sphenoidale –*ssp*–
B'	Extirpation of mucosa of Sinus sphenoidalis

      1 Detachment of mucosa from bone by dissector, if possible throughly, using a **blunt** dissector

      2 Stretching of mucosa by forceps

      1 and 2 To be repeated until the mucosa is removed in as few large pieces as possible.

      If small mucosa pieces remain (i.e. in hidden niches), the danger of a later mucocele exists

C	Opening up of sella floor

      1 Opening up of bony sella floor

      2 Incision of dura lining on sella floor. Watch out for A. carotis int., review angiography!

C'	1 Loosening of tumor by curette

Abbreviations:

asp   Apertura sphenoidalis
av   Ala vomeris
lm   Lamina mediana
ssp   Septum sphenoidale
vo   Vomer

FIG. 24.

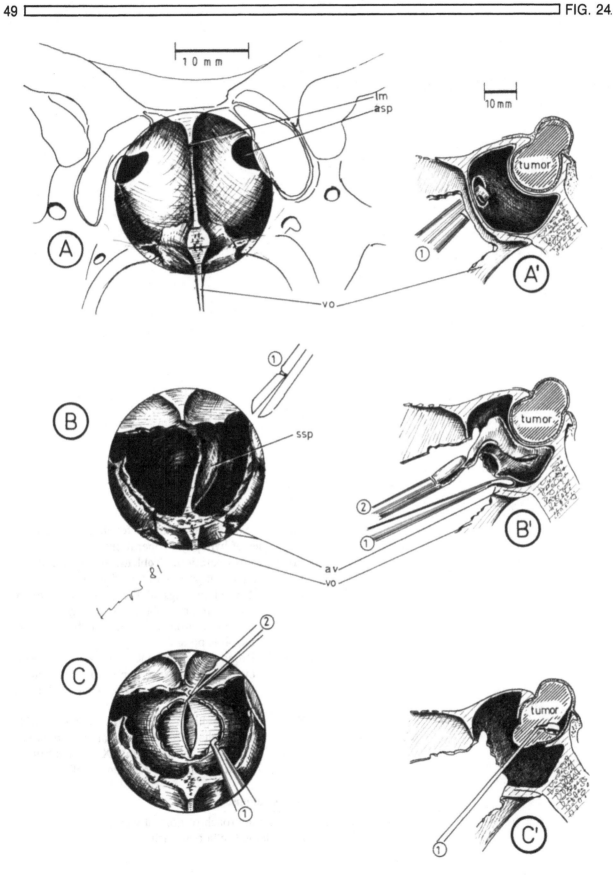

FIG. 25 ⊏━━━━━━━━━━━━━━━━━━━━━━━━⊐ 50

Fig. 25. Special anatomical features and special techniques of hypophysis operations
Principles of operation. **Problems of tumor removal** in the presence of grossly enlarged sella.

A	Typical findings in the presence of hypophysis tumors: sella clearly enlarged; from a narrow approach –*d*– thorough tumor removal is possible
B, C, D	Broad sella, approach –*d*– as in **A.** However, a more rostral approach –**C**–, or more posterior approach –**B** + **D** –, will leave tumor remains
E	Broad sella as in **B** and **D.** Atypically wide approach –**d'**–: tumor can be removed throughly, necessitating X-ray control of curette position in relation to sella wall

Abbreviations:

d Sella approach of normal width
d' Enlarged sella approach

FIG. 25

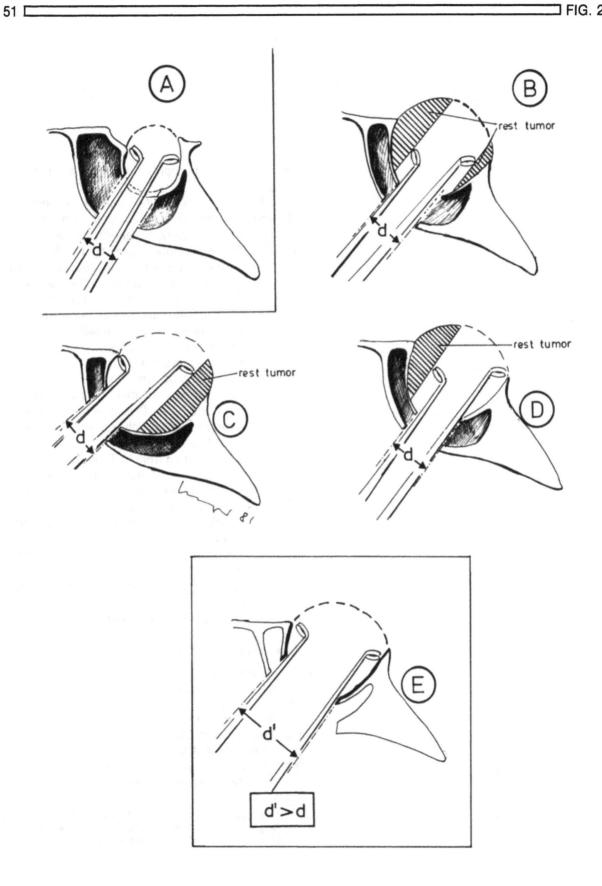

FIG. 26 ⸏══⸎ 52

Fig. 26. Oro-nasal hypophysis operation according to Hardy (modified*)

Clinical example of a chromophobe hypophysis adenoma; preoperative bitemporal hemianopsia, improved postoperatively. Diagnostic procedures

A – B'   Bilateral carotis angiographies. Note the short distance of the Curvatura anterior of A. carotis int. from the midline –*a*– (right side) and –*a'*– (left side). Curvatura post. of A. carotis int. lies farther away –*b*– (right side) and –*b'*– (left side)

C – G   Preoperative CT-findings

C   Section planes of CT

D   Asymmetry of Septum sphenoidale

E   Topographical relation of tumor to A. carotis int. –*cl*–. Processus clinoideus ant. -*pca*-, and mesencephalon –*me*–, as well as to A. basilaris –*bl*–

F'   reconstruction from **F**. Topographical relation of tumor to third ventricle, basal cisterns –*cis*– and Sinus sphenoidalis –*sis*–, frontal section plane

F   Sketch of CT section plane of reconstruction **F'**

G'   Position of tumor in sagittal section, reconstruction from **G**

G   Sketch of CT section plane of reconstruction **G'**

H   Postoperative CT: tumor removed

Abbreviations:

cl   A. carotis int.
cis   Cisternae basales
bl   A. basilaris
me   Mesencephalon
pca   Processus clinoideus ant.
sis   Sinus sphenoidalis
●   Curvatura ant. of A. carotis int.
○   Curvatura post. of A. carotis int.

* I am greatly obliged to Prof. Dr. R. Fahlbusch, Director of the Neurosurgical Clinic, University of Erlangen, Federal Republic of Germany, for suggestions as to operative technique.

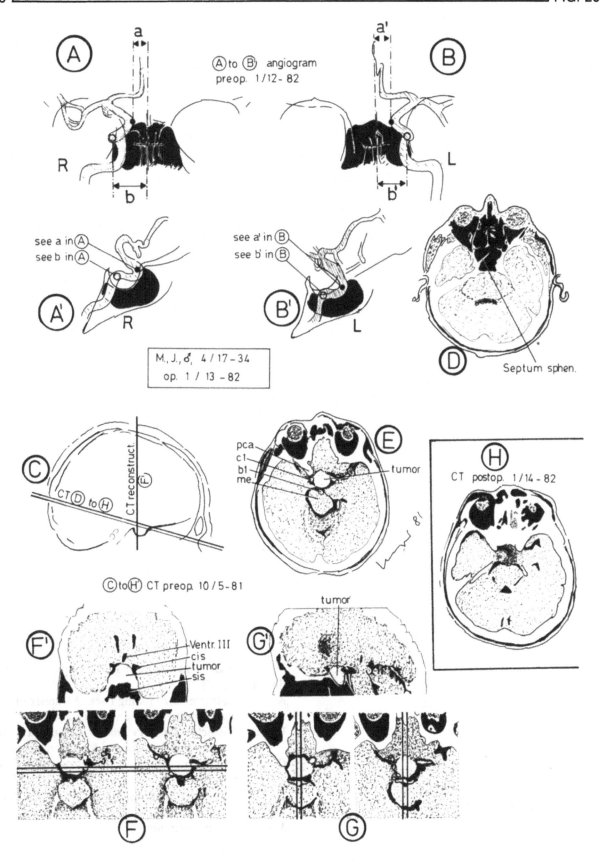

Ⓐ to Ⓑ angiogram
preop. 1/12 – 82

R

L

see a in Ⓐ
see b in Ⓐ

Ⓐ' R

see a' in Ⓑ
see b' in Ⓑ

Ⓑ' L

Ⓓ Septum sphen.

M., J., ♂, 4/17 – 34
op. 1/13 – 82

Ⓒ CT Ⓓ to Ⓗ CT reconstruct. Ⓕ'

Ⓔ pca
c1
b1
me
tumor

Ⓗ
CT postop. 1/14 – 82

Ⓒ to Ⓗ CT preop. 10/5 – 81

Ⓕ' Ventr. III
cis
tumor
sis

Ⓖ' tumor

Ⓕ

Ⓖ

FIG. 27 54

Fig. 27. **Instruments** for oronasal hypophysis operation (HARDY)

A	Retractor for holding back the upper lip
B – D	Instruments for gingiva incision
E + F	Dissector for detachment of mucosa from Septum nasi and floor of Meatus nasalis inf.
G	Spatula for holding back mucosa from Septum nasi
I + H	Shapeable spatulas for holding back torn mucosa s. Fig. 20
J	Hardy speculum

FIG. 27

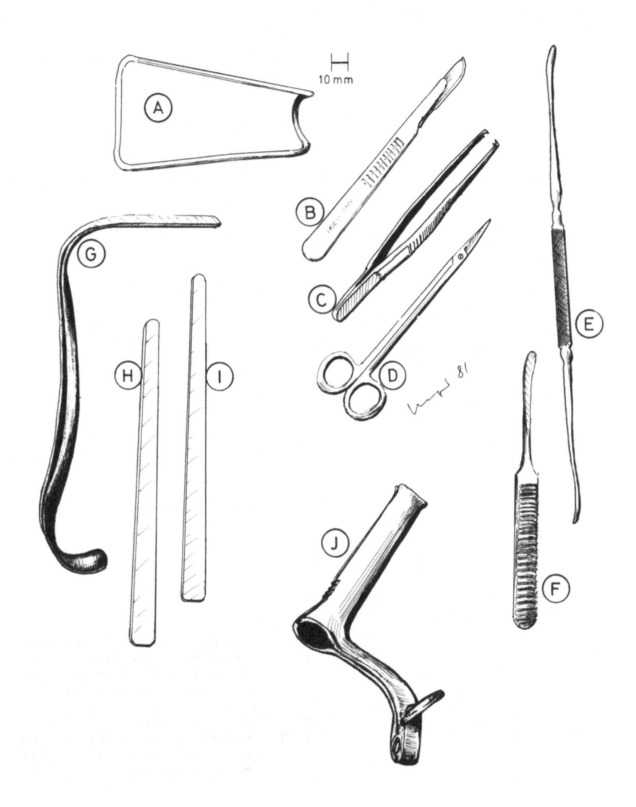

10 mm

FIG. 28 ⊏══⊐ 56

Fig. 28.

A + B Instruments for resection of Septum nasi

C Microdissector for detachment of mucosa from anterior wall of Sinus sphenoidalis (which forms the floor of Sinus sphenoidalis)

D Enlarged detail from **C**

E – H Instruments for opening up sella floor (**G + H**), and for resection of Sinus sphenoidalis floor (**E + F**)

FIG. 28

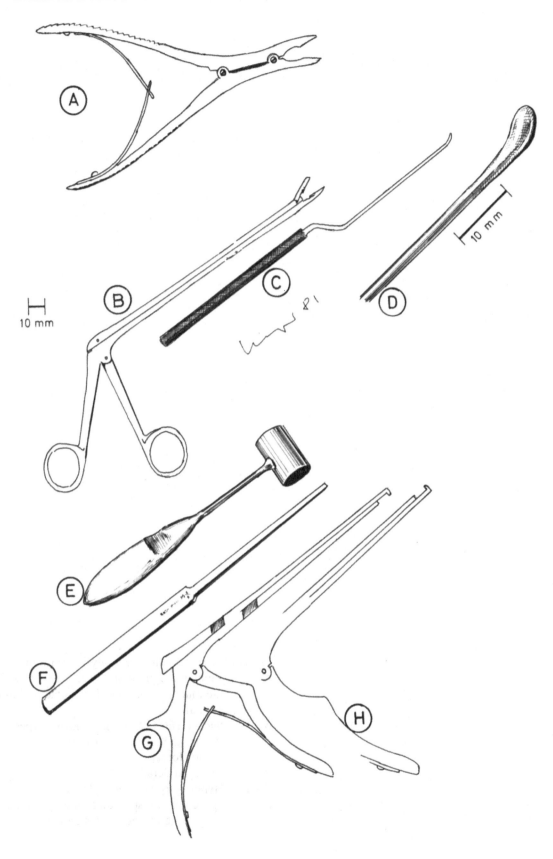

A

B

C

D

E

F

G

H

10 mm

10 mm

FIG. 29 ⊏━━━━━━━━━━━━━━━━━━━━━━━━━━━━━⊐ 58

Fig. 29. **Instruments** for hypophysis operation
A   Bipolar coagulation forceps: to be used in the mucosa area, but, if possible, **not** in the sella area
B   Sucker (maximum size shown, types with smaller lumen also necessary)
C   Tumor forceps
D   Enlarged detail from C
E – L   Hypophysis curettes – Hardy
M   Speculum for spreading nasal opening for tamponage at operation's end

FIG. 29

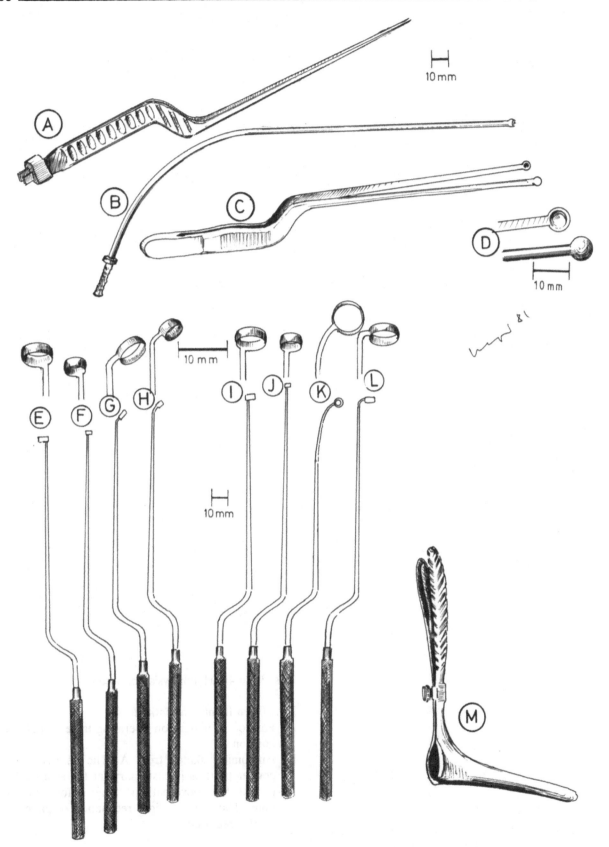

10 mm

10 mm

10 mm

10 mm

FIG. 30 ⊏━━━━━━━━━━━━━━━━━━━━━━━━━━━━━━━━⊐ 60

Figs. 30 to 48. Hypophysis operation

Fig. 30. **Positioning of patient**
A Position of patient on operating table and X-ray position
B Anatomical sketch from **A.** The neurosurgeon does not sit, as is customary, at the side of the patient, but above patient's head as for trepanations. Thus only a slight reclination of patient's head is required

FIG. 30

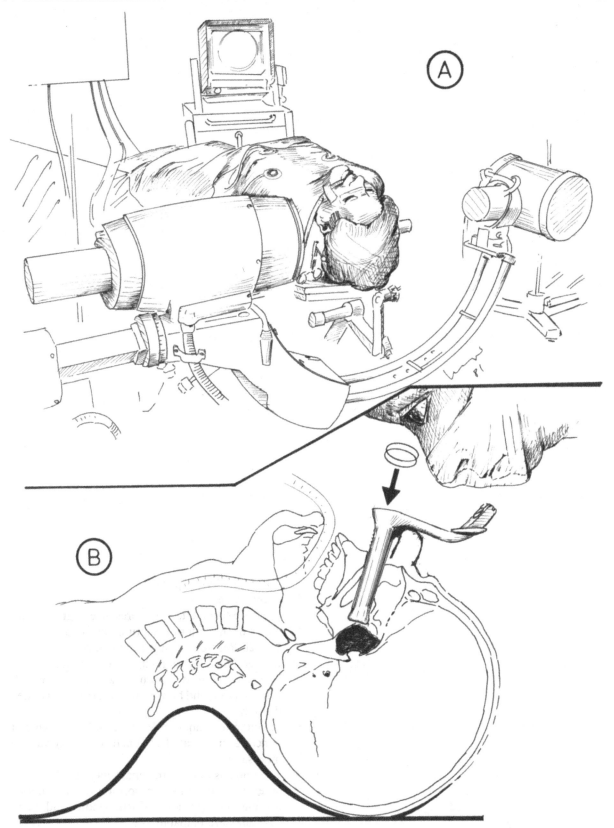

FIG. 31 ⬜═══════════════════════════════════════⬜ 62

Fig. 31. Hypophysis operation
Local anesthesia
A   Injection technique in the presence of gross asymmetry of the anterior Septum nasi area
    1a – 2b Positions of injection needle
    Broken lines: Position change of needle
A' The same as in **A** shown on anatomical model. Cartilaginous and bony structures can be palpated digitally
B   Injection technique in Vestibulum oris. Points of puncture are located at juncture of gingiva and mucosa labii
B' The same as in **B** on the anatomical model. Here an example of a median position of the anterior Septum nasi portions. Cartilaginous and bony structures are palpable

FIG. 31

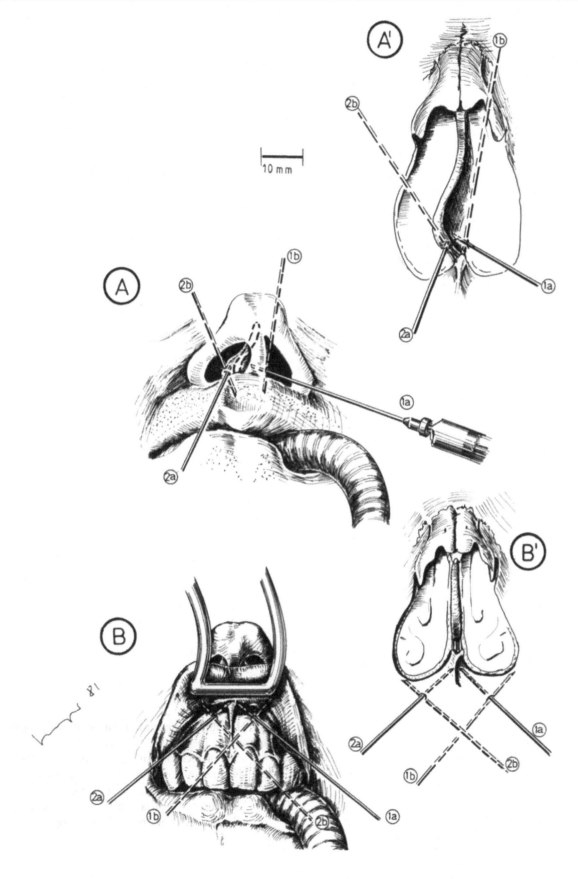

FIG. 32

Fig. 32. Hypophysis operation. **Incision and preparation of mucosa** in Vestibulum oris

A   Mucosa incision just above juncture of gingiva and mucosa labii. Measurements in mm

B + C Detachment of mucosa from Os maxillare

C   Exposure of Spina nasalis ant. and of the inferior medial portion of Apertura piriformis

FIG. 32

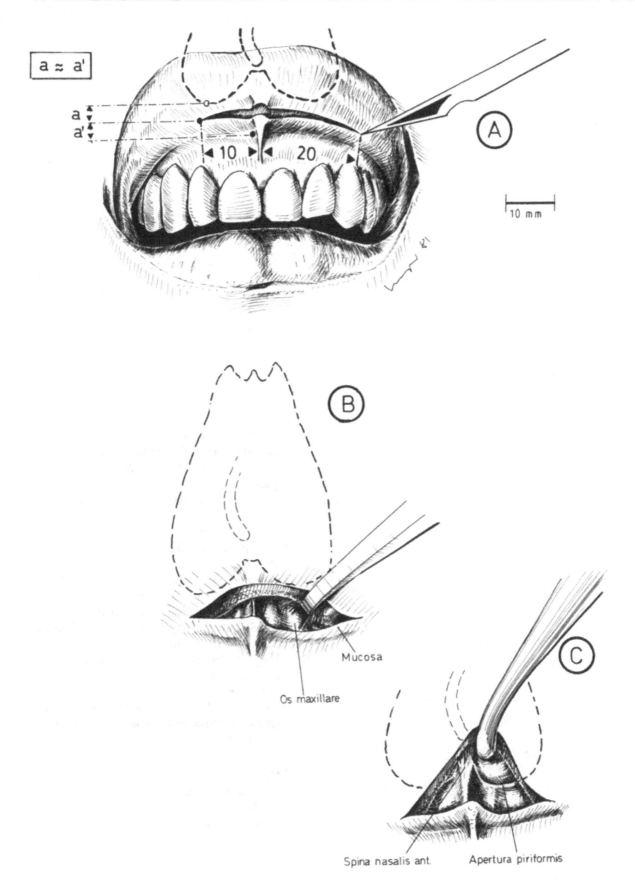

$a \approx a'$

a

a'

◄ 10 ► ◄ 20 ►

10 mm

Ⓐ

Ⓑ

Mucosa

Os maxillare

Ⓒ

Spina nasalis ant.

Apertura piriformis

FIG. 33 ⊏━━━━━━━━━━━━━━━━━━━━━━━━━━━━━━━━━━━━━━━⊐ 66

Fig. 33. Hypophysis operation

D **1a + 1b Detachment of mucosa** upwards

2a Incision over Septum cartilagineum, which is palpable

E **3** **Detachment of perichondrium** –*per*– from Septum cartilagineum –*cart*–

After detachment of perichondrium the incision –*inc*– is extended to Spina nasalis ant. –*spa*–

F **1** Detachment of perichondrium from Septum cartilagineum –*cart*– with spatula

2 Detachment of incised connective tissue between Septum cartilagineum –*cart*– and Spina nasalis ant. –*spa*– with dissector

3 Cutting of fibrous connections between Septum nasi and medial mucosa

G **1 + 3** As in **F**

4 Alternating with **3. At this point there is great danger of perforating the mucosa and opening up Cavum nasi**

Abbreviations:

cart Septum cartilagineum
per Perichondrium
spa Spina nasalis ant.

FIG. 33

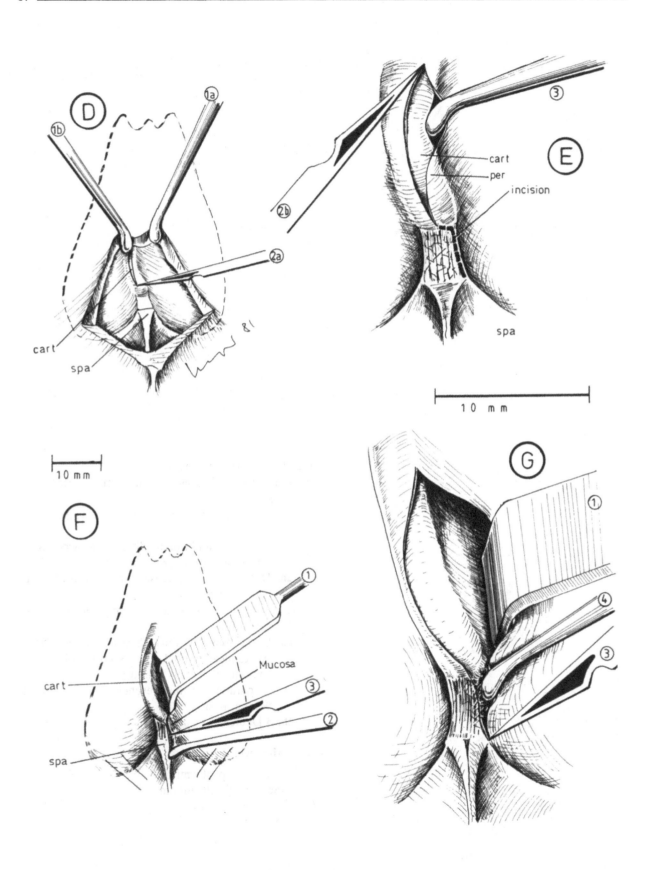

10 mm

10 mm

FIG. 34 ⟾ 68

Fig. 34. Hypophysis operation

H **Detachment of mucosa** from Apertura piriformis
   –api–

   2a Position of dissector. Arrows: movements of dissector

I **1** Cutting of additional adhesions between Septum nasi and mucosa

   2b Detachment of mucosa from Meatus nasi inf. and Septum nasi

H' **2a** Detachment of mucosa from floor of Meatus nasi inf.

   2b Detachment of mucosa from Septum nasi. Anatomical model. S: Section plane of anatomical models **I'** and **I''**

I' + I'' Preparation in the presence of asymmetrical Septum nasi

   2b, 3 Detachment of mucosa

Abbreviations:

api   Apertura piriformis
cart   Septum cartilagineum
lm   Lamina mediana
vo   Vomer

FIG. 34

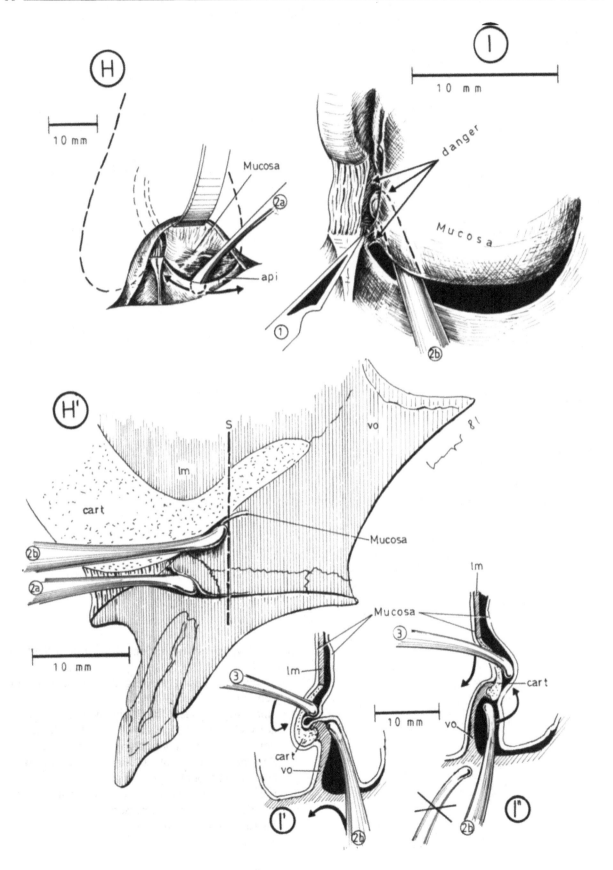

FIG. 35 ⊏━━━━━━━━━━━━━━━━━━━━━━━━━━⊐ 70

Fig. 35. Hypophysis operation. Resection of Septum nasi

A X-ray ap of clinical case, Fig. 26. The deviation of Septum nasi seems slight
B Anatomical model. Cartilaginous Septum nasi – not visible by X-ray – shows considerable deviation. Arrows: possible operative approaches
C **Resection zone (broken line) of Septum nasi,** anatomical model.
   For cosmetic reasons, a 10 mm strip of the anterior Septum nasi is preserved
   Measurements in mm

FIG. 35

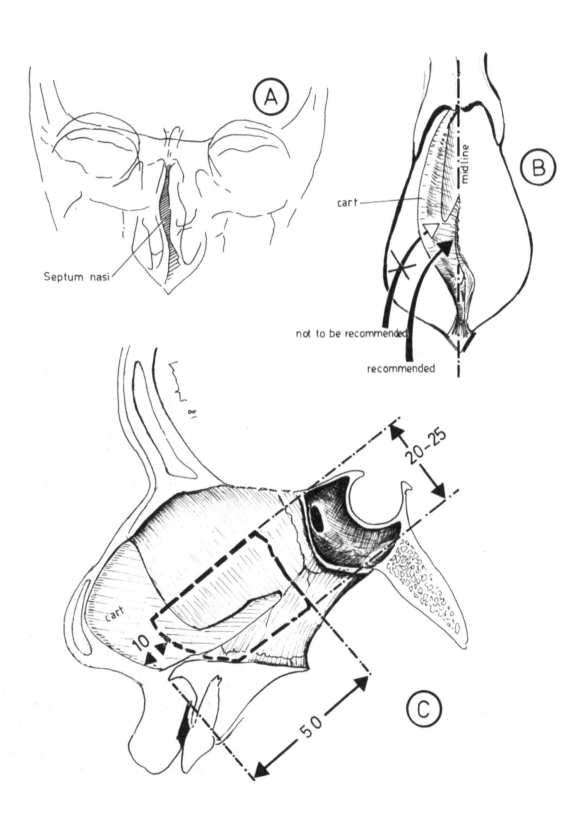

A

B

Septum nasi

cart

midline

not to be recommended

recommended

20-25

cart

10

50

C

FIG. 36 ⊏──⊐ 72

Fig. 36. Hypophysis operation. **Resection of Septum nasi**

A – C   Anterior view
A   1 Lifting up of upper lip and severed mucosa
       2 Insertion of a spatula on Septum nasi
       3 Holding back of mucosa
       4 Incision of cartilaginous Septum nasi
         Broken line: Apertura piriformis
B   Enlarged detail from **A**
       1 – 3 As **A**
       5 Separation of incised cartilage from contralateral mucosa with dissector. Arrows: movements of dissector. See also **C**
       6a + 6b Enlargement of cartilage incision, where the contralateral mucosa has been loosened.
         Dotted line: see **D**
C   Model presentation of procedure **5, B',** frontal section
D   Bone resection, anatomical model
       x: Cartilaginous Septum nasi, already cut through (scissors **6** to be used only for resection of cartilage, not for bone resection)
       y: Dotted line-zone of bone resection using forceps. To begin with, resection does not extend as far as Corpus sphenoidale

FIG. 36

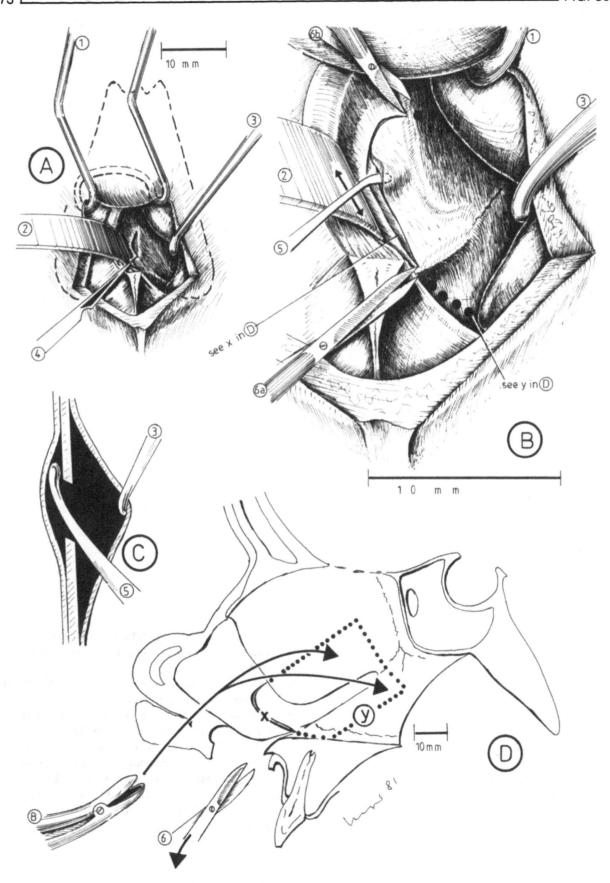

FIG. 37

Fig. 37. Hypophysis operation. Locating **Corpus sphenoidale. Guiding structure** is **Apertura sphenoidalis**

A Anterior to Sinus sphenoidalis, a portion of Lamina mediana is preserved

B Enlarged detail from **A.** In the Apertura sinus sphenoidalis area mucosa is detached from bone surface. This mucosa continues interiorly as mucosa of Sinus sphenoidalis. Since the mucosa of Sinus sphenoidalis is removed, in the typical operative procedure, the only area where the mucosa should be opened is at Apertura sinus sphenoidalis

FIG. 37

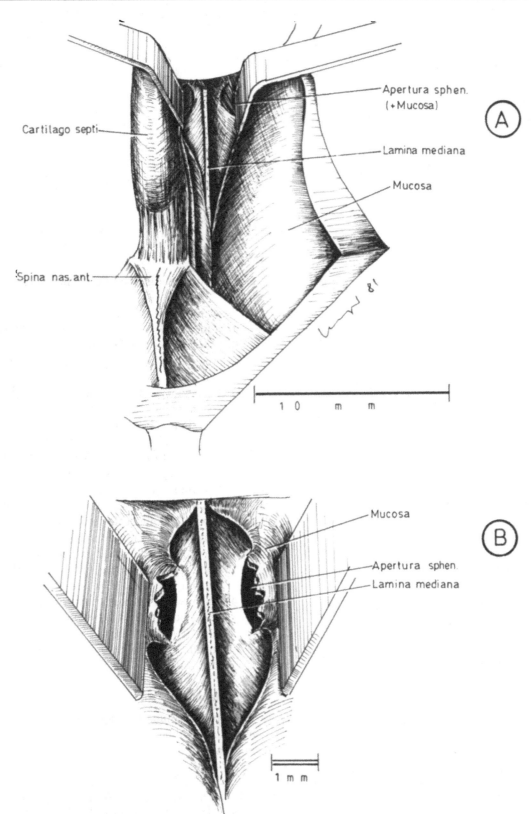

Apertura sphen.
(+Mucosa)

Cartilago septi

Lamina mediana

Mucosa

Spina nas. ant.

1 0   m   m

Ⓐ

Mucosa

Apertura sphen.

Lamina mediana

1 m m

Ⓑ

Fig. 38. Hypophysis operation. Microsurgical operation*

A   Insertion of Hardy-speculum. Residuals of Septum nasi –*lm*– were resected previously with forceps nearly to the Os sphenoidale. Vomer and Ala vomeris are recognizable by their typical thickness

    1 Resection of anterior wall of · Sinus sphenoidalis, starting on both sides at Apertura sinus sphenoidalis –*asp*–

B   **2b** The Sinus sphenoidalis mucosa is detached overall with dissector as thoroughly and cautiously as possible. As far as possible, leave no mucosa remnants in niches, since removal later on is difficult. Mucosa remnants mean the danger of mucocele development. Therefore forceps should not be used as yet –**2a**–

C   **3** The already-detached mucosa is shrunk by electrocoagulation, in order to reach further mucosa portions easily (see **2b** in **B**)

    4 Only when mucosa has been thoroughly detached should it be extracted with forceps. Slight stretching of not yet detached mucosa portions facilitates the detachment by means of dissector

Abbreviations:

asp Apertura sinus sphenoidalis
av Ala vomeris
lm Lamina mediana
vo Vomer

---

* Even the first part of the operation, starting with the mucosa incision, may be carried out microsurgically. Generally one uses the microsurgical technique once the Os sphenoidale is exposed.

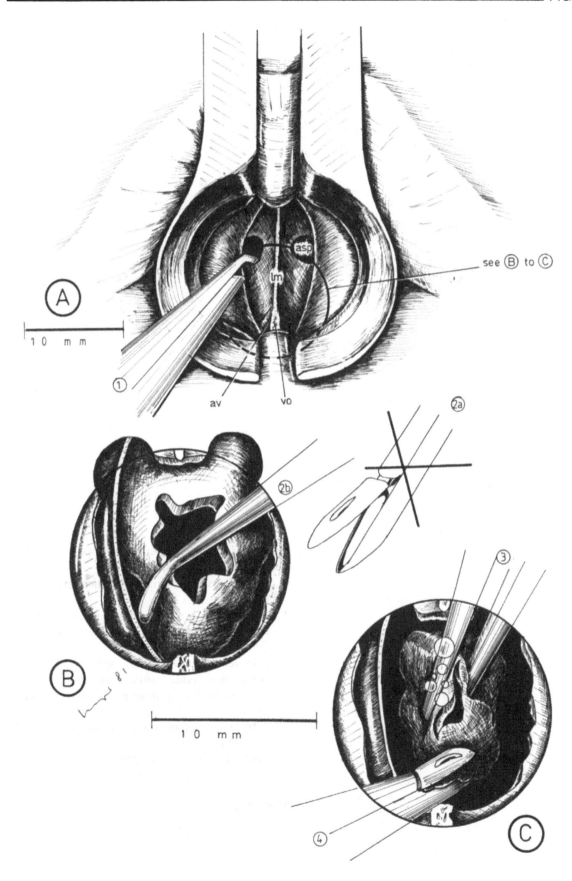

FIG. 39 ⊏══════════════════════════════════════⊐ 78

Fig. 39. Hypophysis operation. Topographical relation of **Septum sphenoidale** *–ssp–*

A Septum *–ssp–* presented in clinical example from Fig. 23

A' Anatomical model corresponding to **A.** The tumor can be reached even without septum resection (arrow)

B Another variant of Septum sphenoidale

B' Anatomical model, frontal section, corresponding to **B.** Without septum resection the tumor can be only partially removed

B'' After septum resection the tumor can be reached on both sides (arrows)

C Anatomical sketch of section planes **A'**, **B'** and **B''**, median section plane

Abbreviation:

ssp Septum sphenoidale

FIG. 39

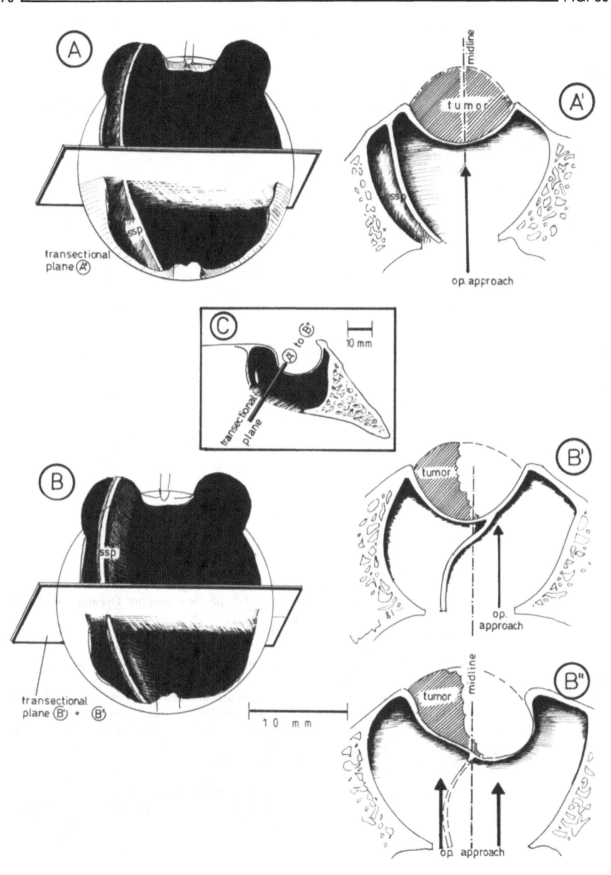

A

transectional plane Ⓐ'

A'
midline
tumor
ssp
op. approach

C
Ⓐ to Ⓑ'
transectional plane
10 mm

B
ssp
transectional plane Ⓑ' + Ⓑ"

10 mm

B'
tumor
op. approach

B"
tumor
midline
op. approach

FIG. 40 ⊏━━━━━━━━━━━━━━━━━━━━━━━━━━━━━━━━━⊐ 80

Fig. 40. Hypophysis operation. **Opening up of sella space**

A Microsurgical site

   1a + 1b Chiseling of bony sella floor

   2 Enlargement of opening by means of a rongeur.

   Open arrow: deep posterior recessus of Sinus sphenoidalis (towards Dorsum sellae)

A' Anatomical model, sagittal section. Situation as in A

B Microsurgical site

   1 Dura incision

   2 Dura detachment with dissector

B' Anatomical model, sagittal section, corresponding to B

FIG. 40

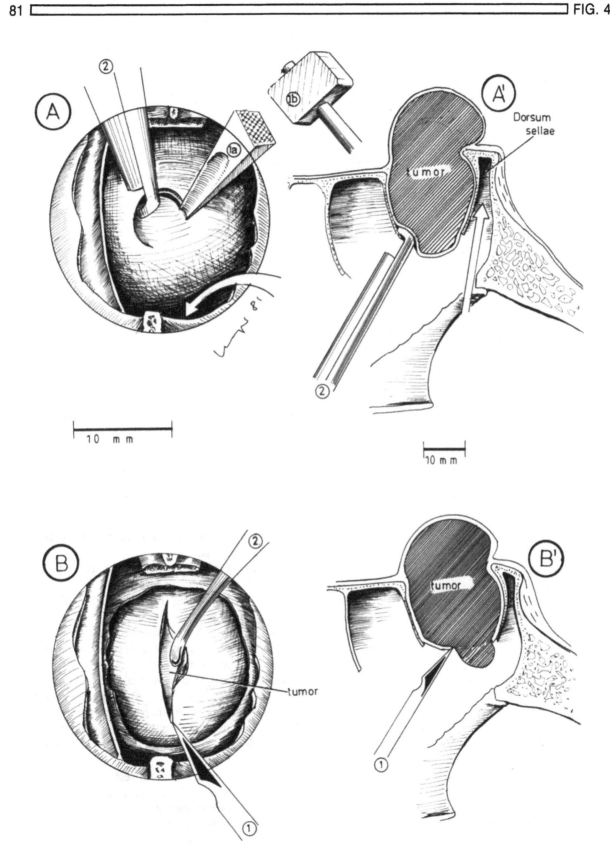

Dorsum
sellae

tumor

tumor

tumor

10 mm

10 mm

FIG. 41 82

Fig. 41. Hypophysis operation. **Tumor extirpation**
A   Microsurgical site
    1a + 1b   Curettage of tumor (various types of curettes see Fig. 29)
    Loosening on both sides of lateral tumor portions
A' Anatomical model, sagittal section
    2a + 2b   Loosening of anterior and posterior tumor portions
B   Main bulk of tumor is removed. Diaphragma sellae becomes visible. If Diaphragma sellae extends deeply in an inferior direction, the risk exists that marginal tumor portions remain
    3a + 3b   Cautious removal of lateral tumor portions
B' Anatomical model, sagittal section
    4a + 4b   Removal of anterior and posterior tumor remnants.
    Arrows: Directions of instrument movements

FIG. 41

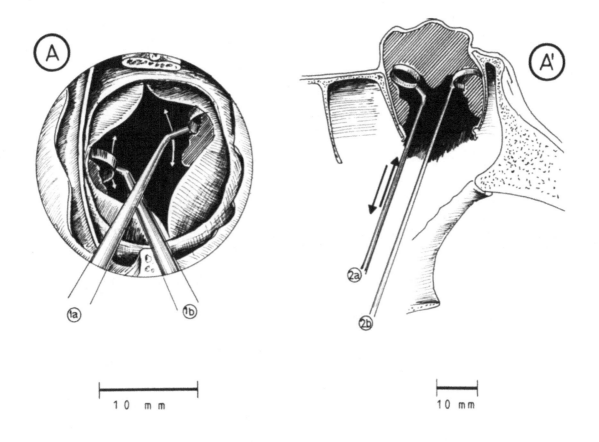

10 mm

10 mm

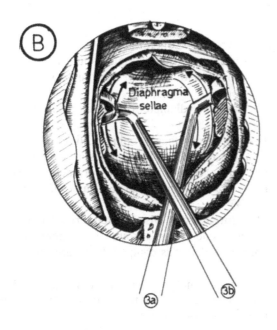

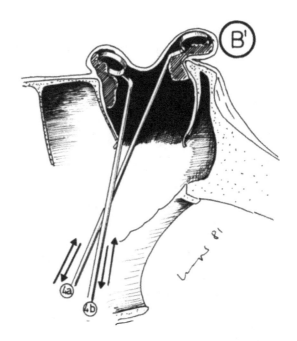

Diaphragma sellae

FIG. 42 ⊏━━━━━━━━━━━━━━━━━━━━━━━━━━━━━━━━⊐ 84

Fig. 42. Hypophysis operation

A Microsurgical site after tumor removal
    d transverse diameter of bone defect in the sella floor
    d" transverse diameter of dura defect in the sella floor

B Disc out of cartilage, lyophilized dura (or bone). Oval piece cut from Septum nasi or from a piece of lyodura, in order to **cover dura defect in sella floor** (see **A**) from inside. Finishing of disc, see Fig. 43

C Microsurgical site. Disc is eased through dura gap to the inside. Open arrows: adjustment of disc until dura defect is completely covered from inside

C' Anatomical model of **C,** sagittal section. The properly fitted disc is fastened with tissue glue (fibrinogen concentrate)

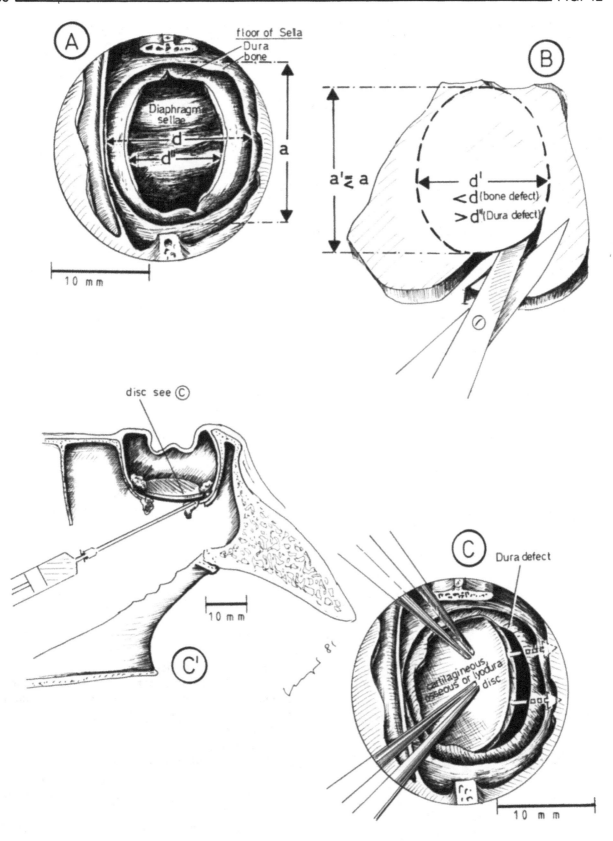

FIG. 43 ⬜==⬜ 86

Fig. 43. Hypophysis operation
Finishing of a disc flap from bone (**A**) or cartilage (**B**).
Technique for **insertion of flap to the inside of dura defect**
A Finishing of flap from bone
B Cutting of cartilage
B' Slicing of cartilage if too thick
B'' Oblique trimming of the cartilage edges, in order to obtain a fine edge, which can be eased through dura opening
C Easing of disc to the inside of sella dura lining –*f*–

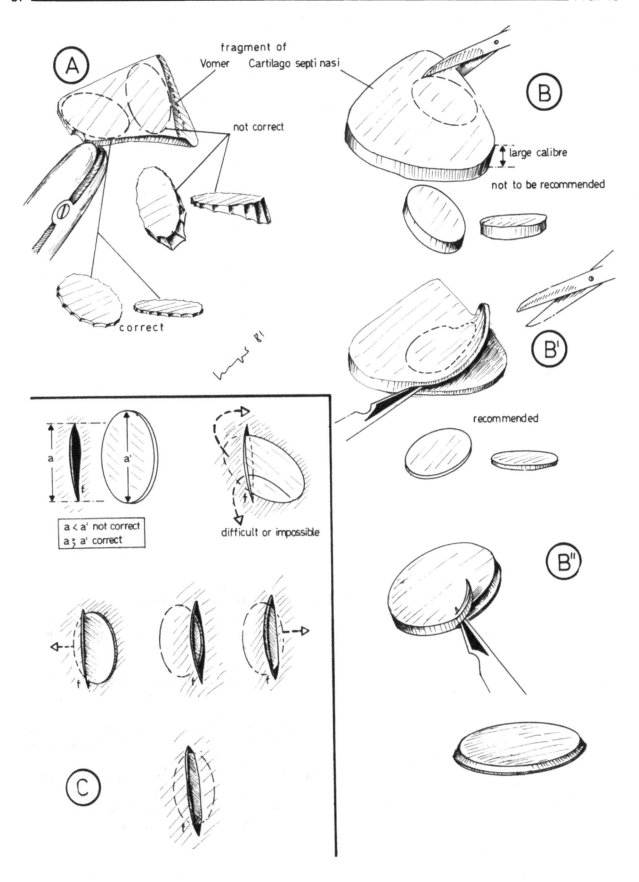

A
fragment of
Vomer   Cartilago septi nasi
not correct
correct

B
large calibre
not to be recommended

B'
recommended

B"

C
a < a' not correct
a ≥ a' correct
difficult or impossible

FIG. 44   88

Fig. 44. Hypophysis operation

Principle of **tamponage of Cavum nasi** with gauze

A **Correct procedure:** Using forceps, grasp gauze away from its end a; and insert it through Meatus nasi inferior

A' **Incorrect procedure:**
- Gauze gripped at its end (danger of gauze end slipping into choane area and narrowing upper respiratory tract, see **B'**)
- Insertion diagonally through Cavum nasi upwards. This prevents tamponage of the posterior portions of Cavum nasi

B Correct tamponage, by which gauze end –arrow a– is pressed against floor of Cavum nasi

B' **Incorrect:** Gauze end has come free, thereby narrowing the upper respiratory tract

FIG. 44

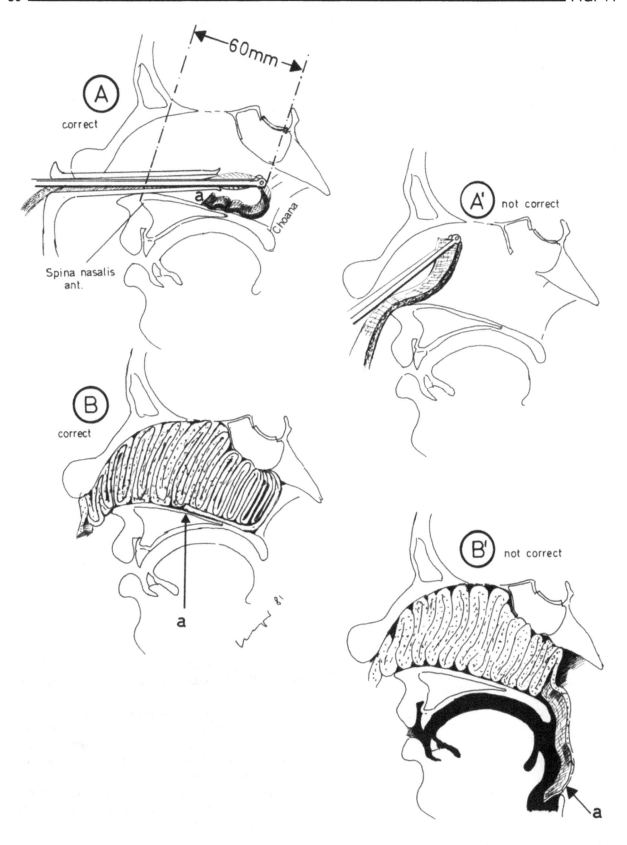

A correct

60mm

Spina nasalis ant.

a

Choana

A' not correct

B correct

a

B' not correct

a

FIG. 45 ⸺⸺⸺⸺⸺⸺⸺⸺⸺⸺⸺⸺⸺⸺⸺ 90

Fig. 45. Hypophysis operation. Tamponage with foam material. Possible mistakes (refer also to gauze tamponage)

A Correct tamponage. Measurements in mm

B Incorrect tamponage: posterior portions of Cavum nasi not packed, creating danger of blood seepage from injured mucosa of Cavum nasi or sinus into naso-pharyngeal space.

C Incorrect tamponage: packing not only Cavum nasi, but also Epipharynx with narrowing of Epi- and Mesopharynx

FIG. 45

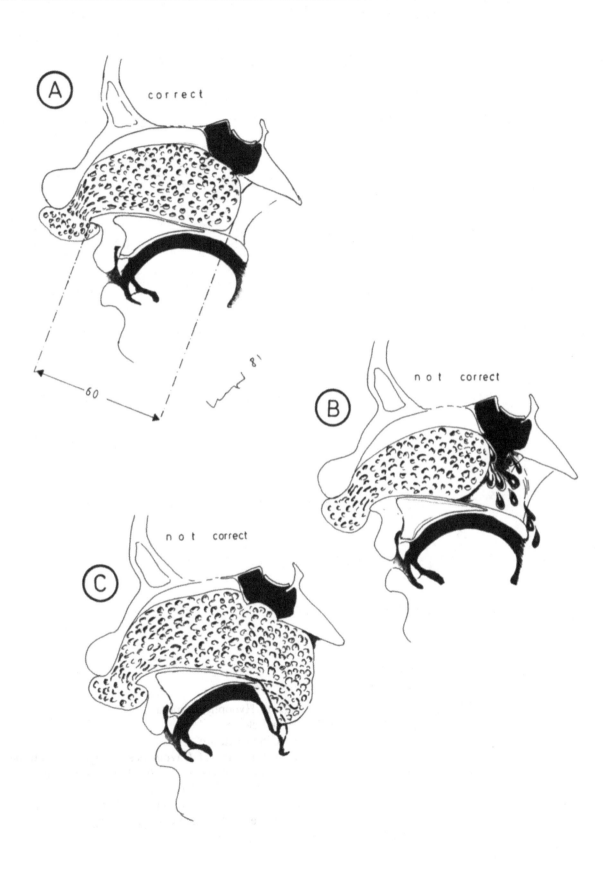

FIG. 46 ⊏▭▭▭▭▭▭▭▭▭▭▭▭▭▭▭▭▭▭▭▭▭▭▭▭▭▭▭▭▭▭▭▭▭⊐ 92

Fig. 46. Hypophysis operation
Wound closure
A Gingiva suture
B Tamponage of Cavum nasi with foam material
–*a*– or with gauze –*b*– (soakend with salve) after
insertion of a speculum
C Situation after tamponage of both nasal openings
D Adhesive bandage over tamponage

FIG. 46

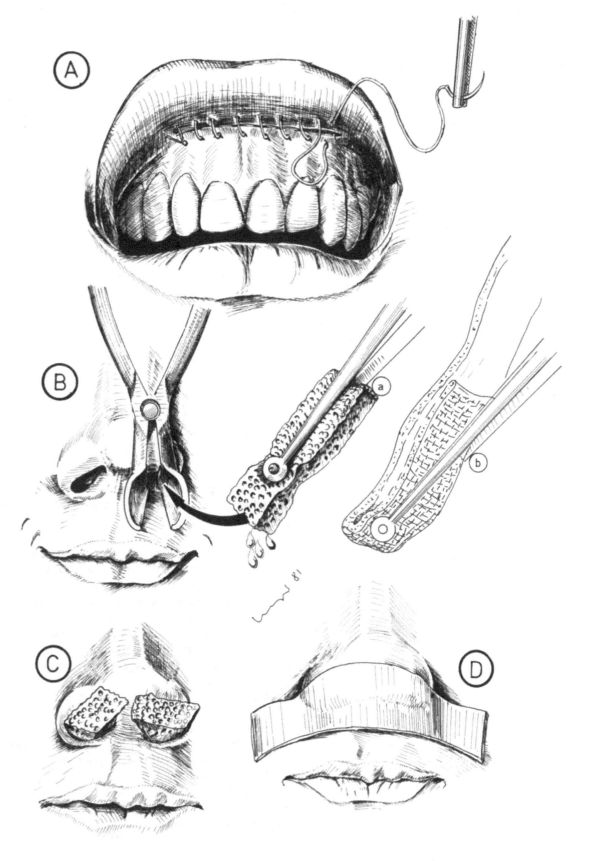

FIG. 47 94

Fig. 47. Hypophysis operation

Special situations: liquorrhea through defect of Diaphragma sellae

A Microsurgical site. One sees defect in Diaphragma sellae and arachnoidea centrally located at penetration area of hypophyseal stalk

A' Anatomical model, sagittal section

B Micorosurgical site after deposition of fatty tissue into sella space

    1 Squirting of tissue glue* (Fibrinogen and activator) around fatty tissue

    2 Pressing of fatty tissue after introduction of tissue glue

B' Anatomical model, sagittal section

    1 + 2 as in B

C Microsurgical site

    1a + 1b Closing of sella floor with cartilagineous or osseous disc cut from Septum nasi

C' Anatomical model

    2 Squirting cartilage disc with tissue glue*

* Immuno-Chemie, Heidelberg.

FIG. 47

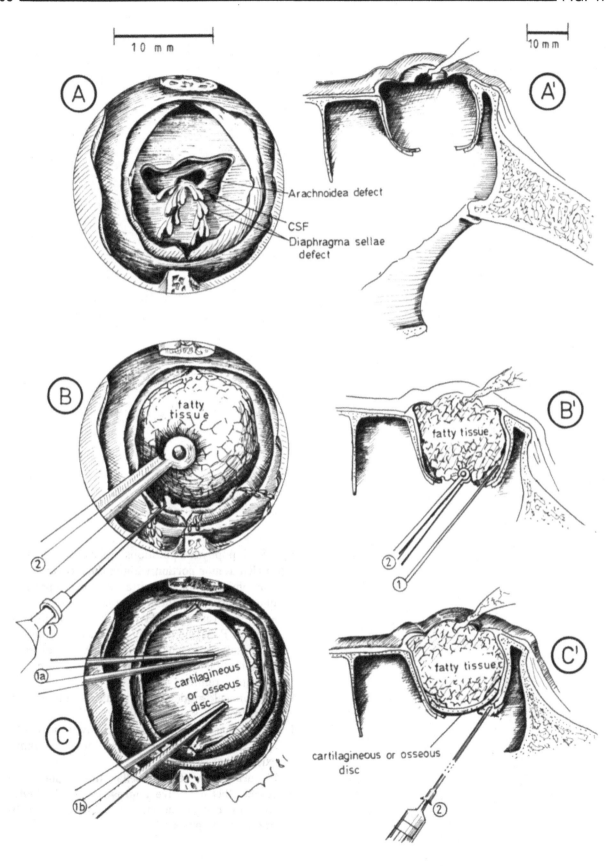

10 mm

10 mm

A

A'

Arachnoidea defect

CSF

Diaphragma sellae defect

B

B'

fatty tissue

fatty tissue

② ②

①

C

C'

fatty tissue

1a

cartilagineous or osseous disc

C

cartilagineous or osseous disc

1b

②

FIG. 48 ⊏⟝ 96

Fig. 48. Hypophysis operations. Special situations:
Suprasellar tumor portion without dura cover

A Anatomical model, sagittal section. Suprasellar tumor portions without dura cover. A. basilaris –*bl*–, N.II (as well as Hypothalamus, perforating arteries, Pons) lie directly against the tumor. By oro-nasal approach, the overview is not sufficiently safe to avoid injuring these structures during tumor removal

A' Anatomical model, continuation and enlargement from **A,** sagittal section

B Microsurgical site. Tumor partially removed. In spite of large residual tumor, liquorrhea shows existence of situation **A'**
If dura cover of suprasellar tumor portion is absent, this operative approach must be halted and tumor removal must be finished later by transcranial approach

FIG. 48

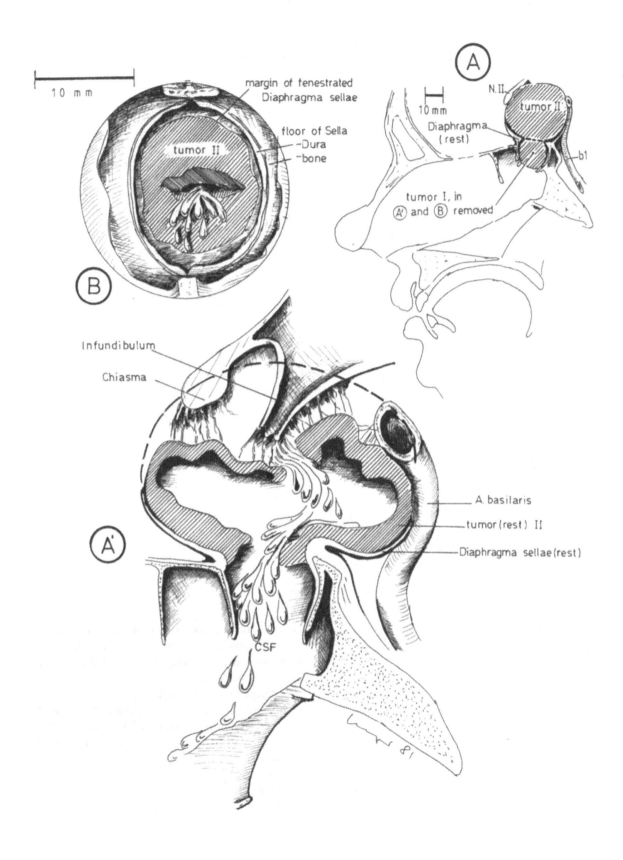

10 mm

margin of fenestrated
Diaphragma sellae

floor of Sella
–Dura
–bone

tumor II

B

A

N. II

tumor II

Diaphragma
(rest)

b1

tumor I, in
A' and B removed

Infundibulum

Chiasma

A. basilaris

tumor (rest) II

Diaphragma sellae (rest)

A'

CSF

10 mm

FIG. 49 98

Fig. 49. Hypophysis operations. Special situations: Normal Diaphragma sellae, **tumor extension predominantly supradiaphragmatical without dura cover**

A   Anatomical model, sagittal section
A' Enlarged detail from **A**
B   Microsurgical site, corresponding to **A** and **A'**
   If dura cover of suprasellar tumor portion is absent, operative approach must be halted for the same reason as in Fig. 48

Abbreviation:

ds   Diaphragma sella, defect

FIG. 49

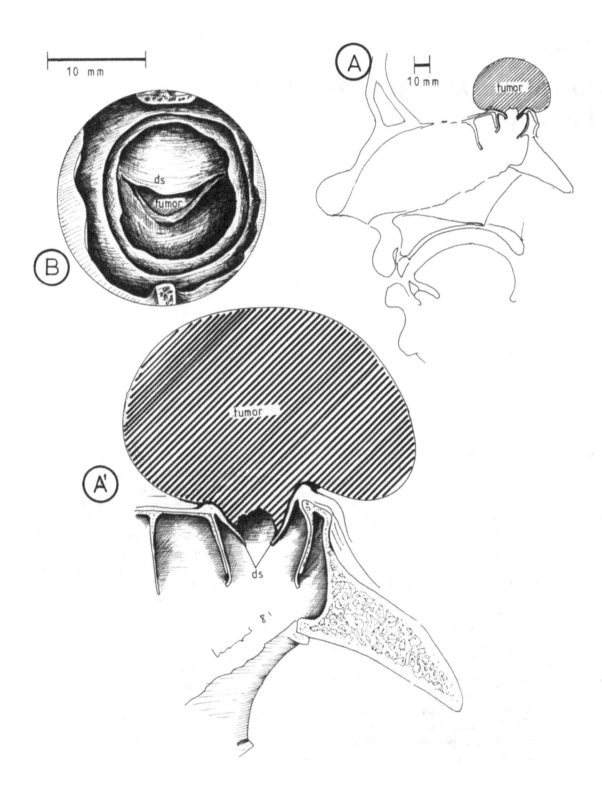

FIG. 50 ⊏━━━━━━━━━━━━━━━━━━━━━━━━━━━⊐ 100

Chapter 2
Operations at Sinus cavernosus
(Figs. 50–99)

Anatomy of Sinus cavernosus (Figs. 50 to 54)

Fig. 50. Operations in the area surrounding Sinus cavernosus.

Anatomy of **intradural path of A. carotis int.** and its branches*

A   View from above: In this sketch: On the left side A. ophthalmica originates intradurally from A. carotis int; on the right side extradurally

A' + A"   A. communicans post. –p5– and A. chorioidea –c5– may originate proximally or distally from A. carotis int.; their points of origin may be close together or far apart

A'''   **In the case of proximal origin of A. communicans post. and A. chorioidea ant. these vessels may be partly covered by the elongated tentorial fold. When clipping A. carotis int. at its penetration point there is danger of closing off these two arteries (especially A. communicans post.) with their perforating branches which run beneath A. carotis int.**

B   Preparation similar to **A,** basal view. In addition to the typical perforating arteries from A. communicans post. and A. chorioidea ant., perforating arteries –x– (running to Hypothalamus) may originate directly from the A. carotis int. (according to Dawson, 1968)

Abbreviations:

c1   A. carotis int.
c5   A. chorioidea ant.
p5   A. communicans post.
te   Tentorium edge
x   Atypical perforating arteries

———————

* Extensive presentation see J. Lang, 1979.

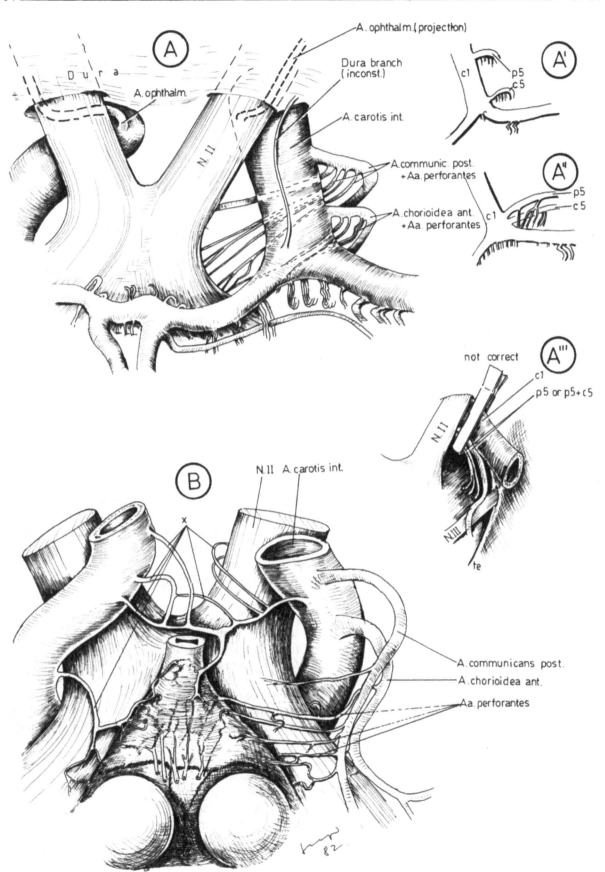

A

A. ophthalm.(projection)

Dura branch
(inconst.)

A. carotis int.

Dura

A. ophthalm.

N. II

A. communic. post.
+ Aa. perforantes

A. chorioidea ant.
+ Aa. perforantes

A'

c1   p5
c5

A''

c1   p5
c5

A'''

not correct   c1

p5 or p5+c5

N. II

N. III

te

B

N. II   A. carotis int.

x

A. communicans post.

A. chorioidea ant.

Aa. perforantes

FIG. 51 [⎯⎯⎯⎯⎯⎯⎯⎯⎯⎯⎯⎯⎯⎯⎯⎯⎯] 102

Fig. 51. Operations in the area surrounding Sinus cavernosus.
Anatomy of the **parasellar area,** example of a skull showing senile bone atrophy
A Overview
B Enlarged detail from **A**

Abbreviations:

ca	Processus clinoideus ant.
fo	Foramen opticum
fos	Fissura orbitalis sup.
flc	Foramen lacerum
fov	Foramen ovale
incl	Incision of Processus clinoideus and Radix of Processus clinoideus ant. anterior to A. carotis int.
rc	Radix of Proc. clin. ant.
rt	Foramen rotundum
sc	Sulcus caroticus
st	Sella turcica
ts	Tuberculum sellae

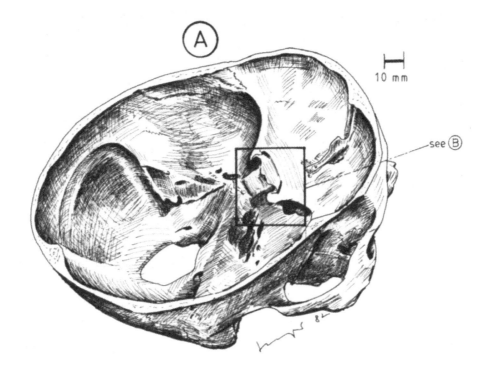

A

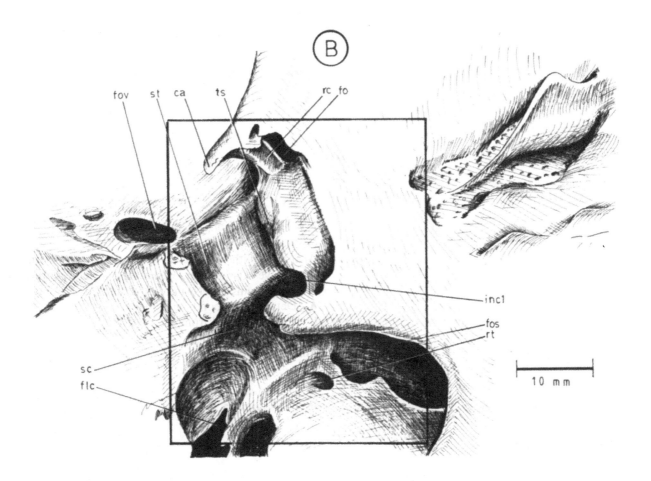

B

FIG. 52 ⬤━━━━━━━━━━━━━━━━━━━━━━━━━━━⬤ 104

Fig. 52. Operations in the area surrounding Sinus cavernosus.

Anatomy of the **parasellar area.** Preparation from Fig. 51, vessels and nerves sketched in. Dura structures with veins and N. maxillaris omitted

A Detail, corresponding to Fig. 51
B Enlarged detail from **A**

Abbreviations:

fos Fissura orbitalis sup.
rt   Foramen rotundum
st   Sella turcica
ts   Tuberculum sellae

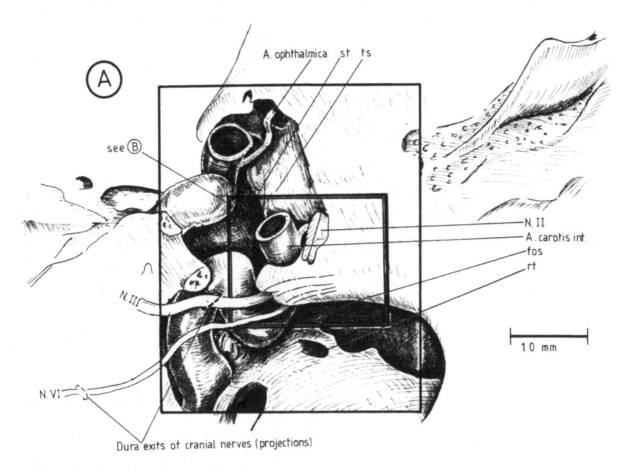

(A)

A. ophthalmica st ts

see (B)

N. II
A. carotis int.
fos
rt

N. III

N. VI

10 mm

Dura exits of cranial nerves (projections)

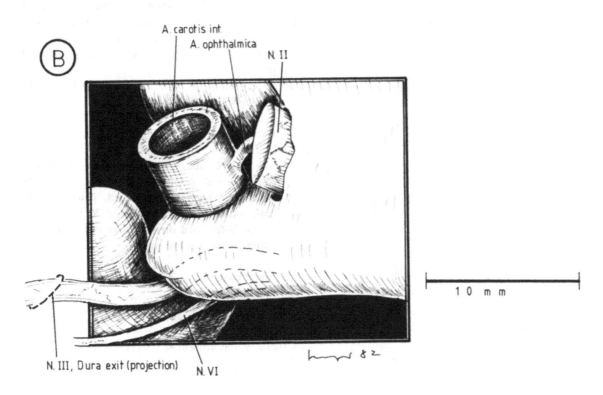

(B)

A. carotis int.
A. ophthalmica
N. II

10 mm

N. III, Dura exit (projection)   N. VI

FIG. 53 ⊏══⊐ 106

Fig. 53. Operations in the area surrounding Sinus cavernosus.

Anatomy of path of A. ophthalmica, variants* (frequency percentage)

Path of A. ophthalmica after resection of Canalis opticus roof (**A, C** and **D**) with additional resection of Processus clinoideus ant. and its covering dura (**A' + B**)

A Typical path of A. ophthalmica

A' Same preparation as **A**, N.III and N.VI sketched in

B Rare variant: A. ophthalmica with its own bony canal. N.III and N.VI sketched in

C Second most frequent variant

D Rare variant: A. ophthalmica is replaced by branch of A. meningea media.

The typical path of A. ophthalmica (see A) is thus characterized: origin –o– is medial anterior from the point where A. carotis int. penetrates dura; path continues laterally behind N. opticus with a loop –an–forward then to leave dura sheath of N. opticus –penetration point _p_ –

Abbreviations:

_c1_ A. carotis int.

_c2_ A. ophthalmica

_____

* After S. S. Haydreh and R. Dass (1962), modified.

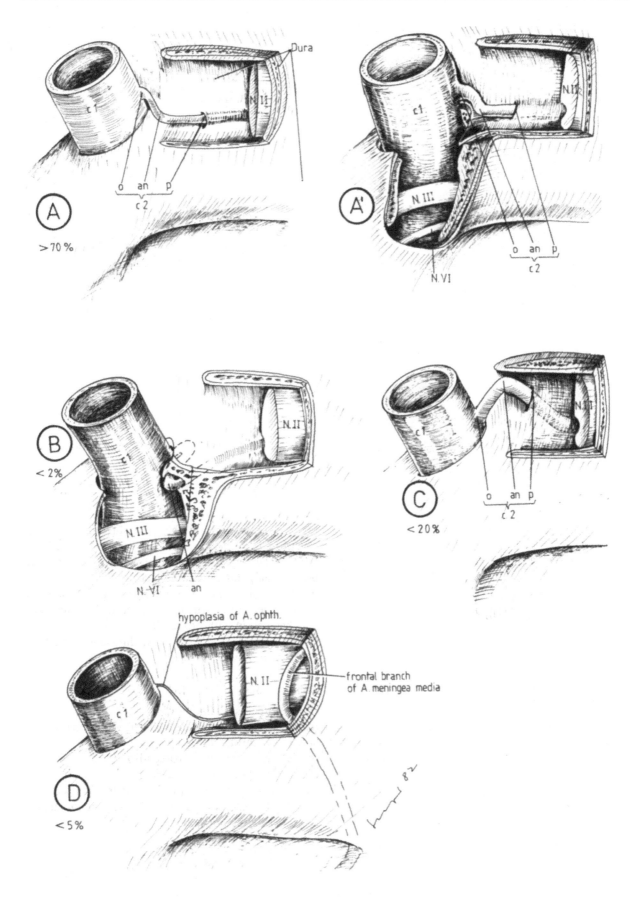

FIG. 54 ⊏━━━━━━━━━━━━━━━━━━━━━━━━━━━━━━━━⊐ 108

Fig. 54. Operations in the area surrounding Sinus cavernosus.

Anatomical topographical relation of **A. carotis int. penetration point** to adjoining structures

A Anatomical sketch, similar to Fig. 52 **B,** dura sketched in. Structures covered by dura are sketched in with broken lines

B Anatomical sketch as in **A,** dura and bone partially removed

Abbreviations:

ca	Processus clinoideus ant.
(ca)	Processus clinoideus ant. (projection)
cl	A. carotis int.
(cl)	A. carotis int. (projection)
(N.VI)	N. abducens (projection)
rca	Pneumosinus in the area of Radix processus clinoidei (protrusion of Sinus sphenoidalis)
ts	Tuberculum sellae

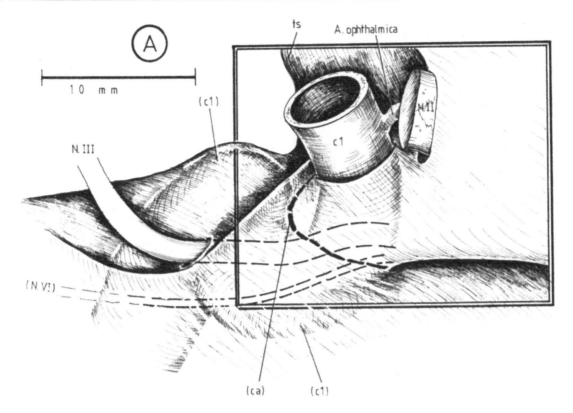

Ⓐ

10 mm

(c1)

N. III

ts   A. ophthalmica

N. II

c1

(N. VI)

(ca)   (c1)

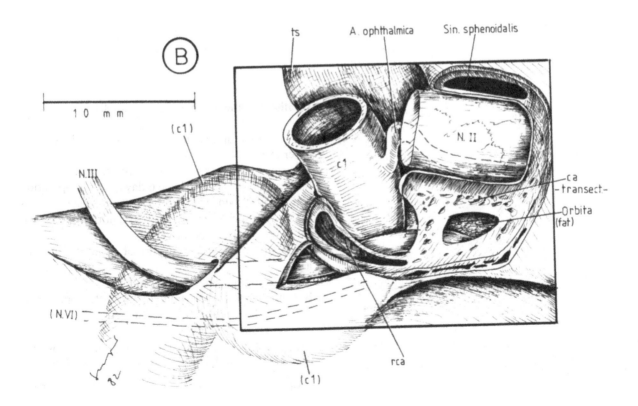

Ⓑ

10 mm

(c1)

N. III

ts   A. ophthalmica   Sin. sphenoidalis

N. II

c1

ca
transect

Orbita
(fat)

(N. VI)

rca

(c1)

FIG. 55 ⊏==⊐ 110

Ophthalmic aneurysms (Figs. 55 to 60)

Fig. 55. Operations in the area surrounding Sinus cavernosus.

Clinical example of an **A. ophthalmica aneurysm** *

Subarachnoidal hemorrhage 6 days prior to operation with slight leftsided hemiparesis, meningism, psychical slowing; oriented. Quick regression of pathological symptoms postoperatively**.

Secondary finding: Aneurysm of A. communicans ant.

A + A' Preoperative angiogram

B + B' Angiography immediately after operation. Both aneurysms are clipped

---

* I am grateful to Prof. Dr. K. Kendel and PD Dr. G. Reinshagen (Neurological Clinic, District Hospital Lahr) for the preoperative angiogram.

** Operation performed by Dr. J. Gilsbach, author's coworker.

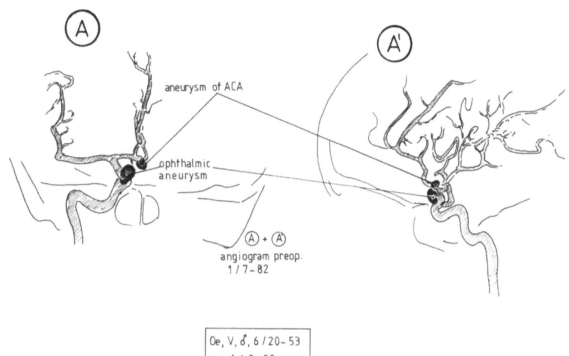

aneurysm of ACA

ophthalmic
aneurysm

Ⓐ + Ⓐ'
angiogram preop.
1 / 7 - 82

Oe, V, ♂, 6 / 20 - 53
op. 1 / 8 - 82

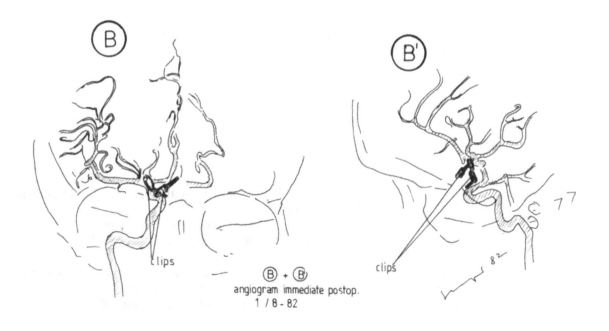

clips

clips

Ⓑ + Ⓑ'
angiogram immediate postop.
1 / 8 - 82

FIG. 56 ☐━━━━━━━━━━━━━━━━━━━━━━━━━━━━━━━☐ 112

Fig. 56. Operations in the area surrounding Sinus cavernosus.

A. ophthalmica aneurysm. Operation

A Location of skin incision and **pterional trepanation**

B Location of trepanation, skull preparation, microsurgical site **C** sketched in

C Microsurgical site after **opening of dura**

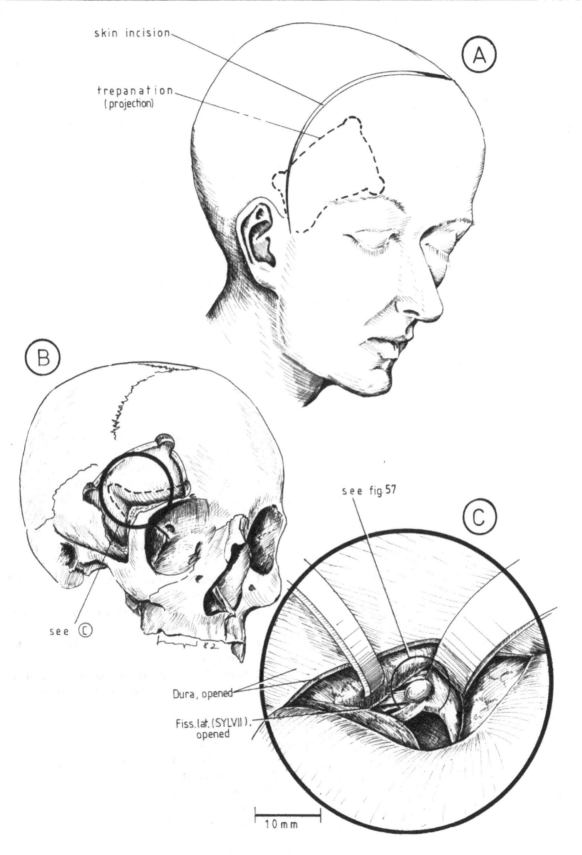

skin incision

trepanation
(projection)

(A)

(B)

see (C)

8 2

see fig. 57

(C)

Dura, opened

Fiss. lat. (SYLVII),
opened

10 mm

FIG. 57 ⊏━━━━━━━━━━━━━━━━━━━━━━━━━━━━━━━━━━━⊐ 114

Fig. 57. Operations in the area surrounding Sinus cavernosus.

A. ophthalmica aneurysm, operation

A Enlarged microsurgical site from Fig. 56 **C,** rotated 90°

    1 Dura incision in front of A. ophthalmica aneurysm

    2 Dura pulled back from Processus clinoideus ant.

B **1** Separation of dura bridge which lies over N.II and aneurysm

    2 Drilling of Processus clinoideus ant. and osseous roof of N.II

C **1** Separation of adhesions from neck of aneurysm

    2 Since clipping is not yet possible, aneurysm is shrunk by bipolar electrocoagulation

Abbreviations:

ap Ala minor
ca Processus clinoideus ant.
cl A. carotis int.
fcm Fossa cranii media
gr Gyri recti
ts Tuberculum sellae

FIG. 57

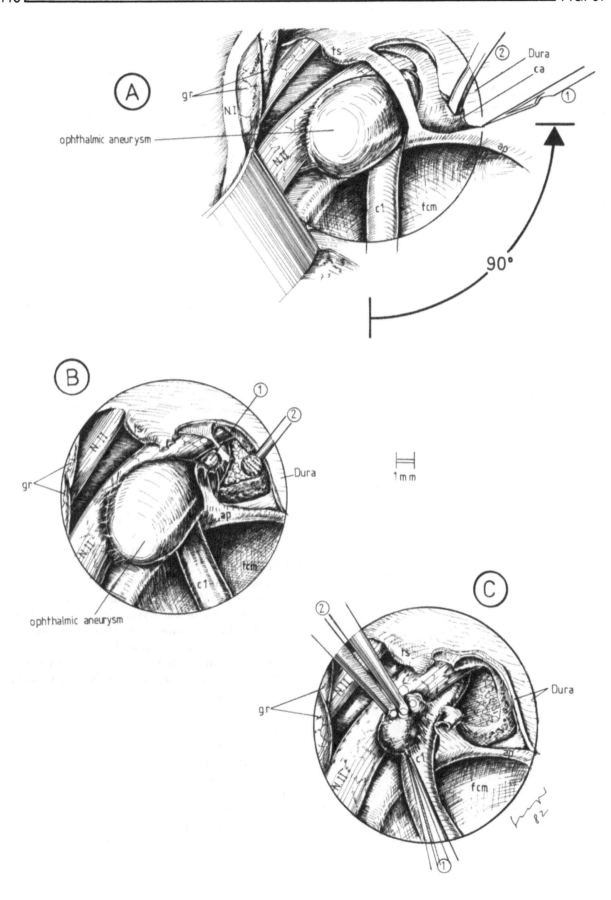

A

gr
N.I
ophthalmic aneurysm
N.II
c1
fcm
ts
② Dura
ca
①
ap
90°

B

①
②
N.II
gr
Dura
ap
N.III
c1
fcm
ophthalmic aneurysm

1mm

C

②
ts
gr
Dura
N.II
c1
ap
N.III
fcm
①

FIG. 58 ━━ 116

Fig. 58. Operations in the area surrounding Sinus cavernosus.

A **A. ophthalmica aneurysm** is clipped

B Aneurysm with clip is folded back laterally. Arrows: neck of aneurysm only partially eliminated. **Clip correction** in direction of arrows

C Situation of final aneurysm clipping.
On A. communicans ant., a second aneurysm was found and eliminated immediately after with the typical technique

Abbreviations:

ap   Ala minor
ca   Processus clinoideus ant. (residual)
cl   A. carotis int.
fcm Fossa cranii media
gr   Gyri recti
ts   Tuberculum sellae

FIG. 58

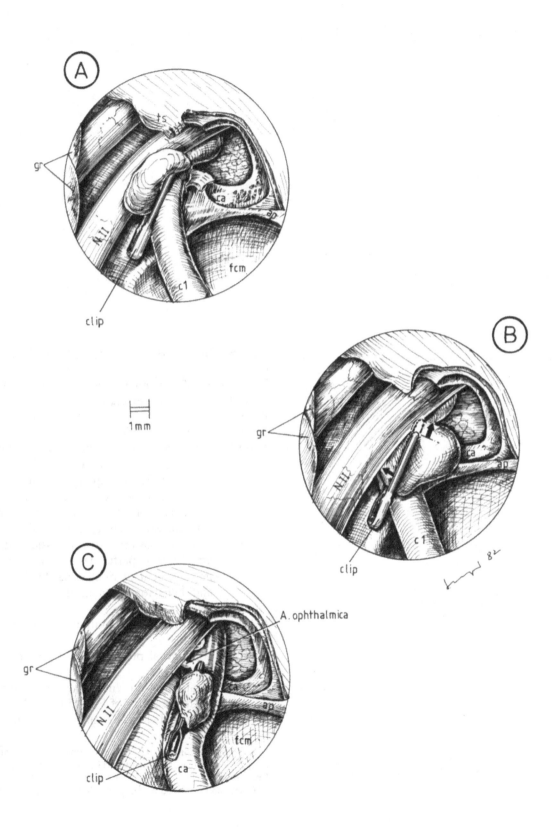

FIG. 59 ☐⸺⸺⸺⸺⸺⸺⸺⸺⸺⸺⸺⸺⸺⸺⸺⸺☐ 118

Fig. 59. Operations in the area surrounding Sinus cavernosus.

Various types of A. ophthalmica aneurysms, anatomical sketches of clinical examples.

Broken lines: path of A. carotis int. in the area of Sinus cavernosus (projection)

A − B'   After subarachnoidal hemorrhage, blind in both eyes; two weeks later, after angiography, acute left hemiplegia, psychical slowing; shortly before operation visual improvement on the left side, on the right side complete nasal hemianopsia, mixed aphasia. Postoperative recession of left arm pareses, partial leg paresis remains, improvement of right visual field, speech and behavior normalized within several weeks*

A + A'   Anatomical presentation of preoperative status

B + B'   Anatomical presentation of postoperative status

C + D   Anatomical presentation of pre- and post-operative status of Fig. 55 to 58**

E + F   No actual clinical example available

---

* Operation performed by author during his time at the Neurosurgical Clinic, University of Giessen, Director Prof. Dr. Dr. h. c. H. W. Pia.
** Operation performed by Dr. J. Gilsbach, author's coworker.

FIG. 59

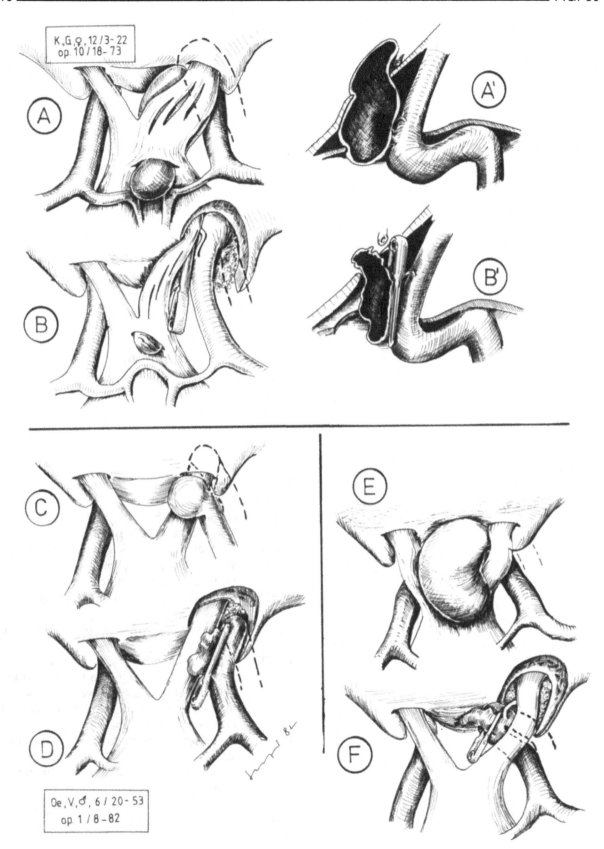

FIG. 60 ⊏────────────────────────────────────⊐ 120

Fig. 60. Operations in the area surrounding Sinus cavernosus.

Various types of A. ophthalmica aneurysms, anatomical sketches of clinical examples

A – B'   For several months gradual diminishing visual acuity and mydriasis on left side, no postoperative worsening*

A + A'   Anatomical presentation of preoperative status

B + B'   Anatomical presentation of postoperative status

C – D'   Within 6 months gradual diminishing of left side visual acuity with temporal visual field defect*. Postoperative visual acuity improvement from 0,6 to 0,8, visual field defects no longer demonstrable

C + C'   Anatomical presentation of preoperative status

D + D'   Anatomical presentation of postoperative status

---

* Operation performed by Dr. J. Gilsbach, author's coworker.

FIG. 60

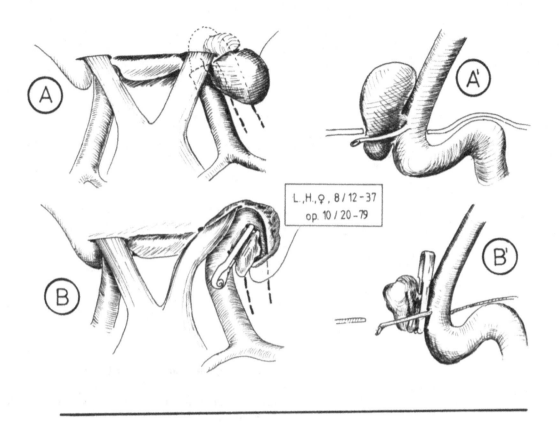

L.,H.,♀, 8 / 12 – 37
op. 10 / 20 – 79

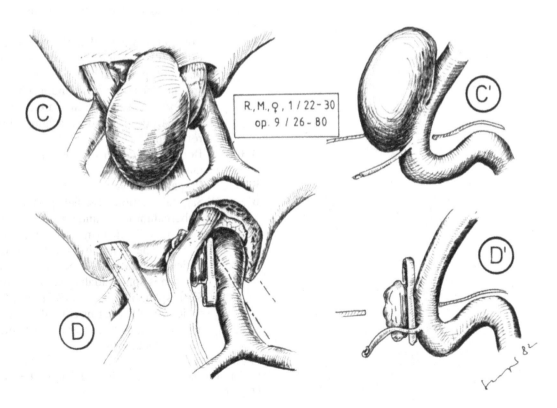

R.,M.,♀, 1 / 22 – 30
op. 9 / 26 – 80

FIG. 61 ⌐══⌐ 122

Pneumosinus dilatans (Figs. 61 to 68)

Fig. 61. Operations in the area surrounding Sinus cavernosus.

Pneumosinus dilatans (of Processus clinoideus ant.), anatomy

A   Position of Sinus sphenoidalis and Canales optici (broken line). Processus clinoideus ant. not pneumatized. Position of Sinus sphenoidalis beneath Planum sphenoidale, Tuberculum sellae, Sella turcica, and Sulcus caroticus, and reaching Foramen rotundum

B + B' Bone preparation with Pneumosinus dilatans*

B   Preparation, view as in **A**

B'   Sagittal section, medial posterior view. Tuberculum sellae and posterior portion of medial wall of Canalis opticus are removed. The remaining portion of Canalis opticus medial wall frequently protrudes into Sinus sphenoidalis. Arrows show that Sinus sphenoidalis extends around Canalis opticus into Processus clinoideus ant., and here surrounds Canalis opticus laterally as well = Pneumosinus dilatans

---

* Skull preparation of Neurosurgical Clinic, University of Freiburg.

FIG. 61

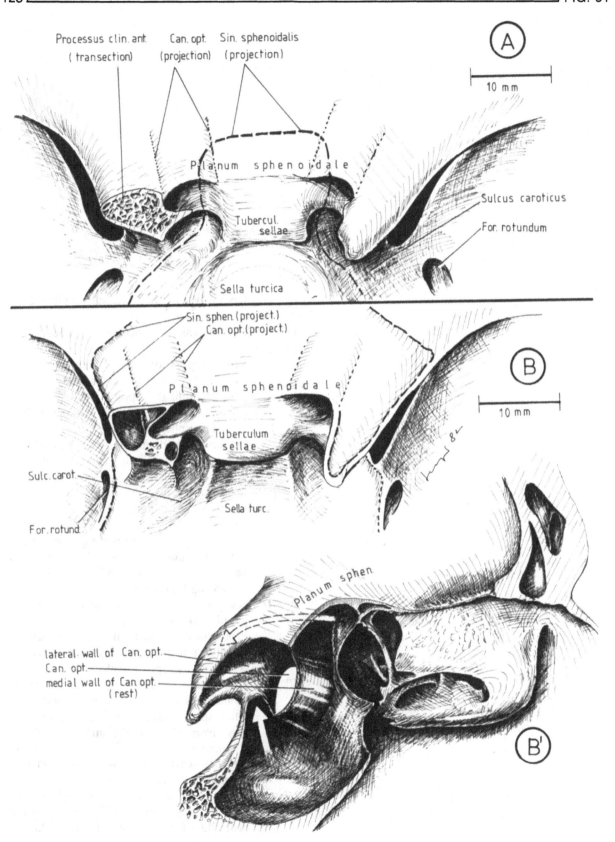

A

Processus clin. ant.
(transection)

Can. opt.
(projection)

Sin. sphenoidalis
(projection)

10 mm

Planum sphenoidale

Sulcus caroticus

Tubercul.
sellae

For. rotundum

Sella turcica

B

Sin. sphen.(project.)
Can. opt.(project.)

Planum sphenoidale

10 mm

Tuberculum
sellae

Sulc. carot.

For. rotund.

Sella turc.

Planum sphen.

lateral wall of Can. opt.
Can. opt.
medial wall of Can. opt.
(rest)

B'

FIG. 62 □⧠⧠⧠⧠⧠⧠⧠⧠⧠⧠⧠⧠⧠⧠⧠⧠⧠⧠□ 124

Fig. 62. Operations in the area surrounding Sinus cavernosus.

Pneumosinus dilatans (of Processus clinoideus ant.), anatomy

A   Skull preparation (detail), superior view, section planes **B – D'** sketched in

B   Normal finding: Topographical relation of Processus clinoideus ant., Canalis opticus and Sinus sphenoidalis

C   Pneumosinus dilatans. Arrows mark the connection of Sinus sphenoidalis into Pneumosinus dilatans, here formed by two recesses of Sinus sphenoidalis –*a* + *b*–

D   Pneumosinus dilatans. Arrows mark connection of Sinus sphenoidalis into Pneumosinus, here consisting of **one** recess only, corresponding to *b* in **C. Pneumosinus** has a **thick wall,** especially **in the presence of Canalis opticus meningiomas**

B' – D'   Section plane somewhat more rostral compared to **B – D (see A)**

B'   Processus clinoideus ant. not pneumatized, Canalis opticus of normal size protruding –*c*– into Sinus sphenoidalis

C'   Pneumosinus dilatans –*a*– and –*b*– corresponding to **C.** Arrows show connection of Sinus sphenoidalis into Pneumosinus dilatans. **Narrowed Canalis opticus** is almost completely surrounded by Pneumosinus, thus lies nearly free in Sinus sphenoidalis

D'   Pneumosinus dilatans –*b*–. Arrow shows connection of Sinus sphenoidalis into Pneumosinus. Canalis opticus very narrow, protruding freely into Sinus sphenoidalis

FIG. 62

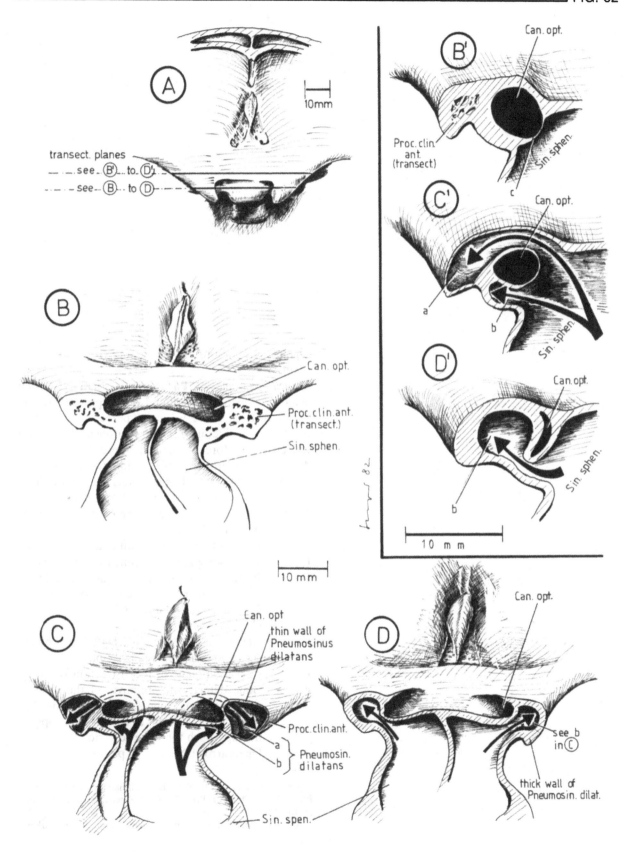

A

10mm

transect. planes
— · — · see (B') to (D')
— · · — · see (B) to (D)

B'

Can. opt.

Proc. clin.
ant.
(transect)

Sin. sphen.

c

C'

Can. opt.

a

b

Sin. sphen.

D'

Can. opt.

b

Sin. sphen.

10 m m

B

Can. opt.

Proc. clin. ant.
(transect.)

Sin. sphen.

10 mm

C

Can. opt

thin wall of
Pneumosinus
dilatans

Proc. clin. ant.

a
b
} Pneumosin.
dilatans

Sin. sphen.

D

Can. opt.

see b
in (C)

thick wall of
Pneumosin. dilat.

FIG. 63 ╠══════════════════════════════════╣ 126

Fig. 63. Operations in the area surrounding Sinus cavernosus.

Clinical example of **Pneumosinus dilatans.** Visual acuity preoperatively diminishing, postoperatively improved from 0,8 to 1,2, color perception improvement on right side; irreversible N. opticus damage on the left*, therefore no operation here**

A – A'   Preoperative X-ray findings (oblique views). Open arrow: Pneumosinus dilatans. Canalis opticus greatly narrowed on both sides

B – C'   CT, preoperative. Open arrows: Pneumosinus dilatans

B   *s:* Section plane of reconstruction **B'**

C   *s:* Section plane of reconstruction **C'**

D   Postoperative X-ray, oblique view. Open arrows: Pneumosinus dilatans. Bony wall of Canalis opticus removed

E – F'   CT, postoperative

E   Reconstruction from **E'**. Defect of Processus clinoideus ant. recognizable

E'   *s:* Section plane of reconstruction **E**

F   Bone defect, after removal of the osseous surrounding of Canalis opticus, recognizable

F'   Enlarged detail from **F**. Black arrow: operative approach for bone resection. Open arrow: N. opticus path

---

* I am grateful to Dr. Unsöld, ophthalmol. Clinic, Univ. Freiburg/Br. (Director: Prof. Dr. Mackensen) for the preop. and postop. findings.
** Operation performed by Dr. W. Hassler, author's coworker.

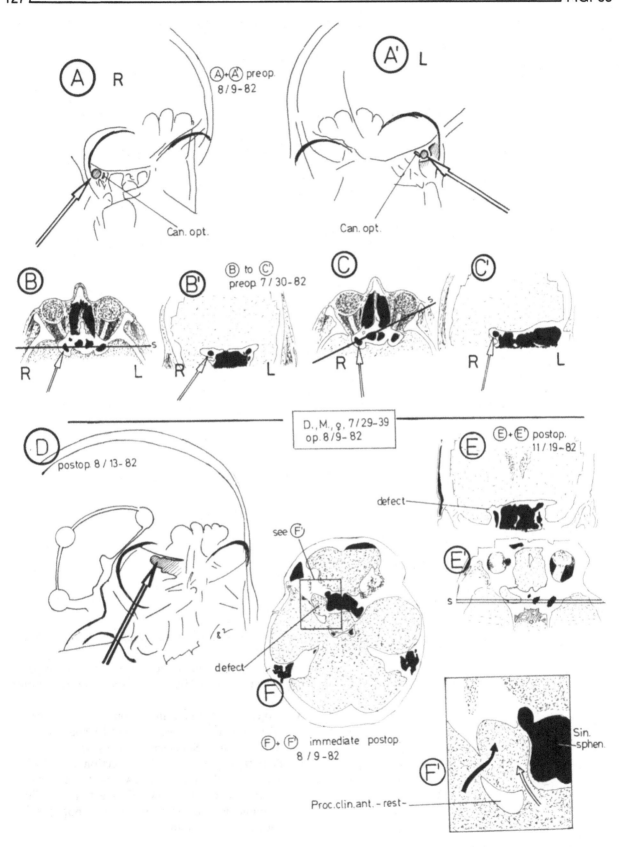

Ⓐ R   Ⓐ + Ⓐ' preop. 8 / 9 – 82

Ⓐ' L

Can. opt.

Can. opt.

Ⓑ   Ⓑ to Ⓒ' preop. 7 / 30 – 82   Ⓑ'   Ⓒ   Ⓒ'

R   L   R   L   R   L   R   L

D., M., ♀, 7 / 29 – 39 op. 8 / 9 – 82

Ⓓ postop. 8 / 13 – 82

Ⓔ   Ⓔ + Ⓔ' postop. 11 / 19 – 82

defect

Ⓔ'

s

see Ⓕ'

defect

Ⓕ   Ⓕ + Ⓕ' immediate postop. 8 / 9 – 82

Ⓕ'

Sin. sphen.

Proc. clin. ant. – rest –

FIG. 64 ⬜━━━━━━━━━━━━━━━━━━━━━━━━━⬜ 128

Fig. 64. Operations in the area surrounding Sinus cavernosus.

Pneumosinus dilatans oblique view of skull preparation (detail). Operative approach along Ala minor sketched in

A Projection (broken lines) on bone surface of **Pneumosinus dilatans,** narrowed Canalis opticus and portion of Sinus sphenoidalis wall

B Preparation as **A** after resection of Canalis opticus wall. Open arrow: path of Canalis opticus. ⸝ Broken arrow: Connection of Sinus sphenoidalis to still remaining portions of Pneumosinus dilatans

FIG. 64

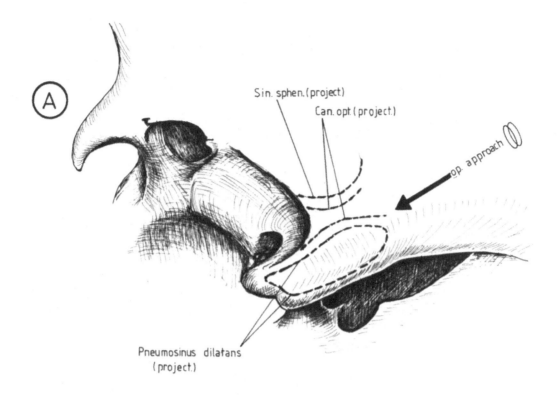

Ⓐ

Sin. sphen. (project.)

Can. opt. (project.)

op. approach

Pneumosinus dilatans
(project.)

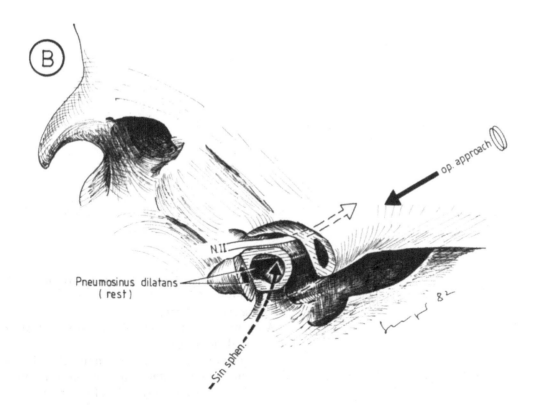

Ⓑ

op. approach

N. II

Pneumosinus dilatans
(rest)

Sin. sphen.

82

FIG. 65 ⊏══⊐ 130

Fig. 65. Operations in the area surrounding Sinus cavernosus.

Pneumosinus dilatans

A Both Nn. optici and right A. carotis int. sketched on skull preparation

B Situation after bone resection. Canalis opticus and Fissura orbitalis sup. form a common space after removing bony walls of N. opticus

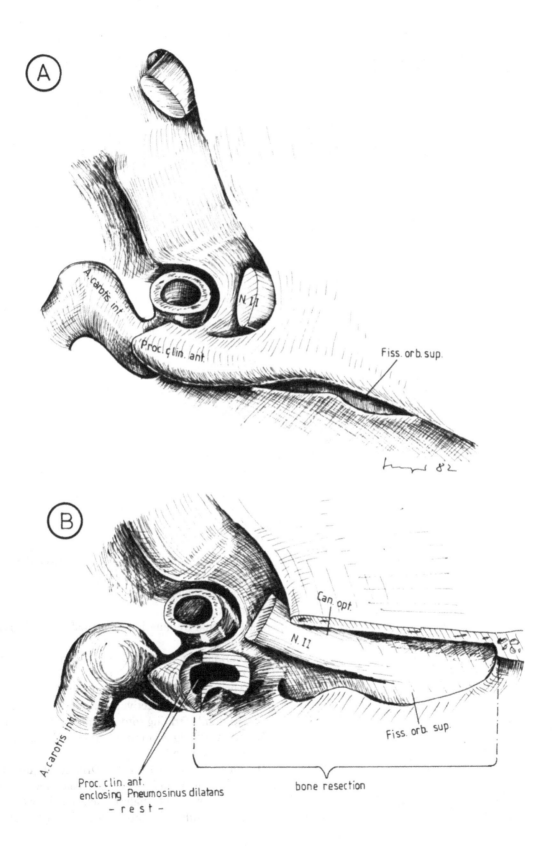

FIG. 66 [=====================================] 132

Fig. 66. Operations in the area surrounding Sinus cavernosus.

Pneumosinus dilatans

Microsurgical site

A Pterional trepanation, sketched on skull preparation

A' Various microsurgical views (arrows), sketched on skull preparation

B Microsurgical site after dura exposure. Because of oblique perspective, Ala minor appears foreshortend. Drilling into Ala major and Ala minor

C After drilling Ala minor, roof of Fissura orbitalis sup. is opened

D Enlarged detail from C. Drilling at juncture of Processus clinoideus ant. and Ala minor remnant. Lateral wall of Canalis opticus partially removed, Pneumosinus dilatans opened in several places

FIG. 66

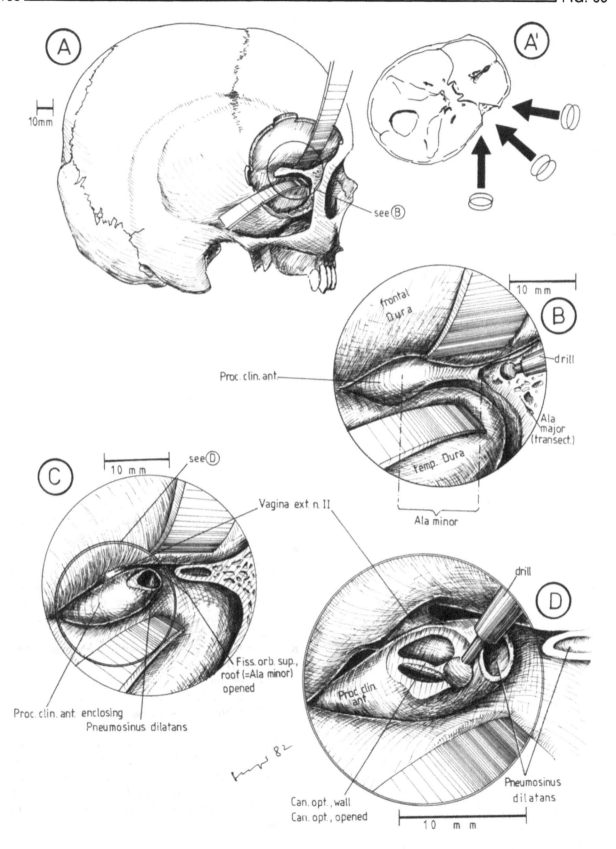

(A)

10mm

(A')

see (B)

(B)

frontal
Dura

10 mm

Proc. clin. ant.

drill

Ala
major
(transect.)

Temp. Dura

Ala minor

(C)

10 mm

see (D)

Vagina ext. n. II

Fiss. orb. sup.,
roof (=Ala minor)
opened

Proc. clin. ant. enclosing

Pneumosinus dilatans

(D)

drill

Proc. clin.
ant.

Pneumosinus
dilatans

Can. opt., wall
Can. opt., opened

10   m m

FIG. 67 | 134

Fig. 67. Operations in the area surrounding Sinus cavernosus.

Pneumosinus dilatans

A Drilling of Canalis opticus wall must be carried out very cautiously (low drill speed, extensive irrigation) in order to prevent negative mechanical and thermal effects to N. opticus already damaged by compression

B Lateral wall of Canalis opticus removed. Stenosed N.II recognizable

   1 Resection of Canalis opticus formed by Planum sphenoidale

   2 Detachment of mucosa in Pneumosinus dilatans

C After mucosa removal from Pneumosinus dilatans, fatty tissue (from abdominal wall) is placed on decompressed N. opticus. Fatty tissue closes entrance of Pneumosinus dilatans, thus preventing communication of Sinus sphenoidalis and epidural space

FIG. 67

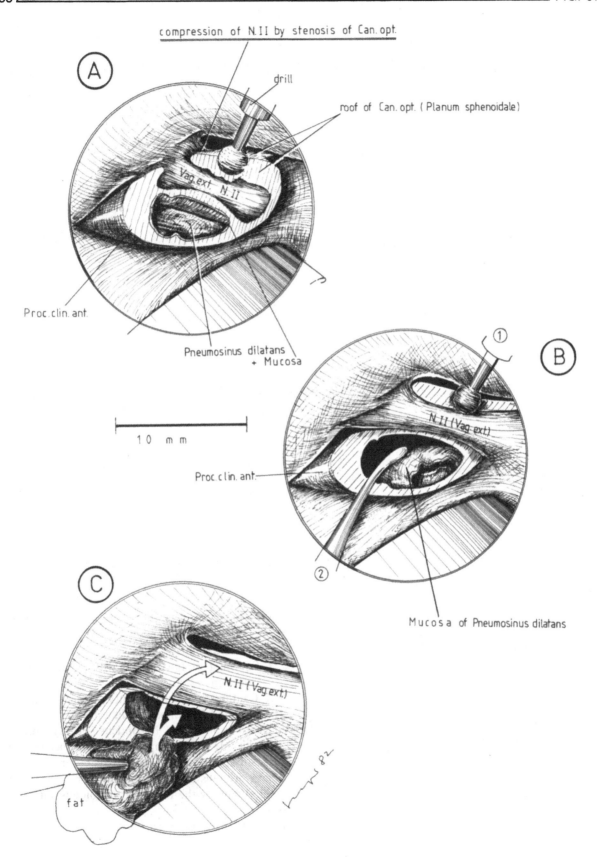

compression of N. II by stenosis of Can. opt.

(A)
drill
roof of Can. opt. (Planum sphenoidale)
Vag. ext. N. II
Proc. clin. ant.
Pneumosinus dilatans + Mucosa

10 mm

(B)
①
N. II (Vag. ext.)
Proc. clin. ant.
②
Mucosa of Pneumosinus dilatans

(C)
N. II (Vag. ext.)
fat

FIG. 68 ⊏▭▭▭▭▭▭▭▭▭▭▭▭▭▭▭⊐ 136

Fig. 68. Operations in the area surrounding Sinus cavernosus.

Pneumosinus dilatans

A 1 Squirting of fatty tissue with tissue glue (fibrinogen + activator)*

2 Cautions pressing of fatty tissue against the stump of Pneumosinus dilatans

B Anatomical model. N. opticus –(N.II)– and A. carotis int. –(c1)– projected on dura surface. One sees that the opened up Canalis opticus and Fissura orbitalis sup. form a common cavity separated only by the Processus clinoideus ant.

---

* Immuno-Chemie, Heidelberg.

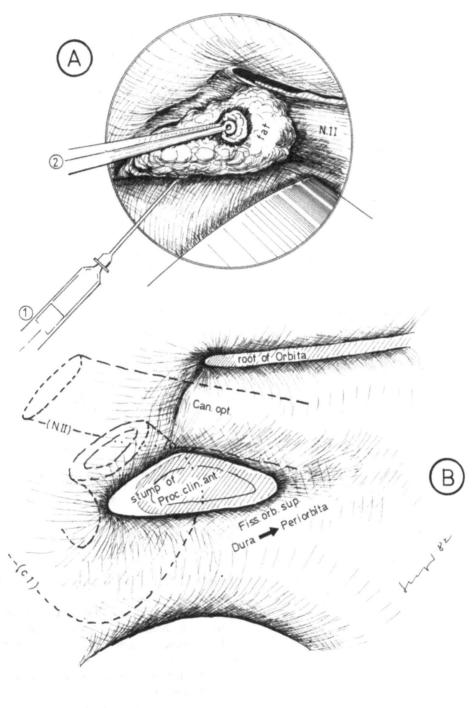

FIG. 69 [==] 138

Tumors (Figs. 69 to 99)

Fig. 69. Operations in the area surrounding Sinus cavernosus.
Flat **meningioma in Sinus cavernosus area** with considerable **bone reaction** of Ala major and minor. Dorso-superior view, right side. Preliminary anatomical remarks
A   Skull preparation, **resection line** sketched in (broken line)
B   Enlarged detail from **A.** One sees that Canalis opticus, Fissura orbitalis sup. and lateral wall of Foramen rotundum will form a common space

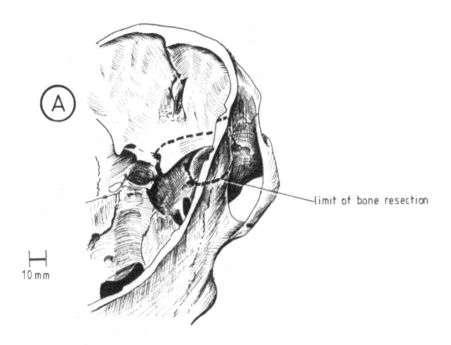

(A)

limit of bone resection

10 mm

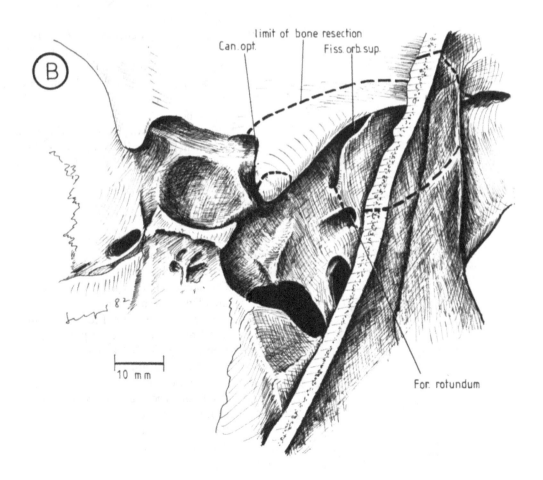

(B)

limit of bone resection

Can. opt.   Fiss. orb. sup.

For. rotundum

10 mm

FIG. 70 ⌐━━━━━━━━━━━━━━━━━━━━━━━━━━━━⌐ 140

Fig. 70. Operations in the area surrounding Sinus cavernosus.

Flat meningioma in Sinus cavernosus area with extensive bone reaction of Ala major and Ala minor

Preliminary anatomical remarks

Topographical **relation of A. carotis int. to bone structures,** from skull preparation; **variants**

A Sulcus caroticus and surrounding structures in skull preparation. Projection of lateral A. carotis int. wall on bone structures (broken line). Medial side of Processus clinoideus ant. shows a deep impression –imp– resulting from A. carotis int. siphon

B Another example, sketched on larger scale. As in **A,** wall of A. carotis int. lies close against Canalis rotundus. Medial side of Processus clinoideus ant. root –ra– shows bone impressions –imp– resulting from A. carotis int. siphon

C In this example one sees that the impression of A. carotis int. is quite deeply sculpted. It impresses Processus clinoideus ant. medially; radix of Processus clinoideus ant. –ra–, Tuberculum sellae –ts– and lateral wall of Sella turcica –st– become impressed too

D Typical bone connection –co1– between Processus clinoideus ant. and Tuberculum sellae –ts–. Thus A. carotis int. siphon is surrounded by bony ring behind Canalis opticus. In this case one could not move A. carotis int. to the side during bone resection

E Similar to **D.** However, sella bridge –co2– is also present here, that is, a connection between Processus clinoideus ant. and Processus clinoideus post., or Dorsum sellae –cp– also

Abbreviations:

ca   Processus clinoideus ant.
cop   Canalis opticus
cp   Processus clinoideus post.
col   Connection between Processus clinoideus ant. and Tuberculum sellae
co2   Connection between Processus clinoideus ant. and Processus clinoideus post.
imp   Impressions by A. carotis int.
lac   Foramen lacerum
ov   Foramen ovale
ra   Radix of Processus clinoideus ant.
rt   Foramen rotundum
st   lat. wall of Sella
ts   Tuberculum sellae

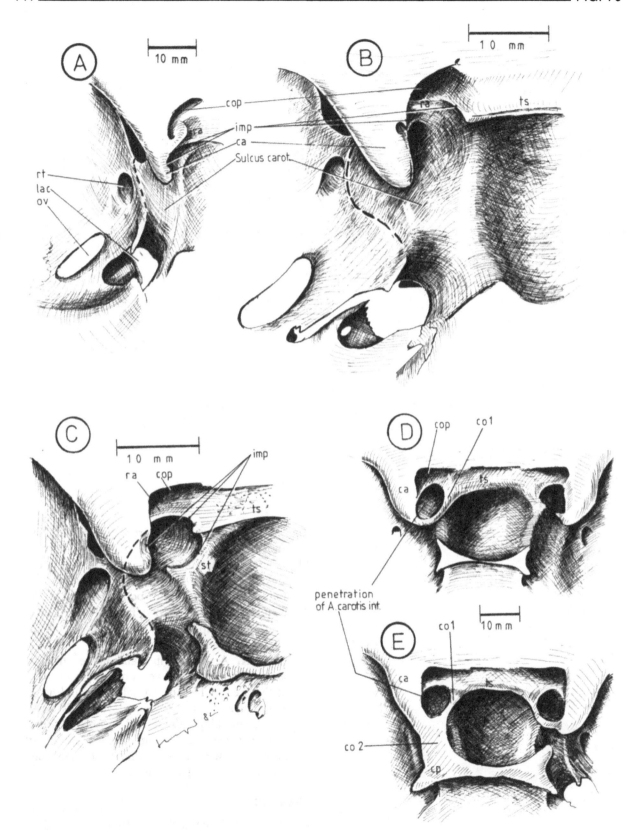

FIG. 71 ⊏▭▭▭▭▭▭▭▭▭▭▭▭▭▭▭▭▭⊐ 142

Fig. 71. Operations in the area surrounding Sinus cavernosus.
Flat meningioma in Sinus cavernosus area with extensive bone reaction of Ala major and Ala minor
Anatomical preparation after bone resection

A **Bone preparation.** Arrow: Path of N. maxillaris after opening up Canalis opticus, Fissura orbitalis sup. and Foramen rotundum

B As in **A**, A. carotis int. and nerve structures sketched in. Dura and veins omitted
In the area of Fissura orbitalis sup. and nearby bone passages for nerves and vessels is a dura sheath, masking nerves and vessels. At these bone passages vessels and nerves are greatly endangered when bone is drilled. Low drill speed with extensive irrigation is required

Abbreviation:

Ggl G Ganglion semilunare (Gasseri)

FIG. 71

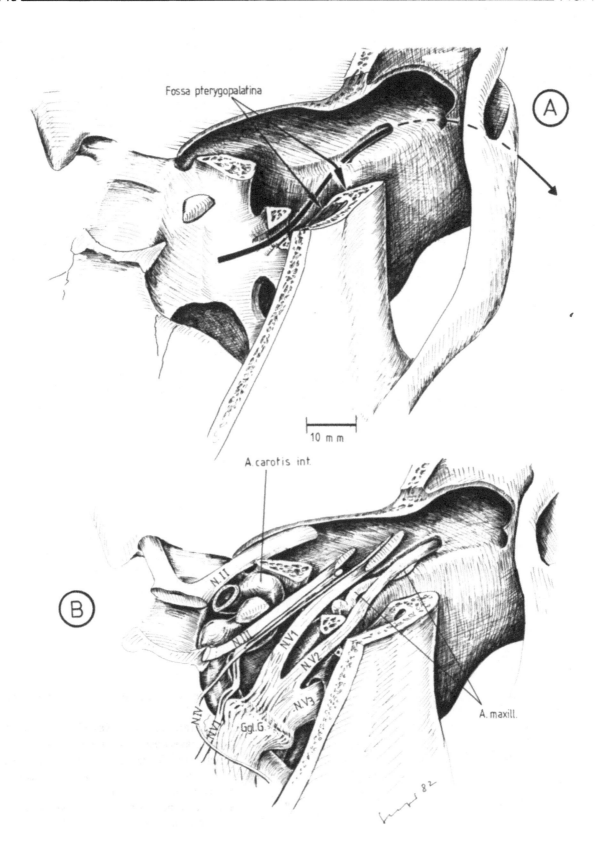

Ⓐ

Fossa pterygopalatina

10 m m

Ⓑ

A.carotis int.

N.II

N.III

N.V1

N.V2

N.V3

N.IV

N.VI

Ggl.G

A. maxill.

FIG. 72 ⊏━━━━━━━━━━━━━━━━━━━━━━━━━━━━━━━━━━⊐ 144

Fig. 72. Operations in the area surrounding Sinus cavernosus.

Anatomical preparation showing vessels and nerves in the area of **Sinus cavernosus.** Dura and veins omitted

A   Skull sketch with A. carotis int. N. abducens is the cranial nerve in closest contact to A. carotis int. in Sinus cavernosus area

B   As **A.** Superficial nerves additionally sketched in, *s1, s2:* Section plane –s– of Fig. 73 sketches

FIG. 72

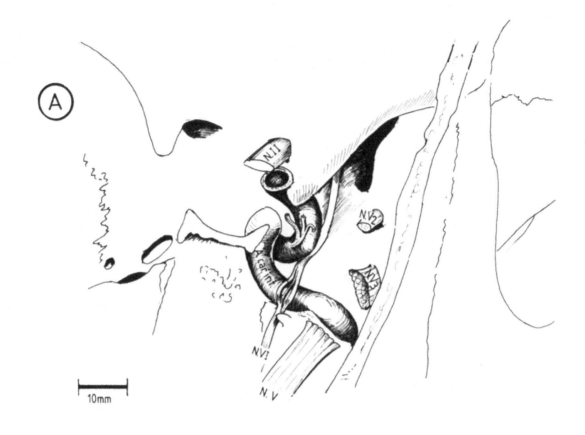

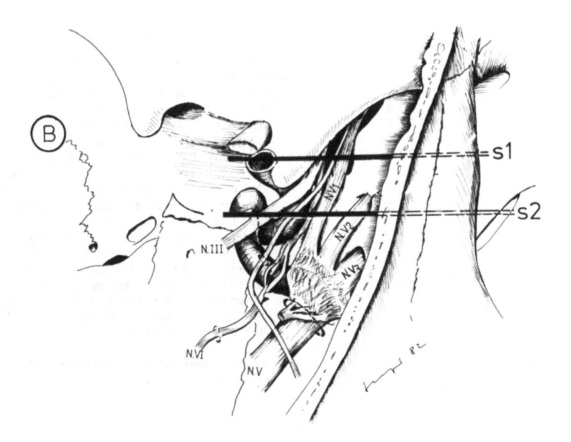

FIG. 73 146

Fig. 73. Operations in the area surrounding Sinus cavernosus.

Frontal section of anterior and posterior **Sinus cavernosus** area (section planes see Fig. 72)

A One sees the close topographical relation of A. carotis int. to N. abducens and N. oculomotorius (deep nerve layer), and to the superficial nerve layer with N. trochlearis, N. ophthalmicus –N.V1– and N. maxillaris –N.V2– in Foramen rotundum. A. carotis int. is sectioned twice in the Curvatura ant. of A. carotis int.

B Section plane at level of Dorsum sellae (Processus clinoideus post.). Here also the close relation between A. carotis int. and N. abducens is seen. Just after dura entry N. oculomotorius still lies in a superficial position. Superficial nerve layer –N. trochlearis and both N. trigeminus branches– lie close under superficial dura layer as in **A**

Sinus cavernosus lies predominantly medial to A. carotis int.

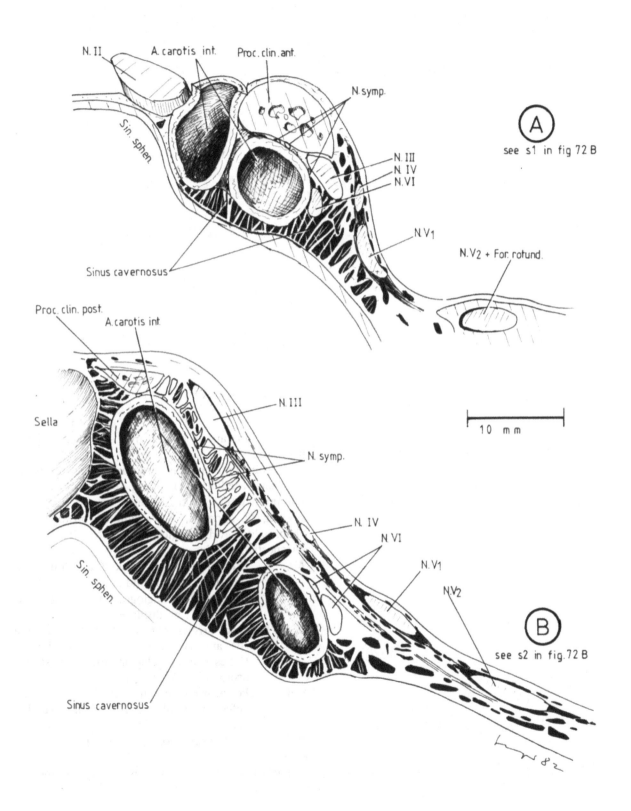

N. II
A. carotis int.
Proc. clin. ant.
N. symp.
Sin. sphen.
N. III
N. IV
N. VI
N. V1
Sinus cavernosus
N. V2 + For. rotund.

A
see s1 in fig 72 B

Proc. clin. post.
A. carotis int.
N. III
Sella
N. symp.
N. IV
N. VI
Sin. sphen.
N. V1
N. V2
Sinus cavernosus

10 mm

B
see s2 in fig. 72 B

FIG. 74 148

Fig. 74. Operations in the area surrounding Sinus cavernosus.

Flat **meningioma in Sinus cavernosus** area with extensive **bone reaction** of Ala major and Ala minor*.

For three weeks Protrusio bulbi on the right with swelling of upperlid. No additional postoperative abnormalities. (Histological finding: Meningioma)

Diagnostic procedures

A	**Preoperative** X-ray of skull, ap. Bone reaction in Ala minor and Ala major area
A'	Preoperative angiography of right A. carotis int.: no displacement
B, B', B''	Black arrows: bone reaction in orbital area (**B**) and Ala major with protrusion of Facies orbitalis alae majoris in posterior orbital area (**B** to **B''**)
C + C'	**Postoperative** findings. Open arrows: bone defect in orbital area, Ala minor (**C**) and in Ala major (**C'**)
D	Lateral skull sketch with CT-planes **B – C'**

* Operation performed by Dr. W. Hassler, author's coworker.

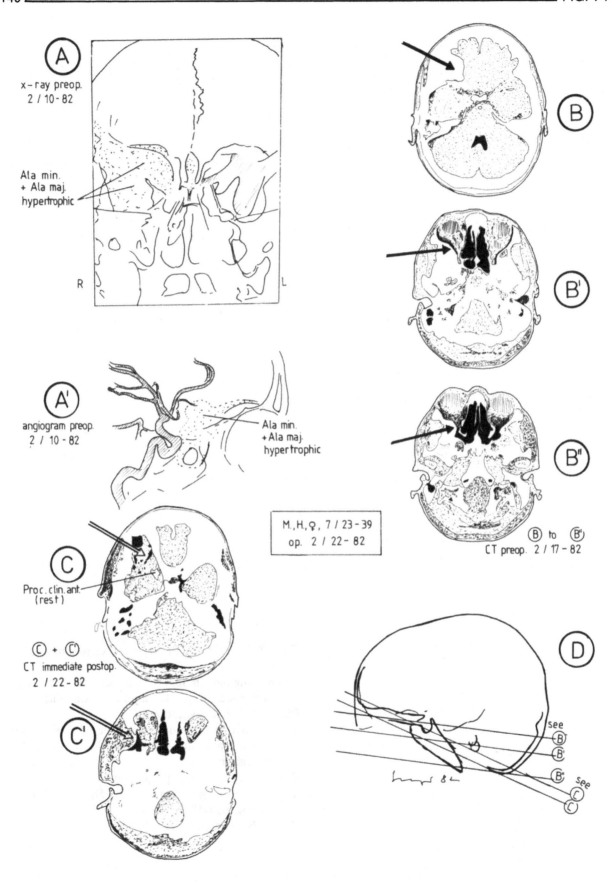

A
x-ray preop.
2 / 10 - 82

Ala min.
+ Ala maj.
hypertrophic

A'
angiogram preop.
2 / 10 - 82

Ala min.
+ Ala maj.
hypertrophic

C
Proc. clin. ant.
(rest)

C + C'
CT immediate postop.
2 / 22 - 82

C'

M., H., ♀, 7 / 23 - 39
op. 2 / 22 - 82

R   L

B

B'

B"

B to B"
CT preop. 2 / 17 - 82

D

see
B
B'
B" see
C
C'

FIG. 75 ⸏=======================================⸏ 150

Fig. 75. Operations in the area surrounding Sinus cavernosus.

Flat meningioma in Sinus cavernosus area with extensive **bone reaction** of Ala major and Ala minor.

Postoperative X-ray findings

A   Arrow: bone defect in area of orbital roof, Ala major and Ala minor. Normal contralateral findings

B + C X-ray, oblique projection

B   Site of operation. Arrow: Defect in Canalis opticus wall

C   Normal contralateral findings

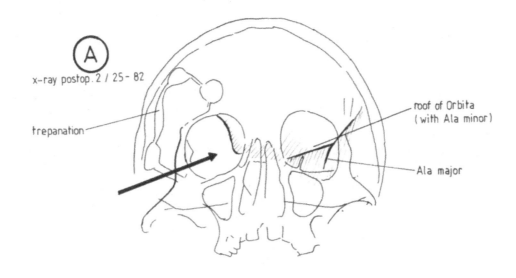

(A) x-ray postop. 2 / 25 - 82

trepanation

roof of Orbita
(with Ala minor)

Ala major

M., H., ♀, 7 / 23 - 39
op. 2 / 22 - 82

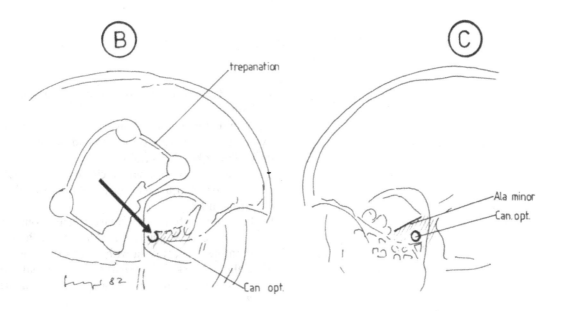

(B) trepanation

Can. opt.

(C) Ala minor

Can. opt.

(B) + (C) x-ray postop. 2 / 25 - 82

FIG. 76 ⊏━━━━━━━━━━━━━━━━━━━━━━━━━━━━━━━━━⊐ 152

Fig. 76. Operations in the area surrounding Sinus cavernosus.

Flat meningioma in Sinus cavernosus area with extensive bone reaction of Ala major and Ala minor.

Principles of bone resection

A Skull preparation, skin incision, immediately in front of Meatus acusticus externus sketched in (broken line)

B Situation after pterional trepanation, after drilling of Ala major and Ala minor. Periorbita (continuation of dura within orbita) exposed

B' Enlarged skull preparation, without dura sketched in, corresponding to anatomical sketch B

Arrow *a:* path of N. opticus

Arrow *b:* path of nerves and vessels, surrounded by Fissura orbitalis sup.

Arrow *c:* path of N. maxillaris

FIG. 76

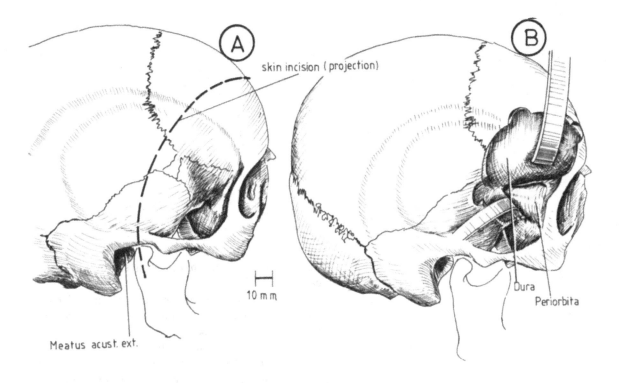

A

skin incision (projection)

10 mm

Meatus acust. ext.

B

Dura

Periorbita

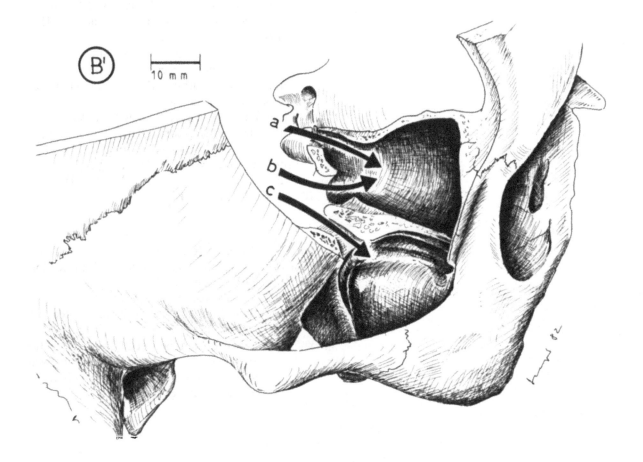

B'

10 mm

a

b

c

FIG. 77 ⌐────────────────────────────────────⌐ 154

Fig. 77. Operations in the area surrounding Sinus cavernosus.

Flat meningioma in Sinus cavernosus area with extensive bone reaction of Ala major and Ala minor.

Principles of bone resection

A   Anatomical sketch showing area of cranio-orbital juncture. Nerves and vessels shown through transparent Dura layer. Dura and Periorbita sketched in; structures enveloped by them are projected upon Dura and periorbital surface. Note close topographical relation of Vagina ext. n.II, Radix processus clinoideus ant., N.III to Curvatura cavernosa ant. of A. carotis int.

−.−.−: level of Fissura orbitalis sup.

Arrows: Topographical relation of Fissura orbitalis sup., Orbita, Fossa cranii media and Fossa pterygopalatina

A'   Anatomical skull sketch, view from **A**

B   Microsurgical site corresponding to anatomical sketch **A.** Due to altered direction of view, orbital roof appears greatly foreshortened. View direction see **B'**

B'   View direction for **B**

Abbreviations:

(ch)   Chiasma (projection)

(Gsem)   Ganglion semilunare Gasseri (projection)

(N.III)   N.III (projection)

(N.VI)   N.VI (projection)

tr   Transition between Dura mater and Periorbita

x   Bone remnant between N.V2 and juncture of Dura to Periorbita, as well as between Orbita (and Fossa pterygopalatina) and Fossa cranii media

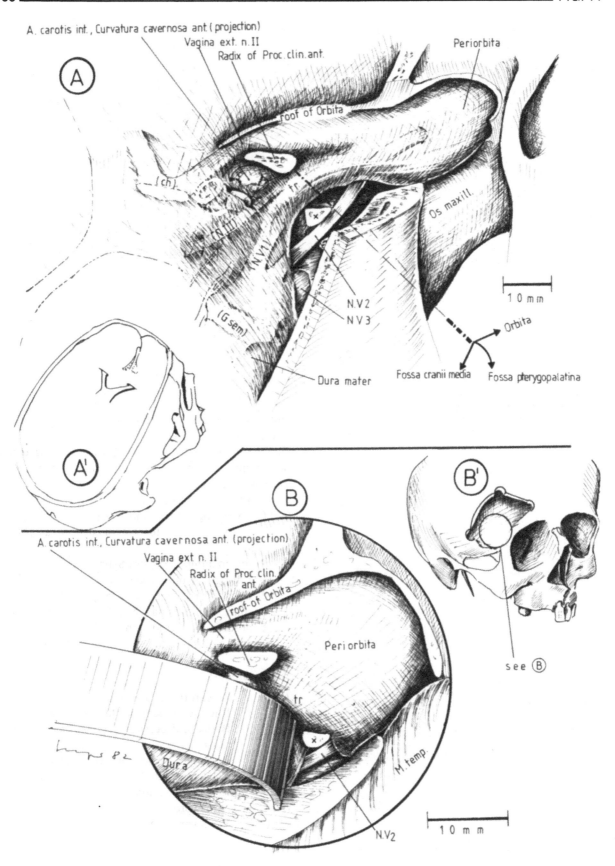

A. carotis int., Curvatura cavernosa ant. (projection)
Vagina ext. n. II
Radix of Proc. clin. ant.
Periorbita

roof of Orbita

(ch)

tr.

Os maxill.

N.VI

N.V2
N.V3

(G sem)

Dura mater

10 mm

Orbita

Fossa cranii media   Fossa pterygopalatina

A. carotis int., Curvatura cavernosa ant. (projection)
Vagina ext. n. II
Radix of Proc. clin. ant.
roof of Orbita

Periorbita

tr.

Dura

M. temp.

N.V2

10 mm

see B

FIG. 78 ⊏━━━━━━━━━━━━━━━━━━━━━━━━━━━━━━━━━━━⊐ 156

Fig. 78. Operations in the area surrounding Sinus cavernosus.

Flat meningioma in Sinus cavernosus area with extensive bone reaction of Ala major and Ala minor.

Microsurgical site

Broken lines = projections

A **Opening up Dura** and posterior portions of Periorbita at the site of opened Fissura orbitalis sup.

B After opening of Fissura Sylvii:

   1 Lifting of frontal lobe

   2 Drawing back of temporal pole. Exposure of small meningioma which lies over Sinus cavernosus area; projection on Dura and meningioma of more deeply lying structures

Abbreviations:

(cl)	A. carotis int. (projection)
ra	Radix of Processus clinoideus ant.
(ra)	Radix of Processus clinoideus ant. (projection)
roo	Resection surface of Orbota roof
(N.III)	N.III (projection)
(N.V1)	N.V1 (projection)
(N.V2)	N.V2 (projection)
(N.V3)	N.V3 (projection)

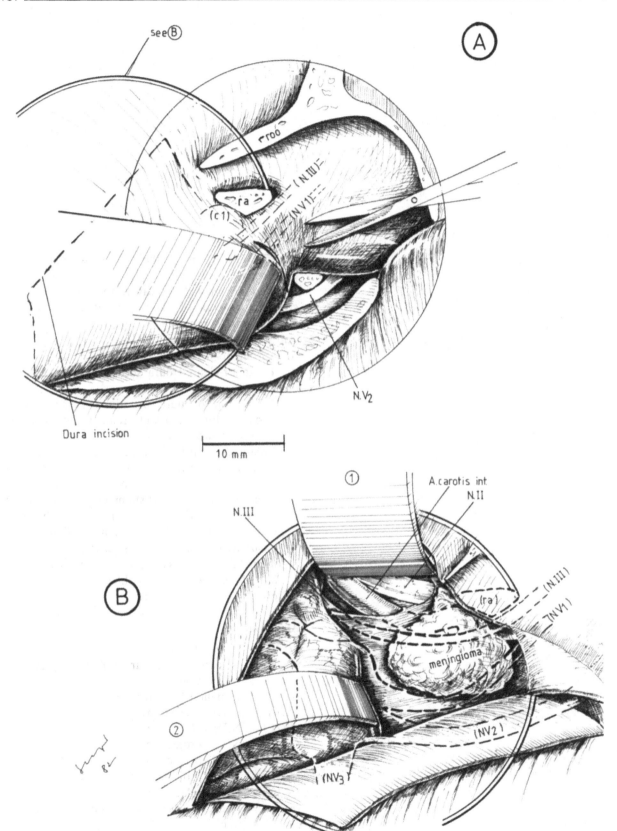

A

see B

rroo

(N.III)

ra

(c1)

(NV1)

N.V₂

Dura incision

10 mm

B

①

N.III

A.carotis int.

N.II

(N.III)

(ra)

(NV1)

meningioma

②

(NV2)

(NV3)

FIG. 79 _____ 158

Fig. 79. Operations in the area surrounding Sinus cavernosus.

Flat meningioma in Sinus cavernosus area with extensive bone reaction of Ala major and Ala minor.

Meningioma is removed, its dura insertion scraped out, with sharp dissector.

Measurements in mm

A **1** Tumor-cleared dura surface is coagulated by means of low amperage

2 Excision of dura insertion of meningioma except for 5 mm wide remnant lateral to N. opticus and A. carotis int.

B Enlarged detail from **A.** After dura fenestration over Sinus cavernosus area, one sees the superficial nerve layer –N.V1 and N.IV–, and then somewhat deeper N.III shimmering through, and A. carotis int. with N. abducens, covered by loose connective tissue. Veins lateral to Sinus cavernosus area normally are less developed than veins medial to A. carotis int. In the case presented, the lateral veins were scarcely bleeding, nearly obliterated by tumor pressure

Abbreviations:

cl	A. carotis int.
(clcc)	A. carotis int., Curvatura cavernosa ant. (projection)
(ggsG)	Ganglion Gasseri (projection)
(N.III)	N.III (projection)
(N.IV)	N.IV (projection)
(N.V1)	N.V1 (projection)
(N.V2)	N.V2 (projection)
(N.V3)	N.V3 (projection)
(N.VI)	N.VI (projection)
(ra)	Radix of Processus clinoideus ant. (projection)

FIG. 79

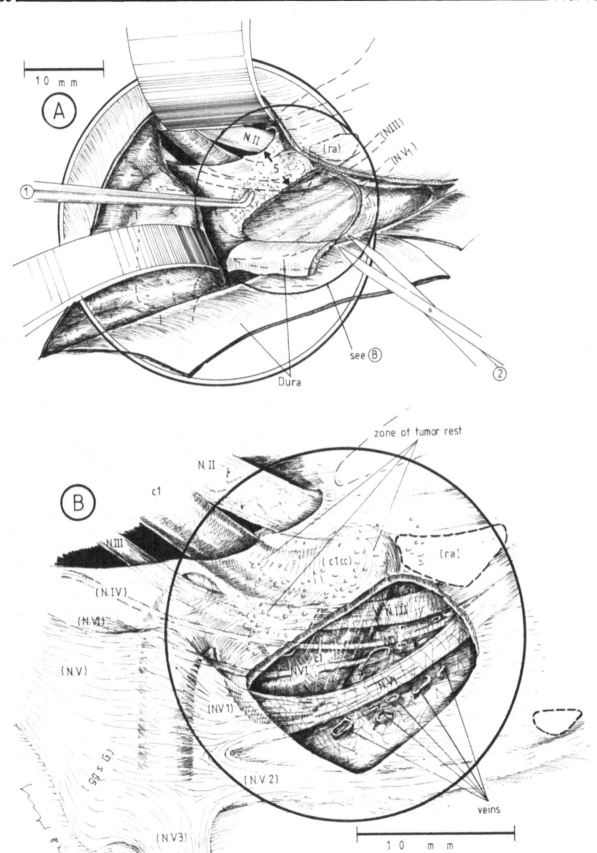

A

10 mm

① ②

N.II

5

(ra)

(N.III)

(N.V₁)

see ⓑ

Dura

B

zone of tumor rest

N.II

c1

N.III

(N.IV)

(N.VI)

(N.V)

(c1cc)

(ra)

N.III

N

c1

N.VI

N.II

(N.V1)

(gg s G)

(N.V 2)

veins

(N.V3)

10 m m

FIG. 80 ⸏ 160

Fig. 80. Operations in the area surrounding Sinus cavernosus.

Tumors of Sinus cavernosus area.

Four tumor types with four operation examples shown. Anatomical transection sketches done according to operation site

A   Sinus cavernosus region, section planes **B** to **E** drawn in. Broken lines = projection

B   Lateral tumor lying outside nerves and vessels of the Sinus cavernosus area = radical operation possible (see clinical example Figs. 81 to 85)

C   Tumor between superficial and deep nerve layer in lateral Sinus cavernosus area (s. clinical example Figs. 86 to 89, here with transition into posterior orbital region) = radical operation possible

D   Tumor in all aeas of Sinus cavernosus except the Sella, but limited to one side (see clinical example Figs. 90 to 93). In most cases radical operation not possible. However, this example shows tumor radically operable, since intraorbital tumor portion caused blindness and led to enucleation of bulbus, whereby all the structures of Sinus cavernosus area could be resected except for A. carotis int.

E   Tumor in all Sinus cavernosus areas extending contralaterally (see clinical example Figs. 99 to 95). Tumor inoperable, except for local nerve decompression, i. e. N.II and N.III

Abbreviations:

cl   A. carotis int.

FIG. 80

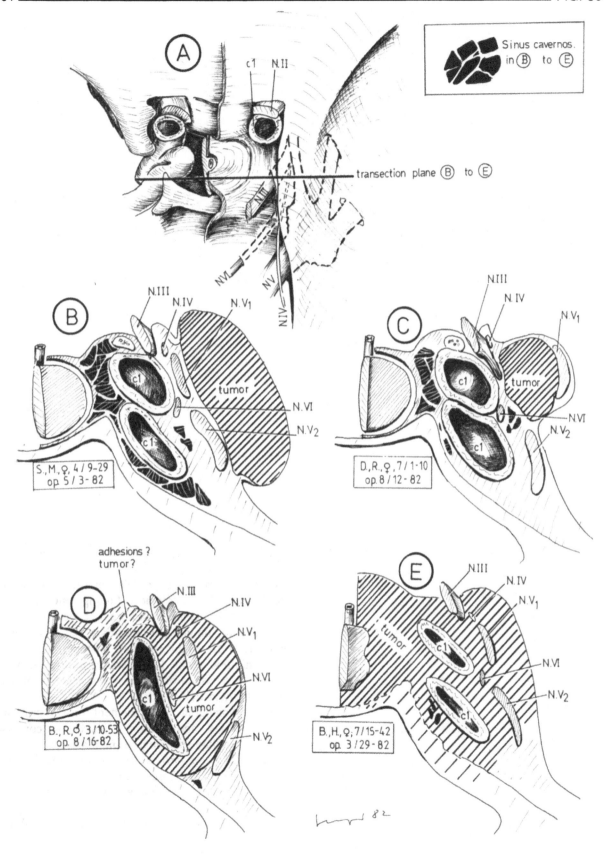

A — c1 — N.II

Sinus cavernos.
in Ⓑ to Ⓔ

transection plane Ⓑ to Ⓔ

N.VI   N.V   N.IV

B
N.III   N.IV   N.V₁
c1
c1
tumor
N.VI
N.V₂
S.,M.,♀, 4 / 9-29
op. 5 / 3-82

C
N.III   N.IV   N.V₁
c1
tumor
N.VI
c1
N.V₂
D.,R.,♀, 7 / 1-10
op. 8 / 12-82

D
adhesions ?
tumor ?
N.III   N.IV
N.V₁
c1   N.VI
tumor
N.V₂
B.,R.,♂, 3 / 10-53
op. 8 / 16-82

E
N.III   N.IV   N.V₁
tumor
c1
N.VI
c1   N.V₂
B.,H.,♀; 7 / 15-42
op. 3 / 29-82

82

FIG. 81 ⊏══⊐ 162

Fig. 81. Operations in the area surrounding Sinus cavernosus.

Clinical example of **superficial lateral Sinus cavernosus tumor***. Histological finding: meningioma. Postoperative incomplete external N. oculomotorius paresis and diminished sensitivity of the three branches N. trigemini; complete postoperative recovery within few weeks. Postoperative improvement of organic psychosyndrome. Passing suspicions of seizure-activity in EEG

A + B Angiogram: displacement of cerebral arteries and tumor, uptake of contrast medium (histological: meningioma)

C – F CT: temporo-medial tumor arising from Sinus cavernosus area

G + H No tumor postoperatively demonstrable

* Operation performed by Dr. W. Hassler, author's coworker.

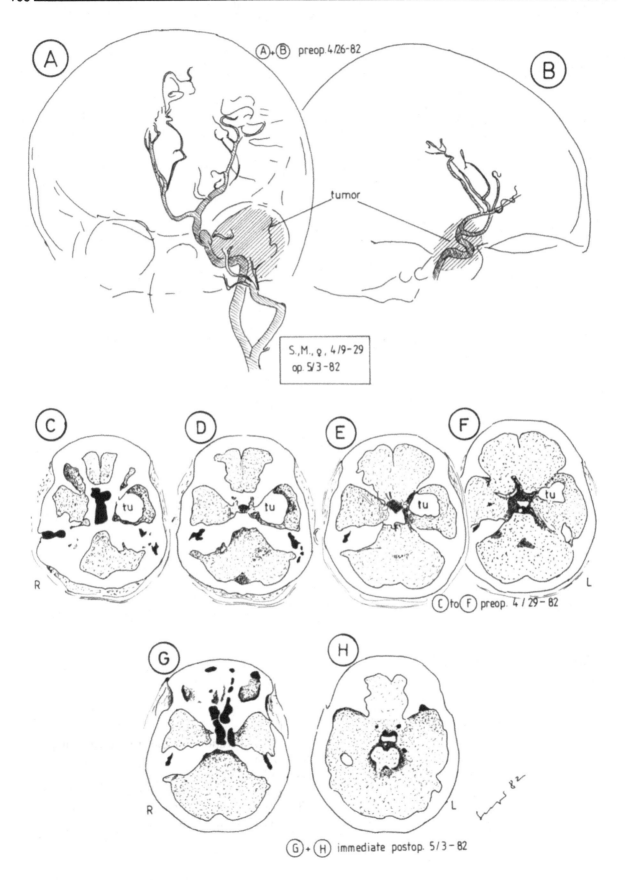

(A)+(B) preop. 4/26-82

tumor

S.,M., ♀, 4/9-29
op. 5/3-82

(C) to (F) preop. 4/29-82

(G)+(H) immediate postop. 5/3-82

FIG. 82 ⬜━━━━━━━━━━━━━━━━━━━━━━━━━━━━━━━━⬜ 164

Fig. 82. Operations in the area surrounding Sinus cavernosus.

Operation site

A **Trepanation** sketched on skull

B Enlarged detail from **A,** microsurgical site of Fig. 83 sketched in

FIG. 82

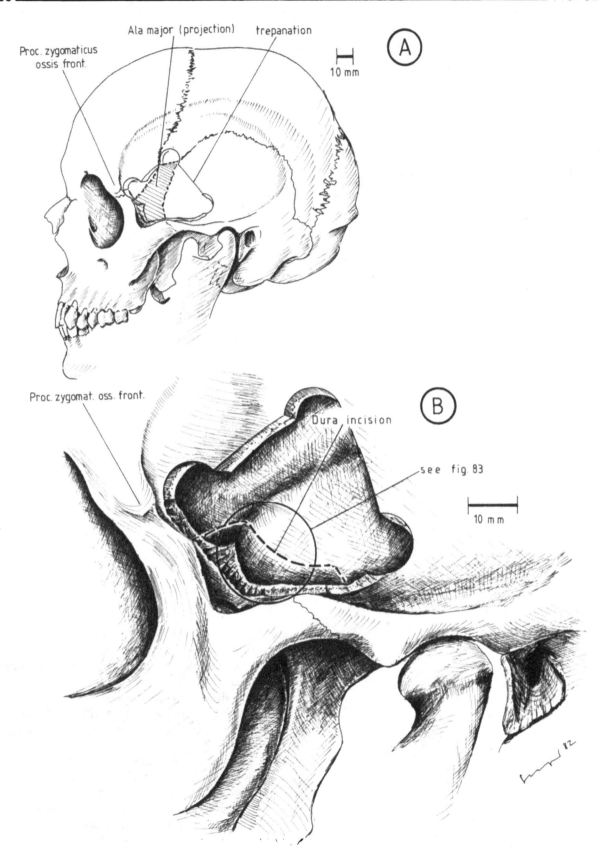

Proc. zygomaticus
ossis front.

Ala major (projection)

trepanation

10 mm

A

Proc. zygomat. oss. front.

B

Dura incision

see fig. 83

10 mm

FIG. 83 ⊏━━━━━━━━━━━━━━━━━━━━━━━━━━━⊐ 166

Fig. 83. Operations in the area surrounding Sinus cavernosus.

Operation site after Dura opening

A 1 Holding back **Arachnoidea** with small hook
2 Opening up Arachnoidea over Fissura lateralis Sylvii

B 1 Retraction of frontal lobe after splitting Arachnoidea of Fissura Sylvii
2 Slight pulling back of temporal lobe
3a Coagulation of tumor insertion in Dura
3b Thorough irrigation and suction

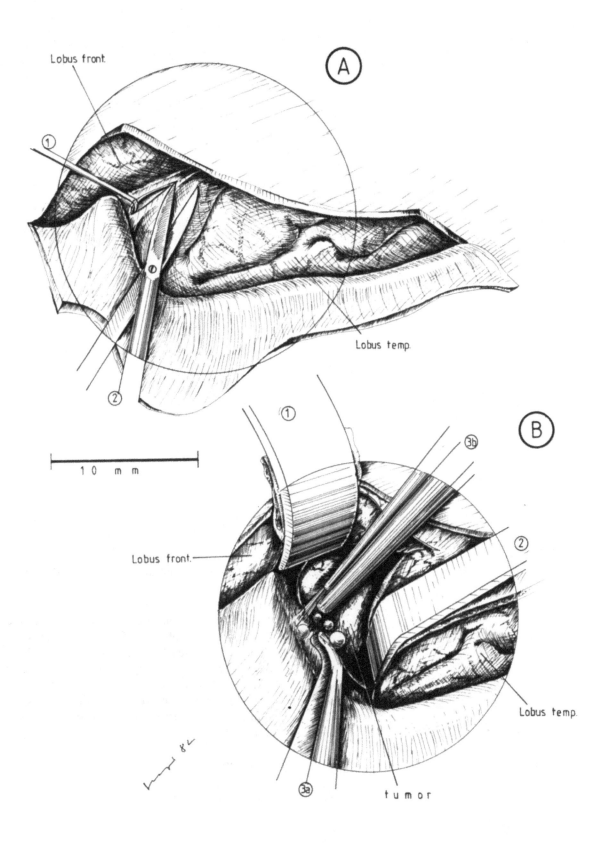

Lobus front.

① ②

Lobus temp.

10 m m

A

①

Lobus front.

③b ②

B

③a tumor

Lobus temp.

FIG. 84 168

Fig. 84. Operations in the area surrounding Sinus cavernosus.

Operation site

A **1** Incision of bipolarly coagulated tumor surface

2 Pushing back of tumor from Ala minor. Open arrow: change of microscopic view, see **B**

3 Squeezing of tumor by forceps, tumor coagulation and removal

B Site after **tumor removal.** Dura still infiltrated by tumor. Black arrow: new microscopic view as opposed to **A**

Abbreviations:

ap Ala minor
cl A. carotis int.

FIG. 84

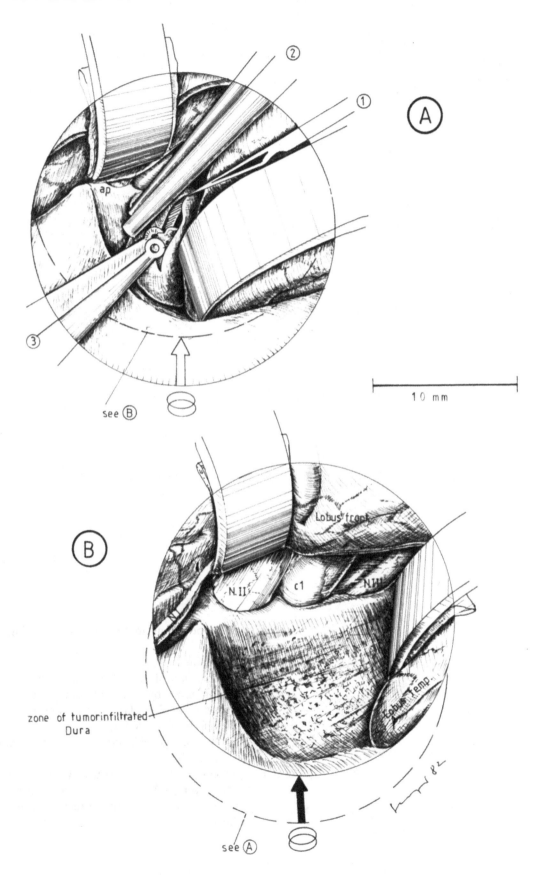

②

①

Ⓐ

ap

③

see Ⓑ

10 mm

Ⓑ

Lobus front.

N. II

c1

N III

Lobus Temp.

zone of tumorinfiltrated
Dura

see Ⓐ

FIG. 85 ⊏══⊐ 170

Fig. 85. Operations in the area surrounding Sinus cavernosus.

Operation site

A 1 Retraction of incised superficial dura layer
   2 Separation, by means of blunt preparation, of superficial dura layer from superficial nerve layer (N.V1 + N.V2)

Arrow: Change of microscopic view as opposed to Fig. 84 **B**

B **Excision of tumor-infiltrated Dura.** Superficial nerve layer (N.V1 + N.V2) is exposed nearly to Ganglion Gasseri. No tumor remnant can now be ascertained

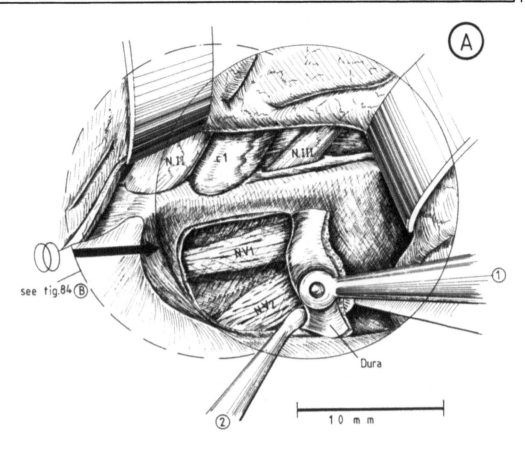

A

N.II c1 N.III

N.V1

N.V2

see fig.84 Ⓑ

①

②

Dura

10 m m

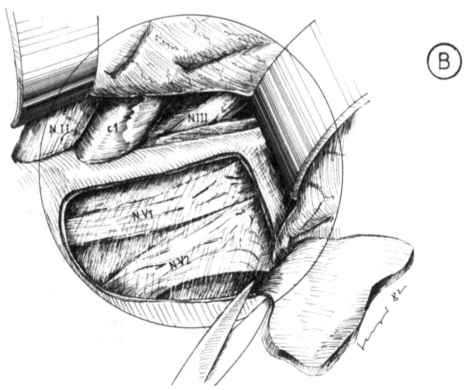

B

N.II c1 N.III

N.V1

N.V2

FIG. 86 ⊏══════════════════════════════════════⊐ 172

Fig. 86. Operations in the area surrounding Sinus cavernosus.

Clinical example of **tumor located between Canalis opticus and Fissura orbitalis sup.*** (histologic: anaplastic meningioma). For 2 months leftsided trigeminal neuralgia, vertical diplopia; neurologica: leftsided ptosis. No additional postoperative deficits, trigeminal neuralgia disappeared

A   Lateral angiogram without tumor uptake of contrast medium

B   CT: Tumor of orbital cavity at orbito-cranial juncture in front of Processsus clinoideus ant. (with Pneumosinus dilatans, an accompanying finding in meningiomas located here)

C + D   CT-reconstructions showing tumor in posterior orbital area

C' + D' Section planes of reconstructions **C + D**

E   Bone resection after complete tumor removal; posterior Processus clinoideus ant. portions remain

* Operation performed by Dr. W. Hassler, author's coworker.

FIG. 86

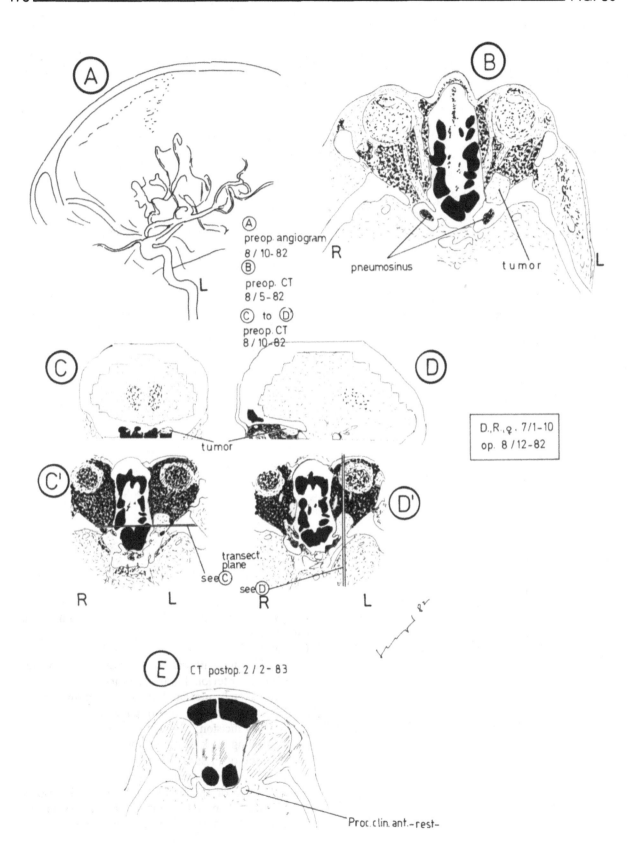

(A)
preop. angiogram
8 / 10 - 82
(B)
preop. CT
8 / 5 - 82
(C) to (D)
preop. CT
8 / 10 - 82

pneumosinus

tumor

tumor

transect.
plane
see(C)   see(D)

D., R., ♀, 7/1-10
op. 8 / 12 - 82

(E) CT postop. 2 / 2 - 83

Proc. clin. ant. -rest-

FIG. 87 [=============================] 174

Fig. 87. Operations in the area surrounding Sinus cavernosus.

Operation site

A   Skull sketch with various microsurgical view possibilities, pterional approach (arrows)

A' Skull sketch, **pterional trepanation** drawn in

B   Microsurgical site after trepanation

   1a Dura incision

   1b Folding back of dura flaps

C   Splitting of Fissura Sylvii

   1 Opening up arachnoidea by small hook

   2 Cutting of arachnoidal filaments with scissors

   3 Gradual spreading apart of Fissura Sylvii

   1 – 3 Fissura Sylvii is widely opened up

FIG. 87

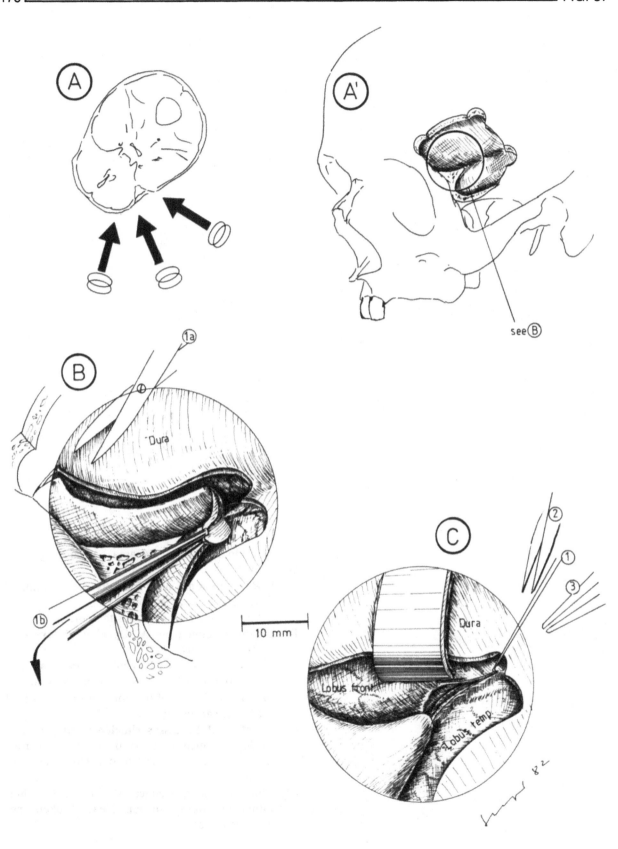

10 mm

see B

FIG. 88 ⊏━━━━━━━━━━━━━━━━━━━━━━━━━━━⊐ 176

Fig. 88. Operations in the area surrounding Sinus cavernosus

A 1 Reclination of Lobus frontalis after opening of Fissura Sylvii arachnoidea

    2 Slight retraction of Lobus temporalis

B Enlarged detail from **A. Opening of dura over Sinus cavernosus** area

    1a Dura incision over N. oculomotorius path and over the palpable Processus clinoideus ant.

    1b + 1c Wedening of incision until close to N.II and A. carotis int. –*c1*–

C Resection of Processus clinoideus ant., a small residual of which is preserved lateral to A. carotis int. –*c1*–; N.III and N.V1 recognizable after dura resection

C' Topographical anatomical sketch for **C.** Thin-dotted line: dura resection. Heavy broken line: tumor localization

FIG. 88

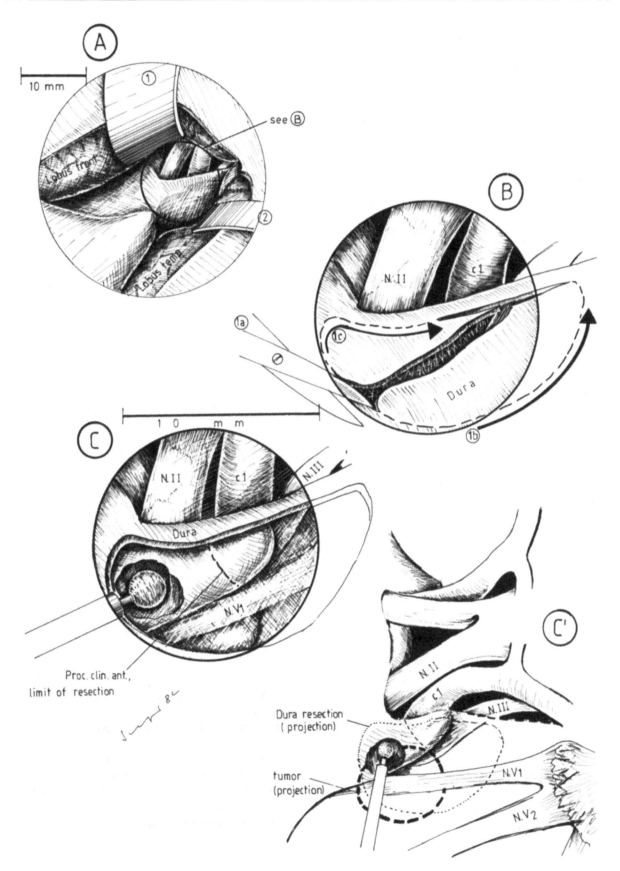

Ⓐ

10 mm

① see Ⓑ

Lobus front.

②

Lobus temp.

Ⓑ

N. II   c 1

①a   ∅

①c   Dura

①b

Ⓒ

10 m m

N. II   c 1   N. III

Dura

N.V₁

Proc. clin. ant.,
limit of resection

Ⓒ'

N. II

c1   N. III

Dura resection
(projection)

N.V1

tumor
(projection)

N.V2

FIG. 89 ⊏━━━━━━━━━━━━━━━━━━━━━━━━━━━━━━━━⊐ 178

Fig. 89. Operations in the area surrounding Sinus cavernosus

A **1a + 1b** Incision of tumor surface above and below N.V1

    2 Hollowing of tumor with curette

    3 Removal of loosened tumor tissue

B **1a + 1b** Removal of loosened tumor bulk from tumor bed

C Site after **tumor removal**

FIG. 89

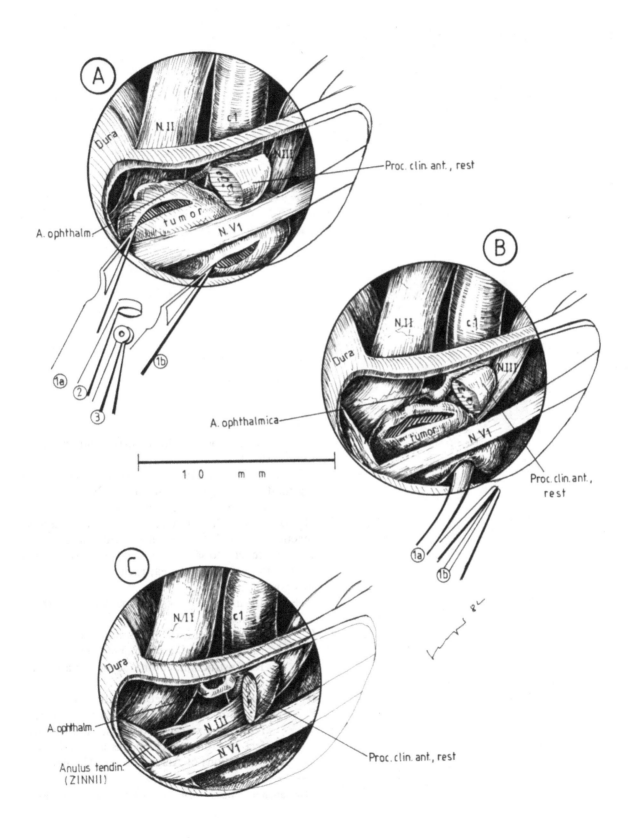

A

Dura
N. II
c1
N.III
Proc. clin. ant., rest
A. ophthalm.
tumor
N. V1

1a
2
3
1b

B

N.II
c1
Dura
N.III
A. ophthalmica
tumor
N.V1
Proc. clin. ant., rest

1a
1b

10   m m

C

N. II
c1
Dura
A. ophthalm.
N. III
N. V1
Proc. clin. ant., rest
Anulus tendin.
(ZINNII)

FIG. 90 ⊏━━━━━━━━━━━━━━━━━━━━━━━━━━━━━━━━⊐ 180

Fig. 90. Operations in the area surrounding Sinus cavernosus.

Clinical example of **meningioma recidivation occupying total left Sinus cavernosus** area*. Normally, this type tumor inoperable. In this case, as patient was already blind, the intraorbital portion of tumor, together with bulbus, was enucleated. Since here it was unnecessary to save the already destroyed nerves of the Sinus cavernosus area, radical tumor removal was possible

A + B　In angiogram: contrast medium uptake by tumor

C　CT, preoperative: basal tumor with exophthalmus (histological: meningioma)

D　Reconstruction, coronal section. Narrowing of basal cisterns by tumor

D'　Section planes of reconstruction **D**

E　Situation after eye enucleation and tumor removal. Extensive bone resection with defect of Processus clinoideus ant. and close-by portions of Ala minor and Ala major

---

* Operation performed by Dr. W. Hassler, author's coworker.

FIG. 90

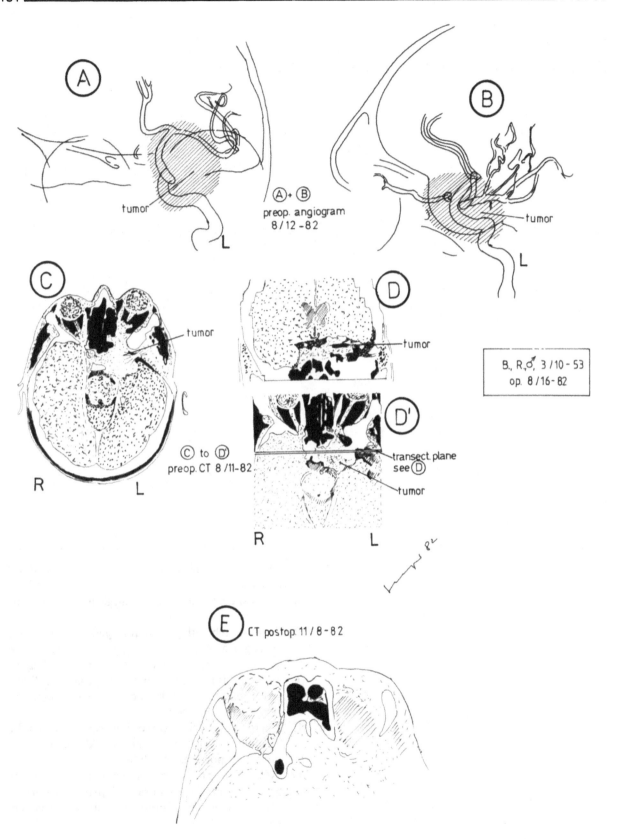

(A)

tumor

Ⓐ+Ⓑ
preop. angiogram
8/12-82

L

(B)

tumor

L

(C)

tumor

Ⓒ to Ⓓ
preop. CT 8/11-82

R   L

(D)

tumor

(D')

transect. plane
see Ⓓ

tumor

R   L

B., R.,♂, 3/10-53
op. 8/16-82

Ⓔ CT postop. 11/8-82

FIG. 91 ⊏━━━━━━━━━━━━━━━━━━━━━━━━━━━━━⊐ 182

Fig. 91. Operations in the area surrounding Sinus cavernosus

A Skull sketch, various microsurgical view positions shown

B Skull sketch with **pterional trepanation** drawn in. Recognizable previous trepanations were more extensive than present ones, corresponding to previous tumor size. In the approach to Sinus cavernosus and to orbital cavity a small pterional approach is sufficient

C Microsurgical site, corresponding to sketch **B. Drilling** of greatly thickened Ala minor and adjoining portions of orbita roof

D After drilling of Ala minor and major, juncture of Fossa cranii, media dura and perorbita dura is exposed medially, Foramen rotundum was not opened

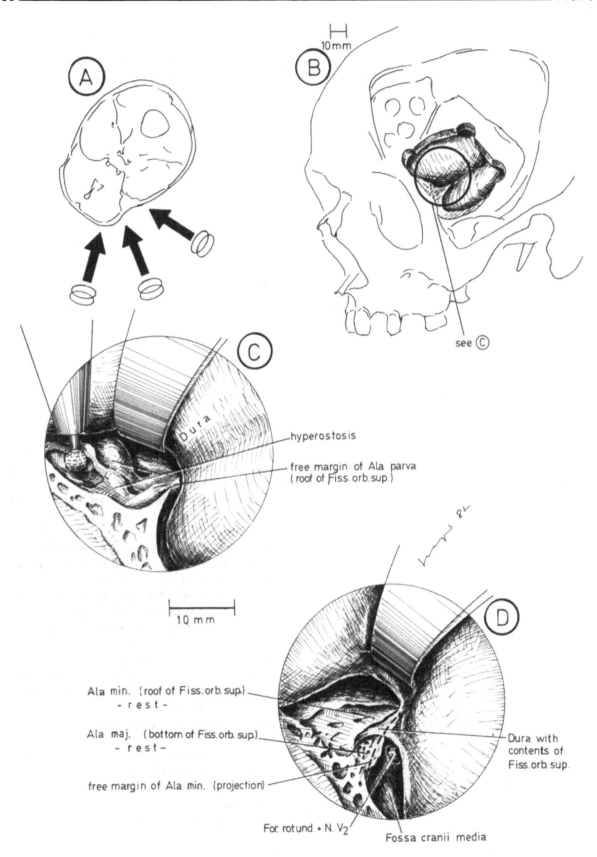

10 mm

10 mm

see Ⓒ

Dura

hyperostosis

free margin of Ala parva
(roof of Fiss.orb.sup.)

10 mm

Ala min. (roof of Fiss.orb.sup.)
- r e s t -

Ala maj. (bottom of Fiss.orb.sup.)
- r e s t -

free margin of Ala min. (projection)

Dura with
contents of
Fiss.orb.sup.

For. rotund.+ N. V₂

Fossa cranii media

FIG. 92 ⬚══⬚ 184

Fig. 92. Operations in the area surrounding Sinus cavernosus

A 1 **Opening of dura**
   2 Separation of adhesions from previous operations, between brain surface and dura
   3 Snaring and pulling out of small basal dura flap

B 1a Stretching of arachnoidal filaments over Fissura lateralis Sylvii by means of small hook
   1b Separation of these adhesions
   2 After **opening of Fissura Sylvii,** insertion of spatula and reclination of frontal lobe
   3 Dura incision over tumor near N.II and A. carotis int. –c1–
   4a + 4b Hollowing of tumor

C 1 Further insertion of spatula and **reclination of frontal brain** after opening of arachnoidea over N.II and A. carotis int.
   2 Slight retraction of temporal pole
   3 Coagulation of dura over tumor
   4 **Incision of tumor** along A. carotis int. path
   5 Stretching of tumor during incision

Abbreviations:

c1   A. carotis int.

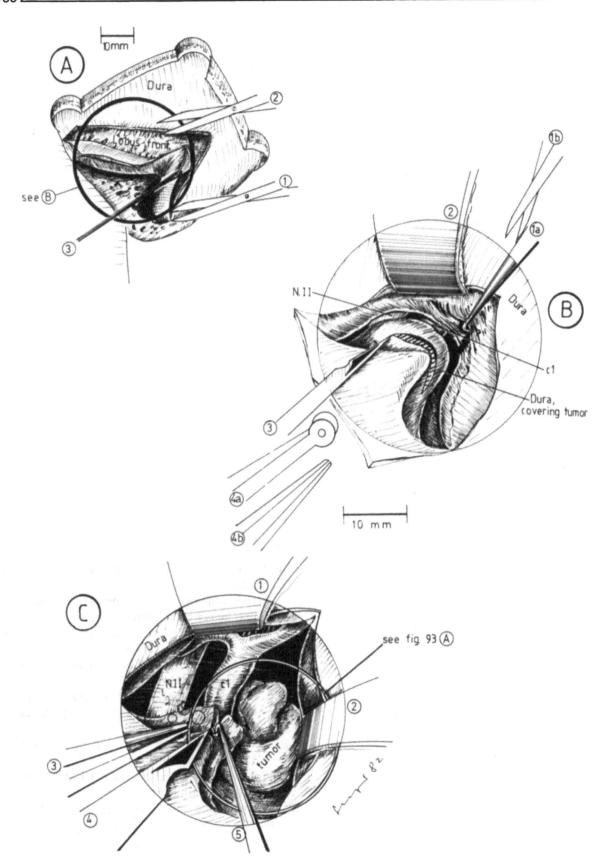

FIG. 93 ⊏━━━━━━━━━━━━━━━━━━━━━━━━━━━⊐186

Fig. 93. Operations in the area surrounding Sinus cavernosus

A Nerves running through Sinus cavernosus area can no longer be identified within tumor. For the already mentioned reasons, care need not be taken to save these nerves

　1 Slight reclination of Lobus temporalis to posterior tumor edge

　2 **Incision of tumor along A. carotis int. path**

B　1 Loosening of tumor from **A. ophthalmica,** which is afterward ligated

　2 + 3 Loosening of tumor remnant from deep dura layer and bone.

　broken lines: cranial nerves N.III, N.IV, N.V1 were not identifiable

B' Topographical anatomical sketch of **B,** left anterior view

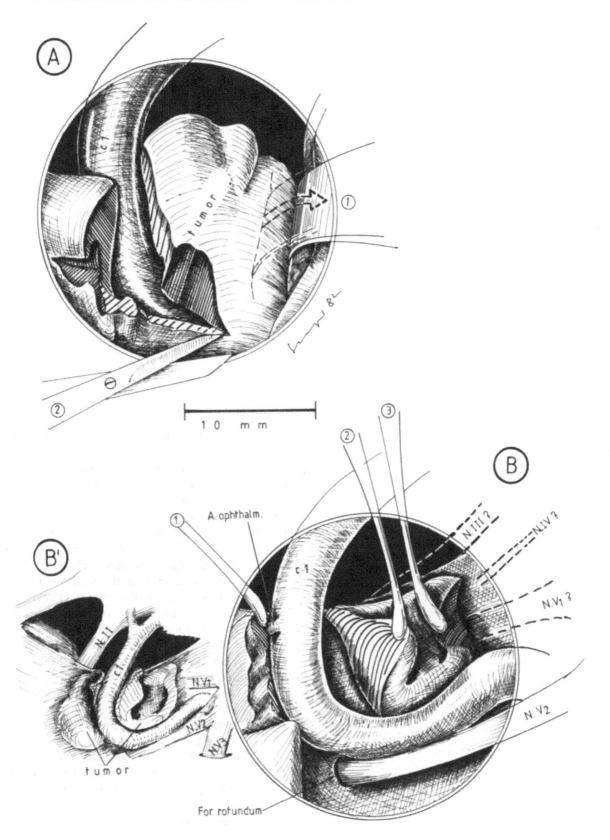

A

c.1

t u m o r

①

②

10 mm

③

②

B'

① A. ophthalm.

N.II

c.1

N.V1

N.V2

N.V3

t u m o r

B

N.III ?

N.IV ?

N.V1 ?

c.1

N.V2

For. rotundum

FIG. 94 188

Fig. 94. Operations in the area surrounding Sinus cavernosus.

Clinical example of **inoperable tumor** (histological: meningioma) with contralateral extension*. In this case only a decompression of N. opticus and A. carotis int. is possible

A + B No contrast-medium uptake by tumor. Arrow: stenosis of A. carotis int. as it passes through Sinus cavernosus. The tumor being inoperable, even a decompression of A. carotis int. is out of the question because of danger to the nerves of Sinus cavernosus area. Carotis externa-interna bypass would be indicated if signs of an imminent cerebrovascular decompensation were present

C Section planes of reconstruction **C'** and **C''** sketched in, showing tumor infiltrating as a thin sheet towards the base

D + E Tumor is limited to Sinus cavernosus area. No sure indication of intradural growth. We have not presented postoperative CT because it was identical to preoperative CT: major portion of tumor was not removed

* Operation performed by Dr. H. R. Eggert, author's coworker.

FIG. 94

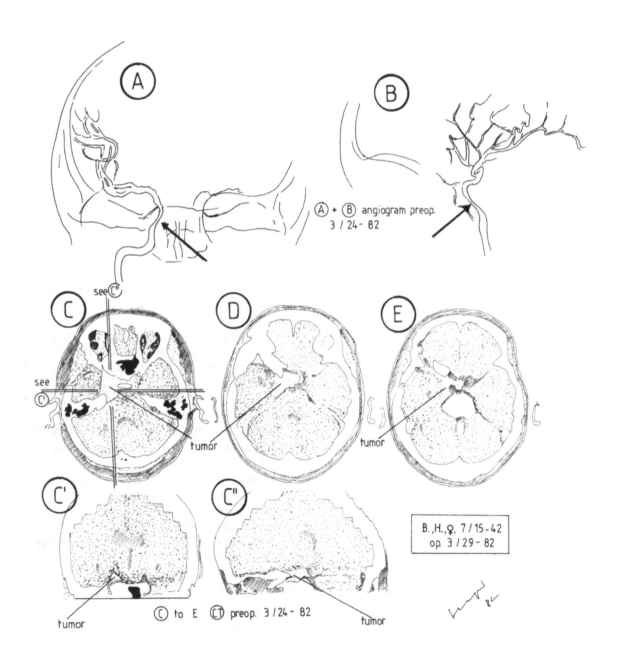

Ⓐ

Ⓑ

Ⓐ + Ⓑ angiogram preop.
3 / 24 - 82

see C"

Ⓒ

see
C'

tumor

Ⓓ

tumor

Ⓔ

tumor

C'

C"

tumor

tumor

Ⓒ to E ⒸⓉ preop. 3 / 24 - 82

B.,H.,♀, 7 / 15 - 42
op. 3 / 29 - 82

FIG. 95 190

Fig. 95. Operations in the area surrounding Sinus cavernosus.

Microsurgical site

A   Spreading of Fissura Sylvii exposes topographical relation of tumor, N. oculomotorius, A. carotis int. –cl–, N. opticus on both sides, as well as Chiasma

B   Coagulation of tumors's dura cover accompanied by extensive irrigation

C   **Tumor slightly shrunken, N.II and N.III are decompressed** at dura penetration points.
Effect of decompression is unsatisfactory, because tumor portions still impinge upon these two nerves at the skull base

B' Anatomical sketch for **B**

C' Anatomical sketch for **C**
Open arrows: Shrinking of tumor by bipolar electrocoagulation

Abbreviations:

ap   Ala minor
cl   A. carotis int.

FIG. 95

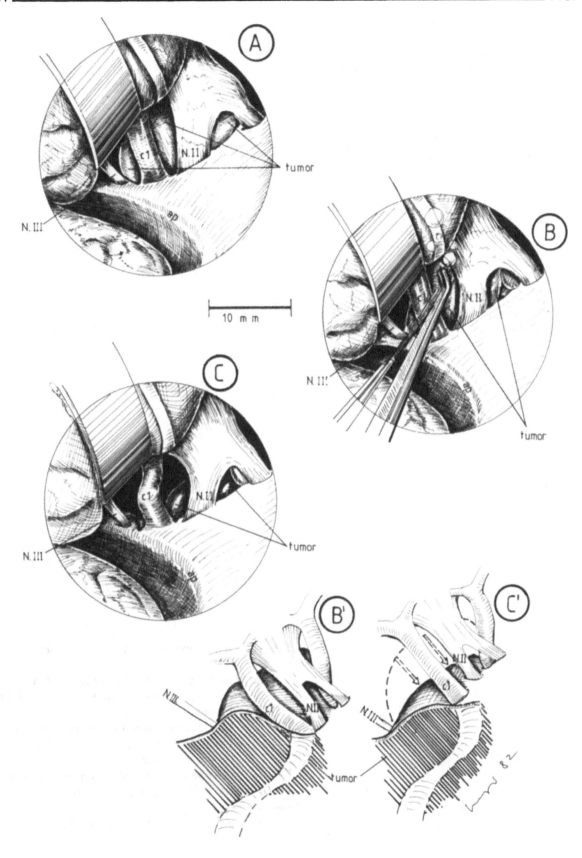

FIG. 96 192

Fig. 96. Operations in the area surrounding Sinus cavernosus.

Clinical example of **Cavum Meckeli-meningioma** *

A + A'   Angiogram shows contrast medium uptake by tumor

B + B'   CT (level see **D**) shows: tumor caused atrophy of Os petrosum tip and Dorsum sellae on the right side

E   CT one day after operation: air marks the site of radically removed tumor

* Operation performed by Dr. H. R. Eggert, author's coworker.

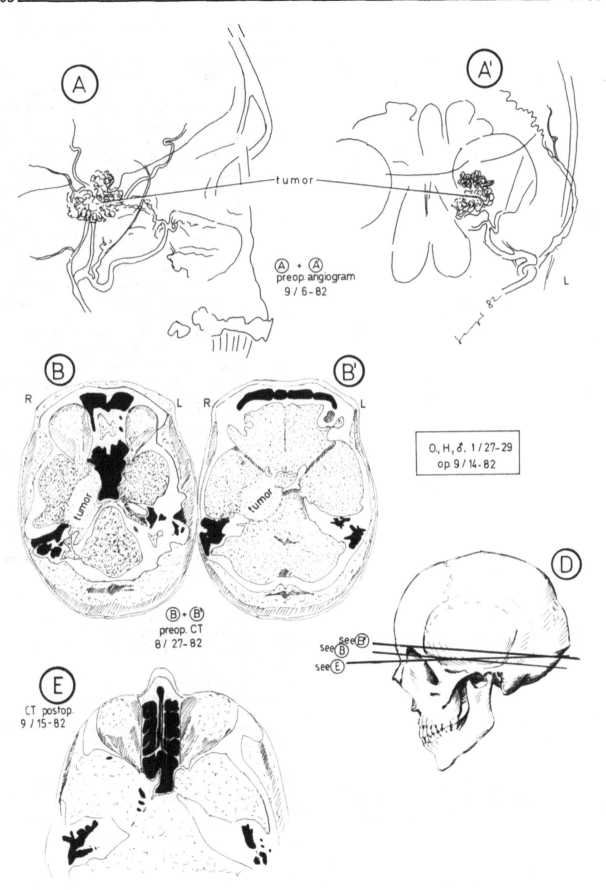

Ⓐ

Ⓐ'

tumor

Ⓐ + Ⓐ
preop. angiogram
9 / 6 - 82

L

Ⓑ

Ⓑ'

R   L   R   L

tumor

tumor

O., H., ♂, 1 / 27 - 29
op. 9 / 14 - 82

Ⓑ + Ⓑ'
preop. CT
8 / 27 - 82

Ⓓ

see Ⓑ'
see Ⓑ
see Ⓔ

Ⓔ

CT postop.
9 / 15 - 82

FIG. 97 ⸻⸻⸻⸻⸻⸻⸻⸻⸻ 194

Fig. 97. Operations in the area surrounding Sinus cavernosus.

Topographical anatomical sketch

A	Skull sketch, overview for **A' + A"**
A'	Detail of skull base with senile bone atrophy. One sees the close topographical relation of Impressio n. trigemini –*imp*–, Foramen lacerum –*lc*– (which surrounds A. carotis int. in the unmacerated skull) and Foramen ovale –*ov*–. Impressio n. trigemini corresponds to position of N.V, Foramen lacerum lies below Cavum Meckeli
A"	Sketch for **A'** with dura, Ganglion Gasseri and several adjoining structures drawn in; broken line indicates site of tumor which, in hourglass form, has distended Cavum Meckeli –*x*– and has penetrated into posterior fossa, with a second tumor lump along path of N. trigeminus –*y*–
B – B"	Another projection, corresponding to **A – A"**. This skull preparation shows two Impressiones trigemini: the smaller one, lying higher –*impn*– caused by N. trigeminus; the larger one, farther lateral, –*impg*– caused by Ganglion Gasseri
C	There are two possible ways for tumor to spread into posterior fossa:

    a dura distension dorsal to N. trigeminus (as operatively verified in this presented case) – the better possibility

    b spreading of tumor along N. trigeminus through its penetration point in tentorium, and growing around N. trigeminus – less advantageous for operation

Abbreviations:

ac	Porus acusticus int.
ca	Processus clinoideus ant.
cv	Cavum Meckeli (transection)
cl	A. carotis int.
ds	Diaphragma sellae
Ggl.G.	Ganglion semilunare (Gasseri)
imp	Impressio trigemini, normal finding
impg	Impression by Ganglion Gasseri
impn	Impression by N. trigeminus
lc	Foramen lacerum
ov	Foramen ovale
ps	Sinus petrosus sup.
te	Tentorium
x, y	Tumor limit, projection

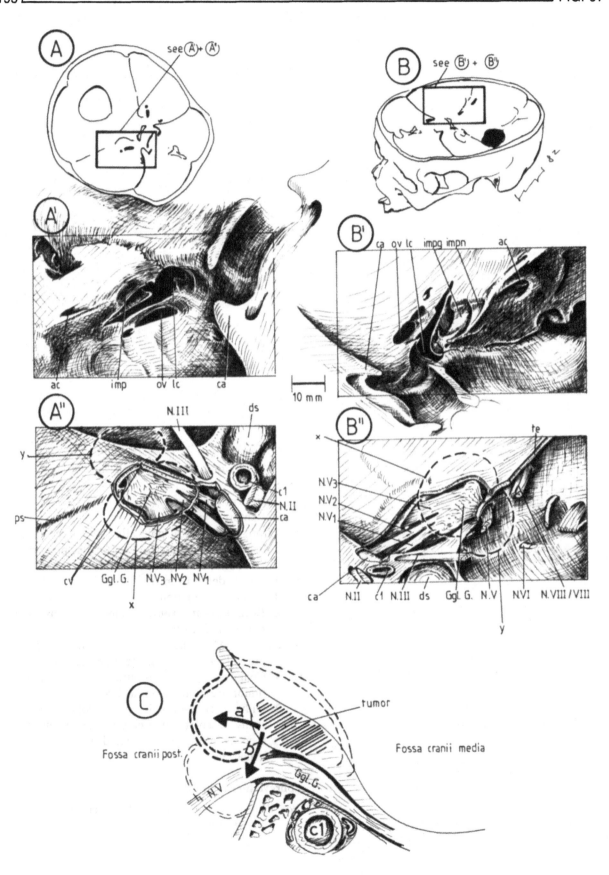

A   see Ⓐ'+ Ⓐ"

B   see Ⓑ'+ Ⓑ"

A'   ac   imp   ov lc   ca

B'   ca ov lc   impg impn   ac

10 mm

A"   N.III   ds
y   c1
N.II
ps   ca
cv   Ggl.G.   N.V₃ N.V₂ N.V₁
x

B"   x   te
N.V₃
N.V₂
N.V₁
ca   N.II   c1 N.III ds   Ggl.G. N.V   N.VI   N.VIII/VIII
y

C   tumor
a
Fossa cranii post.   b   Fossa cranii media
Ggl.G.
N.V
c1

FIG. 98 ⬜══════════════════════════════════⬜ 196

Fig. 98. Operations in the area surrounding Sinus cavernosus.

Microsurgical site

Lateral-anterior view

A   Lifting of temporal pole after spreading Fissura Sylvii. Richly vascularized tumor has penetrated dura at one small spot

B   Enlarged detail from A

   1 Tumor coagulation

   2 Dura incision around tumor as far as Sinus petrosus sup. −sp−

   3a + 3b After incision of dura, its edges are pushed away from tumor (open arrows)

C   **1** Coagulation of tumor surface, outer edges of tumor are pulled from its bed

   2 Only after thorough tumor coagulation, is richly vascularized tumor hollowed out, and then its interior is coagulated, using extensive irrigation

Abbreviations:

(ac) Processus clinoideus ant. (projection)

sp Sinus petrosus sup.

FIG. 98

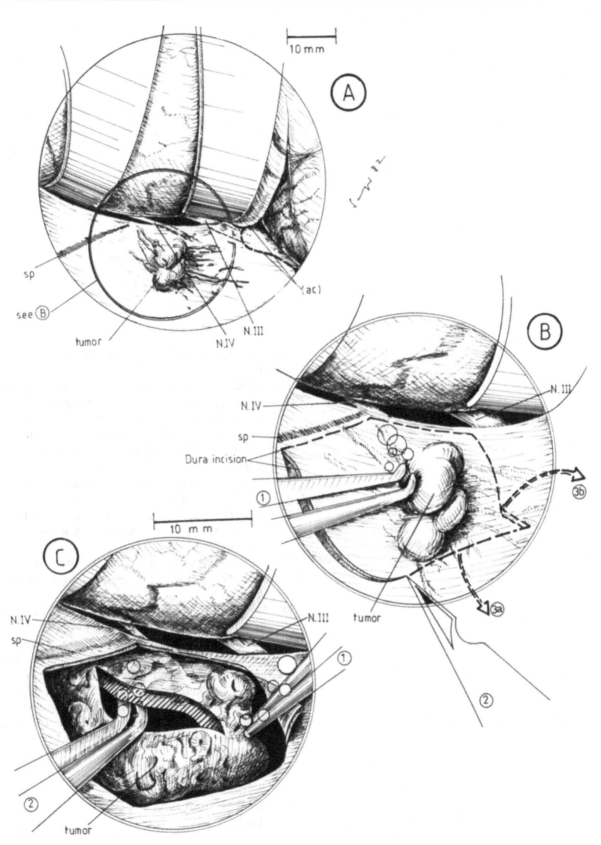

FIG. 99 ⬛══════════════════════════════════════⬛ 198

Fig. 99. Operations in the area surrounding Sinus cavernosus.

Operation site and anatomical model presentations

A Microsurgical site. In front of Sinus petrosus sup. –*sp*–, tumor is severed transversely, and anterior portion, located in Fossa cranii media, is removed

B Anatomical skull sketch, overview for **C + D,** *s* corresponding to section plane **C'**

C Detail of skull preparation, N. trigeminus and its branches drawn in

D As **C,** showing deeply excavated Impressio trigemini. Scalpel and broken line mark site of tumor incision in **A**

C' Section sketch of bone, dura, A. carotis int. and N. trigeminus. Sketch corresponding to section plane –*s*– in **C**

D' As **C,** tumor and tumor incision as in **A** sketched in. Section plane corresponding to *s* in **D**

E Microsurgical site after tumor removal. Ganglion Gasseri and N. trigeminus branches lie in base of tumor bed, covered by translucent dura layer.
(N.V **C'**): Sketch shows original normal path of N. trigeminus preceding tumor development
(N.V **D'**): Path of N. trigeminus, when rotated operation microscope views posterior fossa

Abbreviations:

cl A. carotis int.
sp Sinus petrosus sup.
te Tentorium

FIG. 99

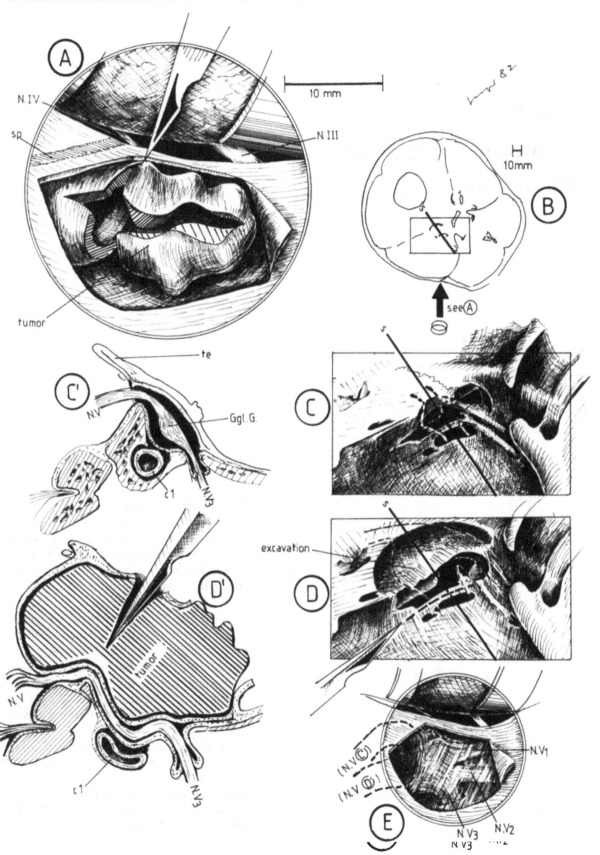

N.IV

sp.

N III

10 mm

tumor

H
10mm

see A

te

C'

N.V

Ggl.G.

c1

N.V3

excavation

D

D'

tumor

N.V

c1

N.V3

(N.V C)

(N.V D)

N.V₁

N V₃
N. V3

N.V₂

E

FIG. 100 ⌐━━━━━━━━━━━━━━━━━━━━━━━━━⌐ 200

Chapter 3
Frontobasal Operations
(Figs. 100 to 134)

Tumor (olfactory groove meningioma) (Figs. 100 to 115)

Fig. 100. Frontobasal operations.
Clinical example of Olfactorius meningioma. For half a year diminishing performance, 2 weeks ago grand mal, bilateral but predominantly left hyposmia. Postoperative bilateral anosmia, no additional deficits, no more seizures; performance improved.
Diagnostic procedures

A – B' Preoperative angiograms show the typical displacement syndrome (arrows). Tumor vascularization mainly from A. ophthalmica through ethmoidal branches. Vessels entry into tumor within a hyperostosis (= enostosis) (see also CT **D – E'**)

C – E' Preoperative CT-findings showing tumor with basal-central hyperostosis. Angiogram shows extensive tumor vascularization. Hyperostosis encloses a **recesse of Sinus sphenoidalis.**
Danger of postoperative liquor fistula!

F Postoperatively, a cavity filled with CS-fluid is seen, instead of tumor

FIG. 100

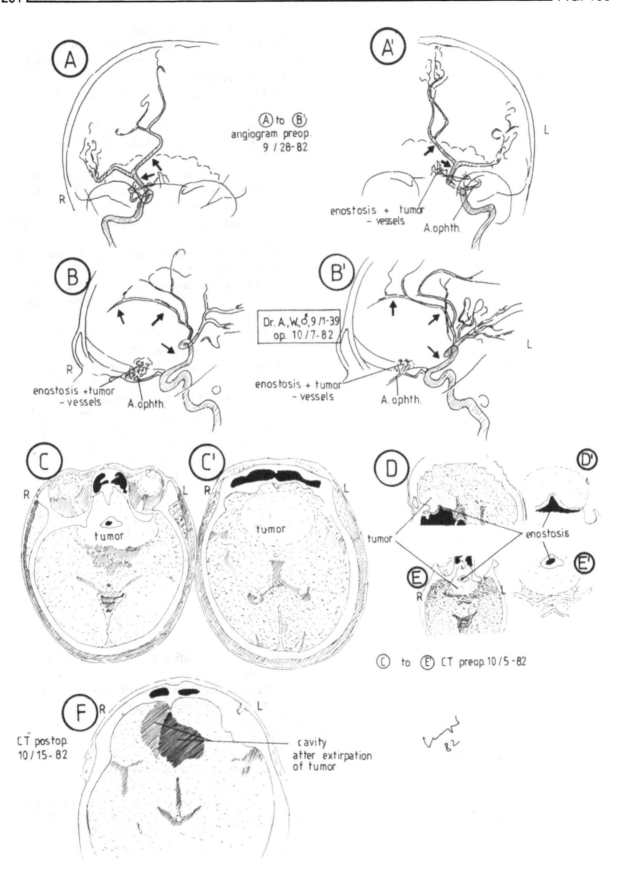

(A) to (B') angiogram preop. 9/28-82

(A')

L

enostosis + tumor - vessels   A.ophth.

(B)

R

enostosis +tumor - vessels   A.ophth.

Dr. A.,W.,♂,9/1-39 op. 10/7-82

(B')

L

enostosis + tumor - vessels   A. ophth.

(C) R   L   tumor

(C') R   L   tumor

(D)   tumor   enostosis   (D')

(E) R   L   (E')

(C) to (E') CT preop. 10/5-82

(F) R   L

CT postop. 10/15-82

cavity after extirpation of tumor

82

Fig. 101. Frontobasal operations.

Olfactorius meningioma, steps from skin incision to trepanation. Broken lines: projection of trepanation and skull structures

A **1** Skin incision. At first periosteum is left on skull surface

A' As **A,** schematic anatomical transection

B Preparation of skin and galea, as well as periosteum

   1 Pushing of skin from periosteum medially as far as nasion, lateraly as far as orbital edge

   2 Periosteum incision

   3 Pushing of periosteum also as far as orbita and nasion*

C Preparation of periosteum and M. temporalis prior to trepanation

   1a, 1b, 1c Galea-skin flap is pulled back by retractors until orbital edges become clearly visible

   2 Only then can periosteum be pushed back as far as orbital edge and nasion

   3 Incision of Fascia and Aponeurosis temporalis at anterior sector of linea temporalis sup.

   4 Pushing away of M. temporalis in the area of incision **3,** in order to place lateral burr hole there (cosmetic result better than burr hole medial of linea temporalis sup.)

   5a Retention of periosteum

   5b Drilling of burr holes

C' As **C,** lateral view

   1 see **C 3**

   2 see **C 4**

   x see **C**

D **1** Loosening dura from inner skull surface in the area of all burr holes, using curved dissector

   2 Drilling of bone

Abbreviations:

cu Cutis

ga Galea aponeurotica (Aponeurosis of M. epicranius)

mf Musculus frontalis (present nomenclature: M. epicranius, Venter frontalis)

p Periost

sk Skull

x Marking of burr hole trepanation in the most anterior area of Fossa temporalis

* Difficult and in some cases incorrect. Better method: Cutis, Galea and periosteum detached from skull in one piece (see Fig. 119).

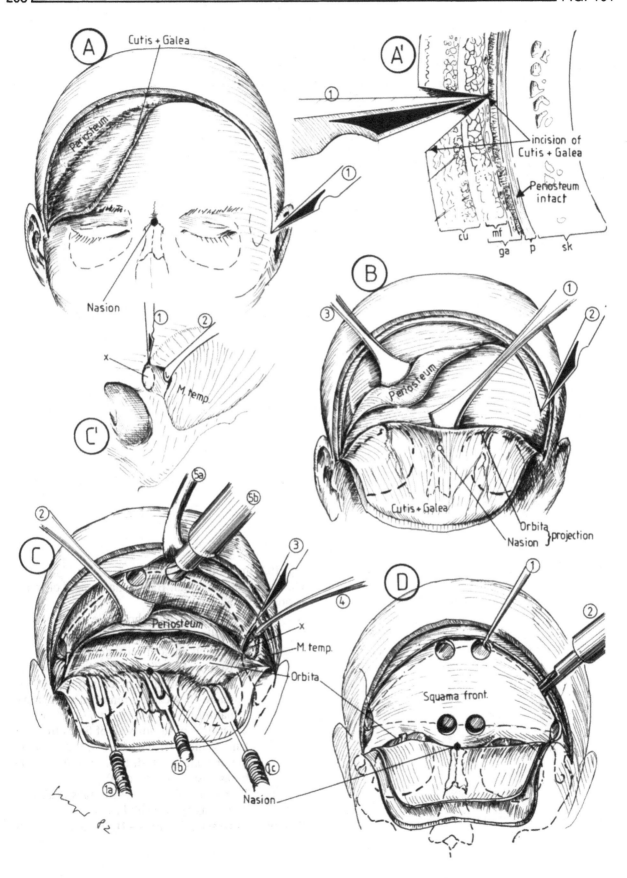

A Cutis + Galea — Periosteum — Nasion

A' ① incision of Cutis + Galea — Periosteum intact — cu — mf — ga — p — sk

C' x — ① — ② — M. temp.

B ③ — ① — ② — Periosteum — Cutis + Galea — Orbita }projection — Nasion

C ② — ⑤a — ⑤b — ③ — ④ — Periosteum — x — M. temp. — Orbita — Nasion — ①a — ①b — ①c

D ① — ② — Squama front. — Orbita — Nasion

FIG. 102 ⊏━━━━━━━━━━━━━━━━━━━━━⊐ 204

Fig. 102. Frontobasal operations.
Olfactorius meningioma. Basal enlargement of trepanation as far as nasion

A   Medio-basal burr holes lie in the Sinus frontalis area above nasion

B   Simplified anatomical sagittal section
   1 Removal of Sinus frontalis mucosa, as far as possible (if mucosa fragments remain, they can be removed after trepanation)
   2 Drilling posterior wall of Sinus frontalis

C   Enlargement of burr hole, on the side of major tumor spread, towards skull base as far as nasion (see **C'** also)

D   Posterior wall of Sinus frontalis is also removed as far as skull base

B' – D' Corresponding to **B – D,** but anterior view

FIG. 102

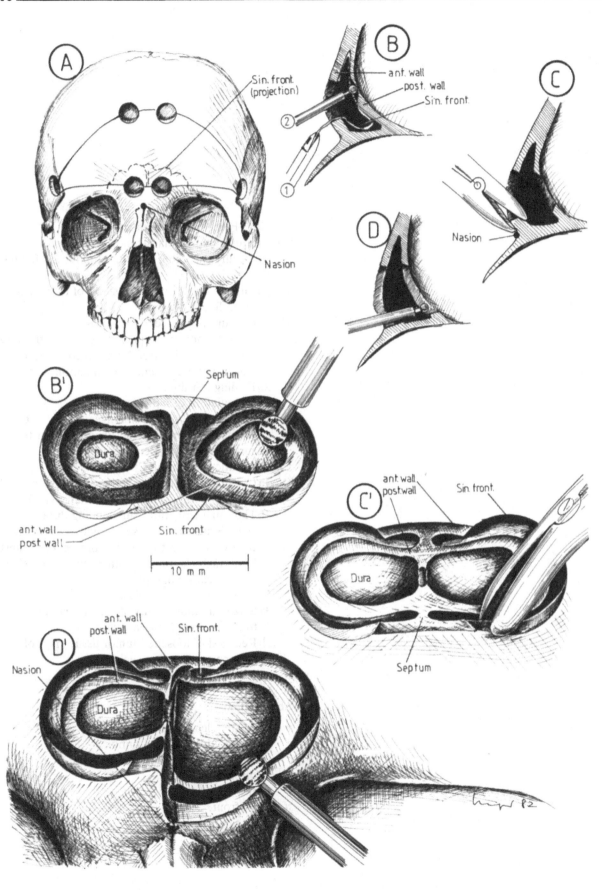

A — Sin. front. (projection) / Nasion

B — ant. wall / post. wall / Sin. front.

C — Nasion

D

B' — Septum / Dura / ant. wall / post wall / Sin. front. / 10 m m

C' — ant. wall / post. wall / Sin. front. / Dura / Septum

D' — Nasion / ant. wall / post. wall / Sin. front. / Dura

FIG. 103 ⸻ 206

Fig. 103. Frontobasal operations.
Olfactorius meningioma. Tumor extirpation

A Microsurgical site of the following figures, sketched on skull

B Enlarged detail from **A.** Position of dura incision (broken lines)

C Small dura flaps folded outwards

  1a + 1b Cotton wool packing of Sinus frontalis after clearing it carefully of mucosa remnants

  2a Covering Sinus frontalis with cotton wool

  2b Folding out dura

  3 Coagulation of leptomeninges

  4 Incision of leptomeninges and fibrous remnants of brain tissue lying between tumor surface and leptomeninges

C' Schematic section for **C**

D **1a** Coagulation of tumor surface (with leptomeninges and thin fibrous brain tissue)

  1b Thorough irrigation; surrounding dura – especially Sinus sagittalis sup. – and brain tissue is covered with cotton wool as protection against heat (sketch omits cotton wool to show anatomical topography)

  2 Incision of tumor surface

  3a Spreading movements of forceps within tumor to loosen tumor parenchyma

  3b Removal of loosened tumor tissue and holding tumor vessels, using sucker

D' Schematic section for **D**

Abbreviations:

a   Arachnoidea, outer layer

a'   Arachnoidea cover of tumor

c   Remnants of fibrous brain tissue

cow Cotton wool

d   Dura

sf   Sin. front.

ss   Sin. sagitt. sup.

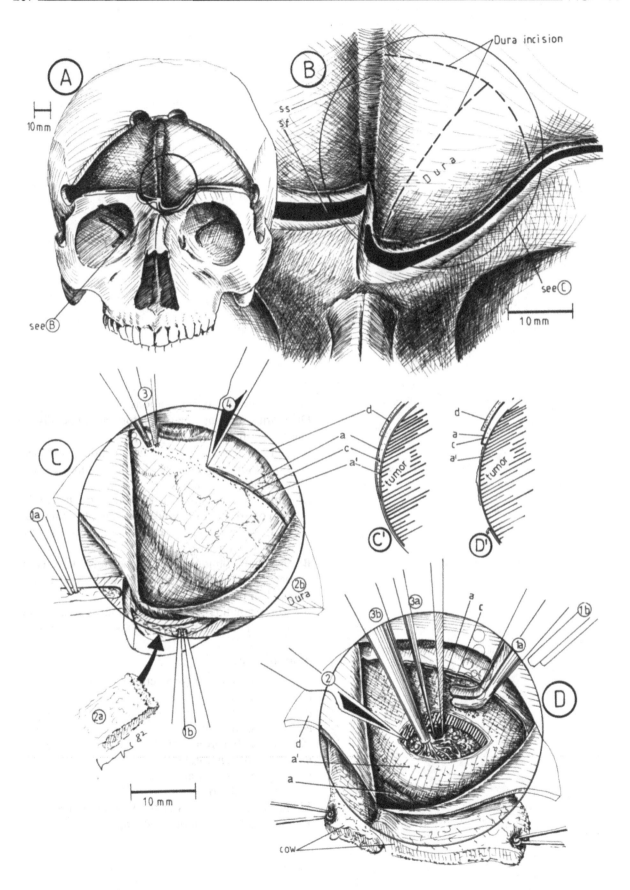

FIG. 104 ⬛══════════════════════════════════════⬛ 208

Fig. 104. Frontobasal operations.
Olfactorius meningioma. Anatomical appendix to microsurgical operation

A Schematic anatomical median section (tumor sectioned somewhat lateral of median plane). *x:* start of tumor hollowing

A' Enlarged detail from **A.** Note topographical relation of excavation to enostosis –*en*–, to projection of Crista galli –*(cg)*– and to projection of posterior falx edge –*(fx)*–.

B Schematic oblique skull transection, sketched-in section planes of tumor *S1, S2* and *S3* parallel to median plane

A" Corresponding to **B** after skull opening and removal of basal tumor portions –*x*–, as in **A + A'**

Abbreviations:

(cg)	Crista galli (projection)
ct	Cutis
d	Dura
en	Enostosis
(fx)	Falx (projection)
mt	M. temporalis
sf	Sinus frontalis
sk	Skull bone
S1, S2, S3	Corner points of transection planes
x	Start of tumor hollowing

FIG. 104

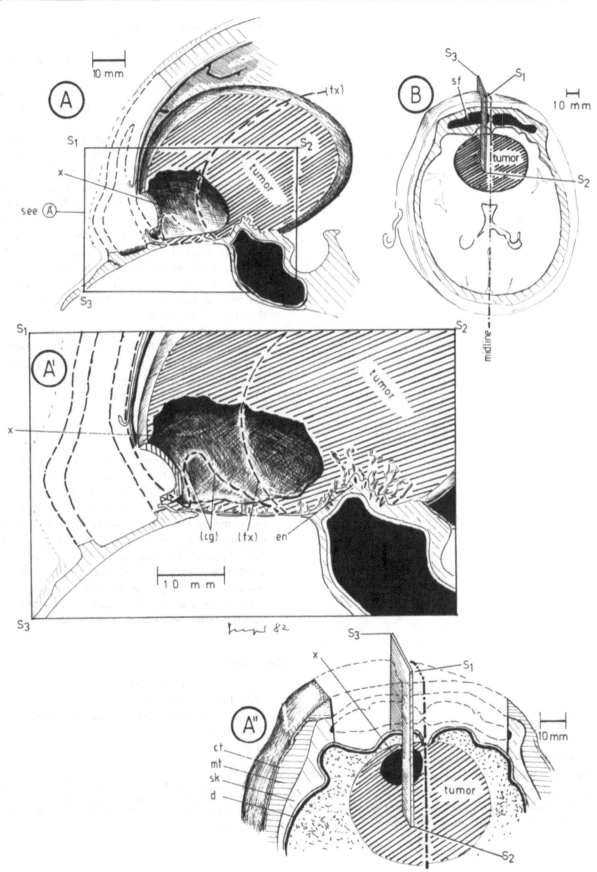

FIG. 105 🗌━━━━━━━━━━━━━━━━━━━━━━━━━━━━━━━🗌 210

2 Electrocoagulation of tumor vessels held by suction

3 Separation of coagulated vessels in enostosis area

Close behind enostosis one can already expect N.II and A. carotis int., on both sides lateral of midline

A' Schematic horizontal section through tumor. Anatomical topographical relation of enostosis, N.II and A. carotis int. −c1− sketched in

B After cessation of tumor bleeding tendency, hollowing of tumor may proceed on a larger scale

C After thorough hollowing of tumor, its outer surface can be loosened from surrounding brain tissue. Preparation has to be carried out exactly between arachnoideal cover of the brain −a− and arachnoidal tumor cover −a'−, to prevent unnecessary traumatization of brain tissue or less than radical tumor removal.

Arrows: tumor and brain tissue may spread apart spontaneously. In this case one must ascertain that this separation has taken place correctly between the arachnoidal layers*

D Microsurgical site for **B + C**

1 Blunt squeezing of tumor using forceps

2 Siphoning off tumor tissue and holding fast of vessels

3 Coagulation of vessels stretched by suction

Principally, when loosening extracerebral tumors from surrounding brain tissue, the preparation must take place between arachnoidal cover of brain and arachnoidal tumor cover. If this is not possible, because one of these arachnoidal covers was ruptured by tumor, then one must seek another site from which correct preparation can proceed. Following this method will result in unprotected brain zones remaining small. This is essential to prevent postoperative epilepsy.

Abbreviations:

a   External arachnoidal layer of brain
a'   Arachnoidal tumor cover
en   Enostosis (main tumor vascularization occurs in this area)
fx   Falx

Fig. 105. Frontobasal operations.
Olfactorius meningioma. Basal tumor hollowing with early elimination of tumor vessels

A 1 Holding tumor vessels by sucker after siphoning off loosened tumor parenchyma

---

* The author thanks Prof. Dr. G. Yaşargil, Zürich, for his reference to this principle of arachnoidal preparation in cases of acoustic meningioma, which can be applied to all operations of extracerebral tumors.

FIG. 105

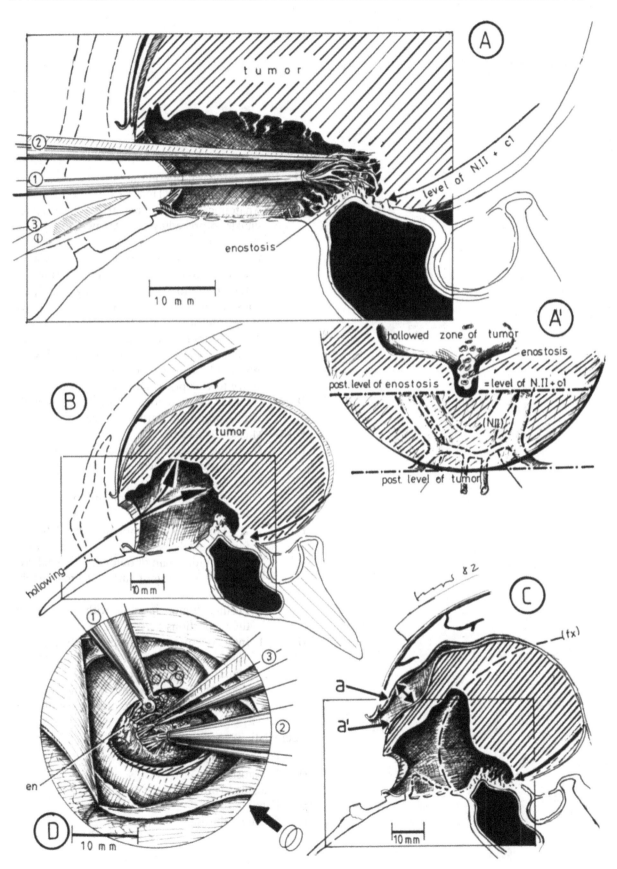

A

tumor

② ① ③ ⑦

level of N.II + c1

enostosis

10 mm

A'

hollowed zone of tumor

enostosis

post. level of enostosis = level of N.II + c1

(NII)

post. level of tumor

B

tumor

hollowing

10 mm

C

82

(fx)

a a'

10 mm

D

① ③ ②

en

10 mm

FIG. 106 212

Fig. 106. Frontobasal operations.
Olfactorius meningioma. Tumor extirpation

A Anatomical longitudinal transection sketch similar to preceding fig. Arrows: tumor collapse

 1 Collapsing tumor portions are removed by cutting around original tumor incision

B After further hollowing, collapsing tumor portions are circularly sliced away (*s1 – s4*), see microsurgical sites **E – G**

C After further tumor hollowing, falx *–fx–* becomes visible medially. Basal hollowing must not be done yet because of the danger of injury to N. opticus and/or A. carotis int.

D If tumor shows tendency to collapse, spatula can be positioned into tumor cavity

E – G Microsurgical sites

E   1 Pulling back arachnoidal layer of brain from tumor surface

  2 As **1**

  3 Circular tumor resection around previous incision

F   1, 2, 3 Hollowing of tumor and coagulation of tumor vessels as before

  4 Preparation again of outer arachnoidal layer away from tumor surface (tumor arachnoidea)

  5 Further tumor incision with removal of tumor portions

G   1 Insertion of spatula to prevent sinking of tumor and of Lobus frontalis lying above tumor. Falx *–fx–* exposed

  2 Tumor hollowing extends into the opposite side, however not quite as far as skull-base

Abbreviations:

(cg) Crista galli (projection)
en Enostosis
(en) Enostosis (projection)
fx Falx
lc Lamina cribrosa

FIG. 106

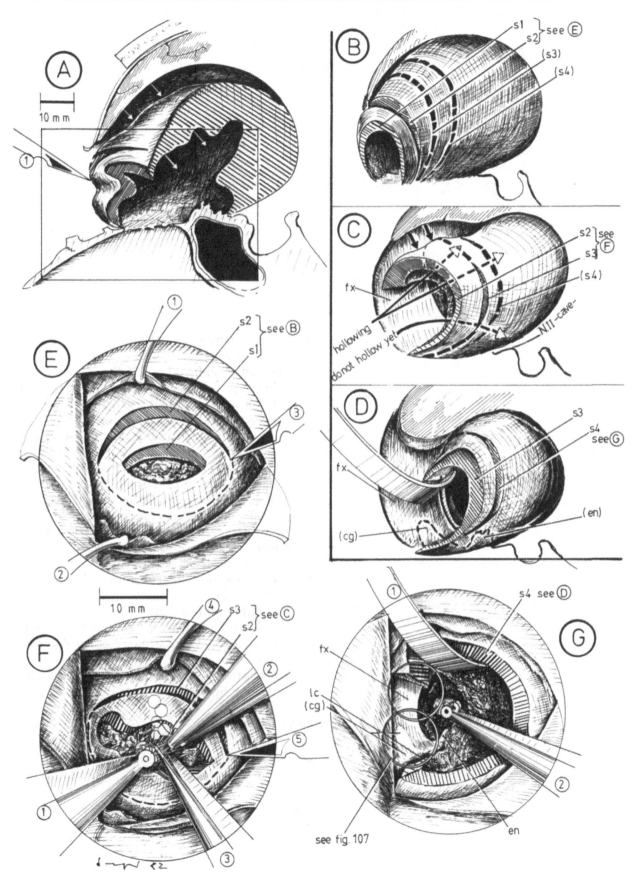

see fig. 107

FIG. 107 ⌐==⌐214

Fig. 107. Frontobasal operations.

Olfactorius meningioma. Tumor extirpation

A Enlarged detail from Fig. 106 **G**

    1 Incision of falx leaf around Crista galli on tumor side along Sinus sagittalis sup. –*ss*–

    2 Resection of Crista galli

    3 Transcision of falx nearly as far as Sinus sagittalis sup. –*ss*–

A' Schematic horizontal section through tumor and neighboring structures. Arrow: direction of microscopic view. *p:* due to oblique microscopic view projection, falx appears foreshortened

A" Anatomical section sketch of **B,** to show topographical relation of incised falx leaf –*i*–, Crista galli and Sinus sagittalis sup. –*ss*–

B **1a** Loosening of contralateral tumor from incised falx portion

    1b Stretching of falx (both leafs)

    2 Incision of contralateral falx leaf after Crista galli removal. White arrows: excision of incised falx portion

C Bleeding from incised falx portion is controlled by suture (not by clip) *

Abbreviations:

en   Enostosis

p   Seemingly foreshortened falx

ss   Sinus sagittalis sup.

---

* For this suggestion I thank PD Dr. A. M. Landolt, Neurosurgical Clinic, University of Zürich, Switzerland.

FIG. 107

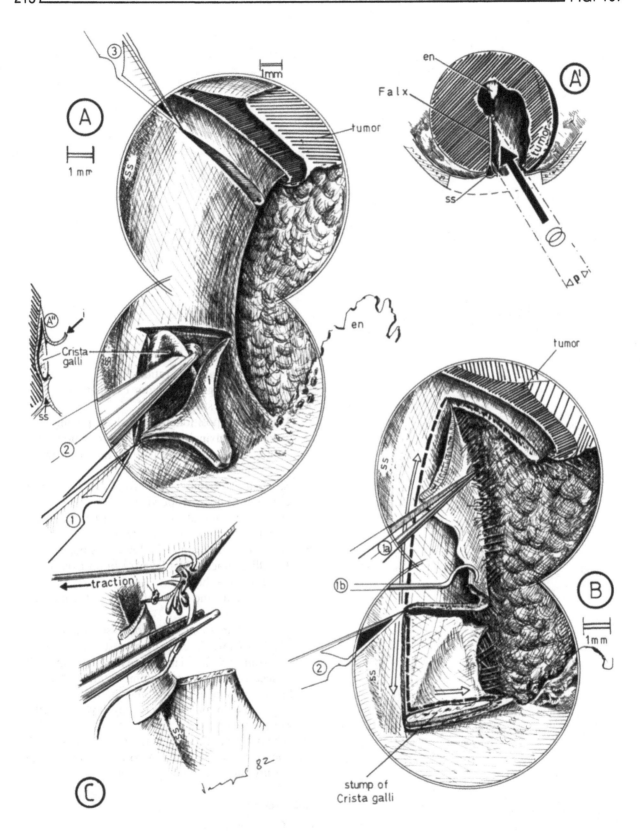

FIG. 108 ⸺⸺⸺⸺⸺⸺⸺⸺⸺⸺⸺⸺⸺⸺ 216

Fig. 108. Frontobasal operations.
Olfactorius meningioma. Tumor extirpation
A   Microsurgical site
    1 Spatula repositioned, then slight pulling
    2 Further falxincisions and falx-resections (broken line) until contralateral tumor surface is reached
A' Schematic horizontal anatomical section. Arrow: direction of microscope view
A'' Schematic sagittal anatomical section, corresponding to microsurgical site **A**
B   **1a + 1b** Further tumor hollowing as before
    2 Pulling arachnoidal layer of brain from tumor arachnoidal layer
    3 Resection line (broken line) of superficial tumor portions
B' Schematic anatomical horizontal section for situation **B.** Arrow: direction of microsurgical view in **B**
C   Microsurgical site. Tumor greatly diminished. Its surface can also be seen contralaterally dorsally. Spatula no longer lies in tumor lumen, but rather underneath brain (protected by layer of cotton wool –*cow*–)
C' Schematic anatomical horizontal section, situation corresponds to **C.** Arrow: direction of microsurgical view, corresponding to **C**

Abbreviation:

cow Cotton wool

FIG. 108

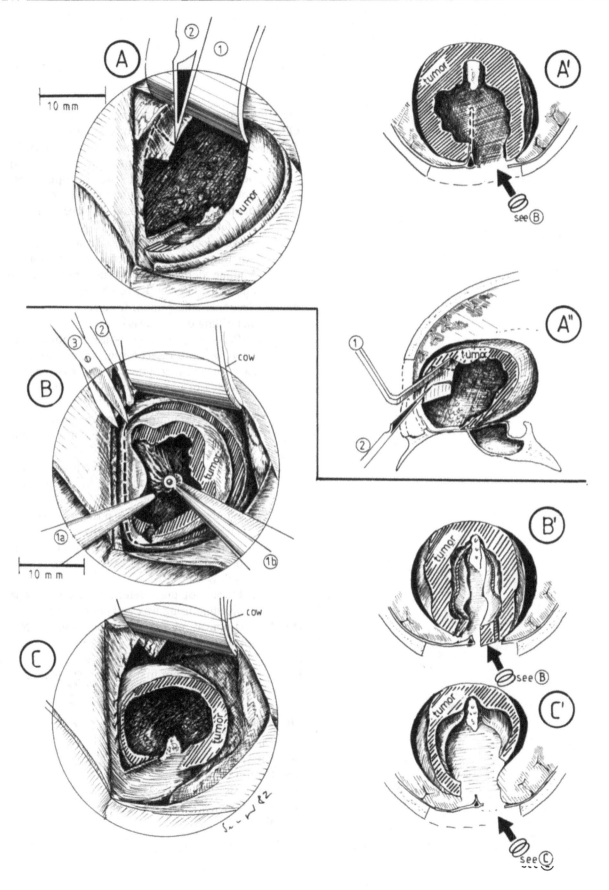

FIG. 109 ⊏━━━━━━━━━━━━━━━━━━━━━━━━━━━━━━⊐ 218

Fig. 109. Frontobasal operations.

Olfactorius meningioma. Tumor extirpation

A	Microsurgical site. Tumor removed exept for a bowl-shaped remnant deep basally. Until now, Aa. carotis intt. and Nn. optici were not yet visible. Over tumor one can see, in the depth of Fissura mediana, Aa. cerebri antt. and left A. frontopolaris
A'	Anatomical horizontal section sketch for **A**
A''	Anatomical sagittal section sketch for **A**. Midline defined first by falx remnant and enostosis, later by A. cerebri ant.
B	Sectional enlargement from **A**
	1a Drilling of enostosis –en–
	1b Pressing of wax –wx– using cotton wool –cow– onto resection surface of enostosis
	2a + 2b Pushing tumor away from arachnoidea of Cisterna optica –co–, from N.II and from Chiasma –ch–
C	**1a + 1b** Scraping off tumor remnants in the area of Tuberculum sellae and Planum sphenoidale
	2 Cautions coagulation of bleeding points in the area of Planum sphenoidale und Tuberculum sellae
	3 Blind coagulation at posterior edge of Tuberculum sellae. Hypophyseal stalk may lie close by; danger of unnoticed opening of Sinus sphenoidalis exists if anterior Sella wall is thin
	4 In case of dura defects, control of bone bleeding using wax and cotton wool
D + E	Anatomical model of preparation in Nn. optici area
D	Marking of midline (see also **A'**)
E	Pushing off tumor first from midline area, and only then, from Nn. optici

Abbreviations:

ch	Chiasma
co	Cisterna optica (arachnoidea)
cow	Cotton wool
en	enostosis
fx	Falx remnant
wx	Wax

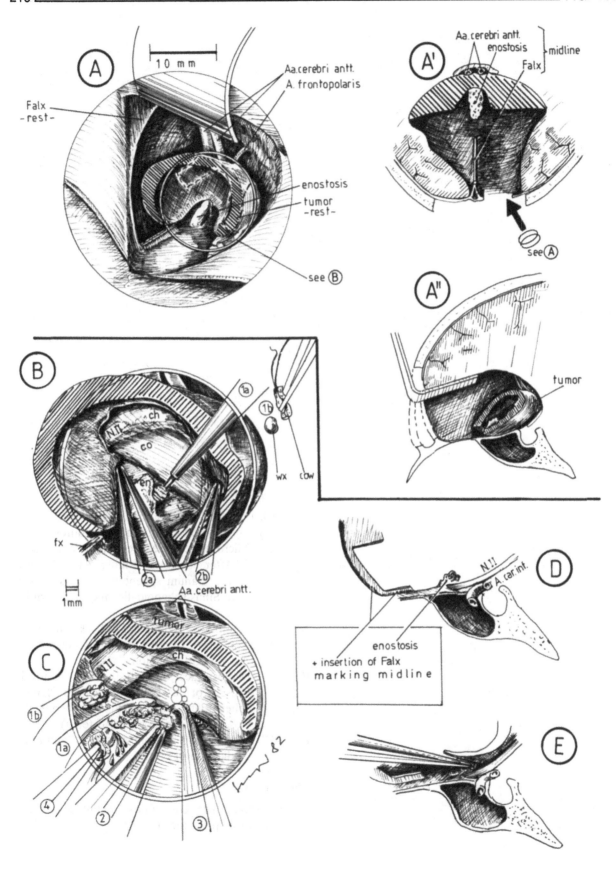

A

10 mm

Falx -rest-

Aa.cerebri antt.
A. frontopolaris

enostosis

tumor -rest-

see Ⓑ

A'

Aa.cerebri antt.
enostosis
Falx
} midline

see Ⓐ

A''

tumor

B

ch
N.II
co
①a
①b
wx   cow
en
fx
②a   ②b
Aa.cerebri antt.
1mm

C

tumor
ch
N.II
①b
①a
④
②
③

D

N.II
A. car. inf.

enostosis
+ insertion of Falx
marking midline

E

FIG. 110 ⬛══════════════════════════════════════⬛ 220

Fig. 110. Frontobasal operations.
Olfactorius meningioma. Grafting procedures

A	Microsurgical site after tumor removal
	1 After enostosis, drilling defect of dura and Planum sphenoidale exists. Injury to Sinus sphenoidalis mucosa cannot be seen
A'	Anatomical topographical sketch (view from above), of microsurgical site **A**
A''	As **A,** sagittal section
B	Microsurgical site after tumor removal. Closure of dura and bone gap in Planum sphenoidale (roof of Sinus sphenoidalis closed by stitching on periosteum)
B' + B''	Enlarged detail from **A''** before and after application of graft

Abbreviations:

co Cisterna optica, covered by arachnoidea
(en) Enostosis (projection)

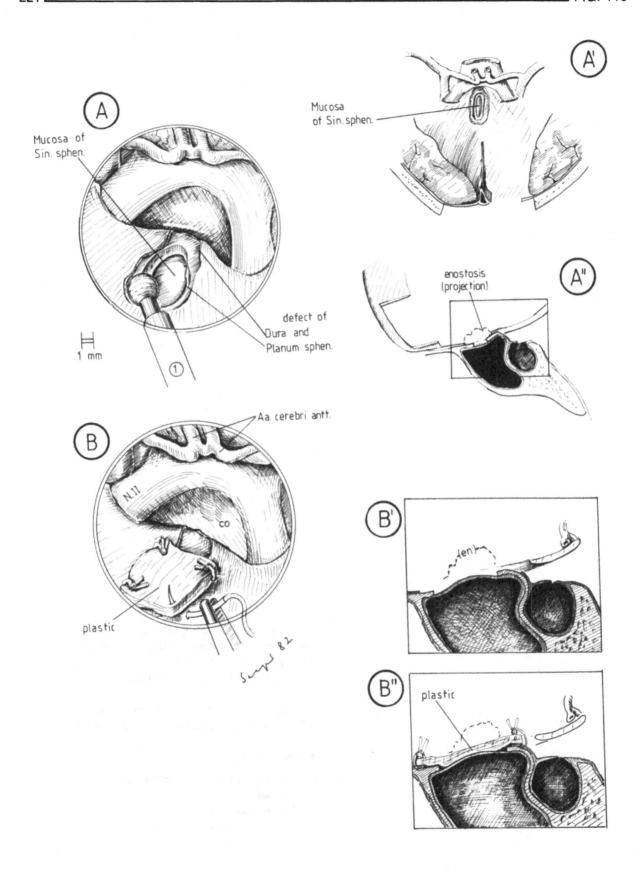

A

Mucosa of Sin. sphen.

1 mm

①

defect of Dura and Planum sphen.

A'

Mucosa of Sin.sphen.

A"

enostosis (projection)

B

Aa. cerebri antt.

N.II

co

plastic

B'

dent

B"

plastic

FIG. 111 ⌐━━━⌐ 222

Fig. 111. Frontobasal operations.
Olfactorius meningioma. Grafting procedures
A Graft closure of dura
A' Anatomical section sketch for **A**
B Dura closed
B' Anatomical horizontal section sketch for **B**
B'' Anatomical sagittal section sketch for **B**

Abbreviations:

a Dura graft (galea or periosteum)
b Medial dura flap
c Latero-basal dura flap
d Dura of convexity

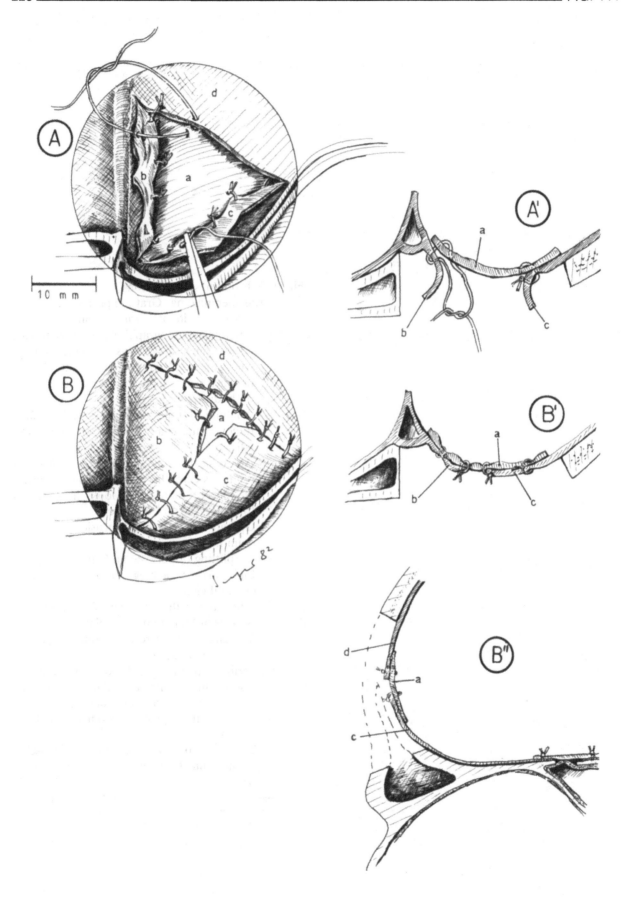

FIG. 112 224

Fig. 112. Frontobasal operations.
Olfactorius meningioma. Grafting procedures

A   Operation site after dura closure

B   Anatomical topographical sketch, view from above, mucosa portions of Sinus frontalis still preserved. Light arrows: epidural cleft, in which periosteum graft is placed later on, on both sides

C   Anatomical topographical sketch. **1, 2, 3** removing mucosa remnants from Sinus frontalis

C'   Anatomical topographical sketch. Mucosa remnants carefully removed from all niches of Sinus frontalis. One looks into Ductus fronto-nasalis on both sides

D   Operation site. Median incision of periosteum flap
      1 Splitting of periosteum flap.
      Light arrow: tucking periosteal flap into epidural cleft *

E – E" Schematic anatomical sagittal sketches

E   A piece of M. temporalis is placed into Sinus frontalis. Light arrow: tucking of periosteum into epidural cleft

E'   Periosteum is fastened to dura by suture

E"   Tissue glue ** injected from beneath into periosteum layer and musculature
      1 Injection of tissue glue from lateral direction
      2 Pressing of periosteum flap and muscles into Sinus frontalis

---

* This method is not applicable in frontalbasal fractures (see appropriate chapter).
** Fibrinogen concentrate, Immuno.

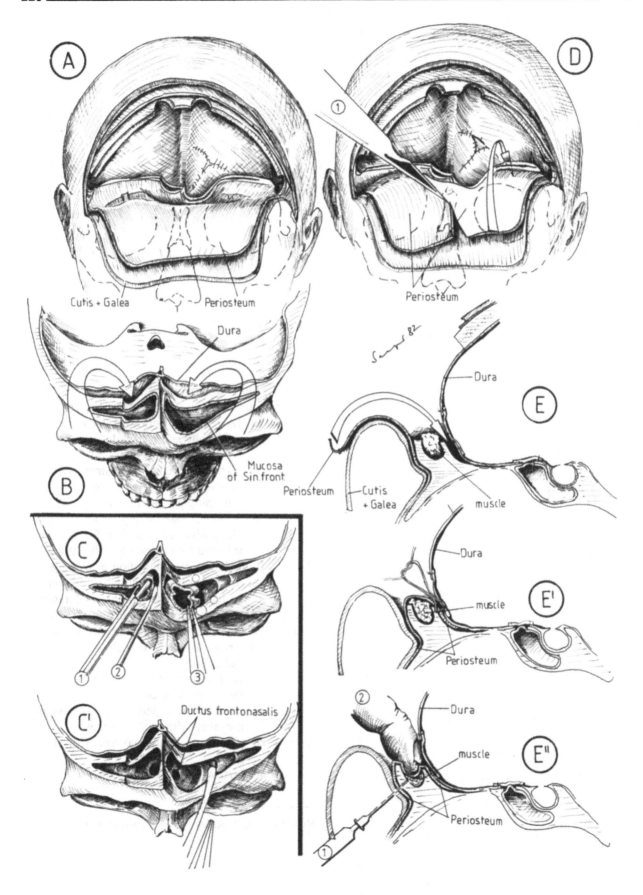

A

Cutis + Galea — Periosteum

Dura

Mucosa
of Sin. front.

B

C

① ② ③

C'

Ductus frontonasalis

D

Periosteum

Sanpe 82

Dura

Periosteum — Cutis
+ Galea

muscle

E

Dura

muscle

Periosteum

E'

②

Dura

muscle

Periosteum

①

E''

FIG. 113 226

Fig. 113. Frontobasal operations.
Olfactorius meningioma. Grafting procedures

A **1a** (Arrow): left periosteal flap positioned epidurally and fastened (see preceding figure)

   1b (Arrow): right periosteal flap is positioned in the same way

A' **2** Fastening periosteal flap to dura

   3a + 3b Periosteum flap, as well as muscle, positioned into Sinus frontalis, are injected from beneath with fibrin glue

A" Immediately after injection of tissue glue, periosteum graft, and muscle positioned in Sinus frontalis, are firmly compressed. Graft forms a depression in Sinus frontalis.

B – B" Periosteum graft can be fastened to lateral bone edge at base with nails*

C Wound closure

   1 Reinsertion of bone flap, then attached by sutures

   2a Burr holes, especially above nasion, are filled with bone shavings

   2b Gluing of bone shavings with fibrin glue

   3 (arrow) placing of drain, suture of Galea and skin

---

* Method of Prof. T. Riechert, author's predecessor.

FIG. 113

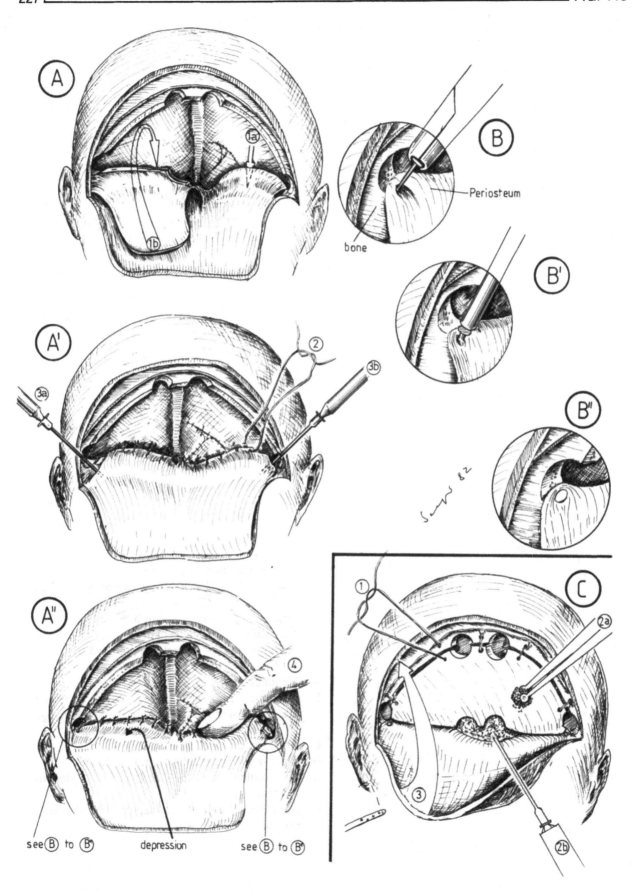

Periosteum

bone

see Ⓑ to Ⓑ"   depression   see Ⓑ to Ⓑ"

FIG. 114 ⊏══════════════════════════════════════⊐ 228

Fig. 114. Frontobasal operations.
Olfactorius meningioma. Grafting procedures
Appendix to Fig. 113: Riechert's technique of bone nailing

A   Nail holder, overview, with hammer
A' Nail holder with nail, greatly enlarged
      Arrows: grooves for holding nailhead
A" Nail
B   Hammer
C   Instrument for deeper nailing. Nail is partly hammered in using holder **A,** then holder is changed for instrument **C** to enable firm nailing
C' Enlarged detail of **C**
D   Thick-walled corticalis cannot be nailed
D' Thin-walled corticalis should not be nailed too forcefully
E   Nailing is possible in strong spongiosa, whether or not thin compacta is present

FIG. 114

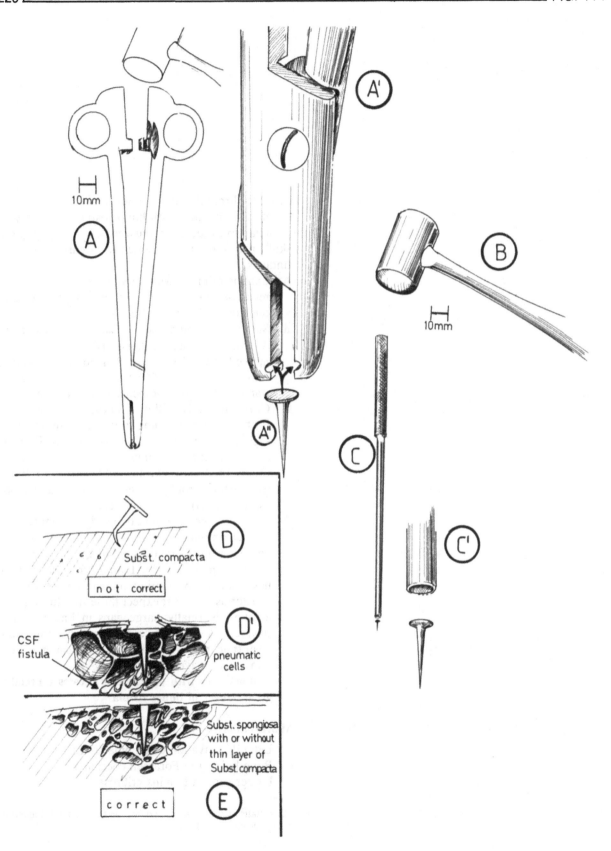

A

10mm

A'

B

10mm

A''

C

C'

D

Subst. compacta

not correct

D'

CSF
fistula

pneumatic
cells

Subst. spongiosa
with or without
thin layer of
Subst. compacta

correct

E

FIG. 115 ⊏══════════════════════════⊐ 230

Fig. 115. Frontobasal operations.

Frontobasal fracture with liquor fistula. Anatomy of Lamina cribrosa, four enlargements, details from skull preparations*, frequently occurring normal findings

A Lamina cribrosa with varying excavations, Foramen coecum not exactly in mid-line, but lying to the side of Sulcus sagittalis

B Similar asymmetry –x– of Lamina cribrosa as in **A**. Foramen coecum unusually voluminous with marked bony edges –y– circling Foramen coecum, contrary to **A** where foramen edges diverge frontwards in two bony branches from Crista galli

C Crista frontalis without Sulcus sagittalis sup.. Probably corresponding to lack of anterior Sinus sagittalis sup. portion (according to Kaplan, atresia of anterior Sinus sagittalis sup. portion occurs in 7% of normal individuals). In skulls with senile atrophy larger gaps are found especially in anterior Lamina cribrosa area –z–

D Small Foramen coecum, bone edge structures –y– neither ring-like as in **B,** nor surrounded by two diverging bony branches as in **A** and **C.** Behind foramen, most anterior Lamina cribrosa portion lies quite deep. During preparation of Bulbus olfactorius one must expect these structural irregularities. Normally, large gaps in Lamina cribrosa (z in **A** + **C**) are covered only by a thin dura layer (and in the area of Meatus nasi superior by a thin mucosa layer).
Contact here with instruments creates especially great danger of liquor fistula

Abbreviations:

x Lateral excavation of Lamina cribrosa
y Bone bulging in Foramen coecum area
z Larger gaps in Lamina cribrosa

---

* Schematic presentations of variants can be found in J. Lang (in: Lanz – Wachsmuth, 1979).

FIG. 115

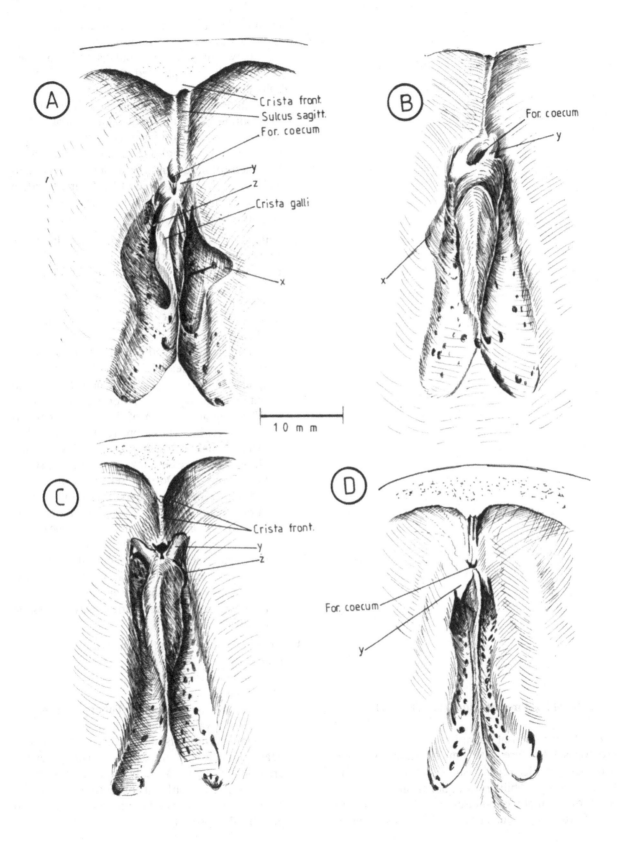

Crista front.
Sulcus sagitt.
For. coecum
y
z
Crista galli
x

For. coecum
y
x

10 mm

Crista front.
y
z

For. coecum
y

FIG. 116 ⌐━━━┐232

ethmoidales remains nearly constant, Sinus frontales vary greatly. Anatomical topographical relation between Sinus sphenoidalis and skull base can be quite complicated. In rare cases, Sinus sphenoidalis is missing. Most often it is located beneath Planum sphenoidale and Sella; it may incorporate Dorsum sellae and Clivus. Frequently Processus clinoidei antt. are also pneumatized (see also Pneumosinus dilatans). Foramen rotundum may lie in Sinus sphenoidalis wall. Then the medial wall of Foramen rotundum protrudes into Sinus sphenoidalis (see chapter on Hypophysis)

A' Enlarged detail from **A'**, bone relief drawn in. Localization of liquor fistula
- **a** Lamina cribrosa, most frequent localization for liquor fistula
- **a'** Planum sphenoidale
- **b** Tuberculum sellae, liquor fistula difficult to identify (see **B**)
- **c** Drilling roof and medial wall of Canalis opticus may easily lead to opening of Sinus sphenoidalis (i. e. as in operations for A. ophthalmica aneurysms or N. opticus tumors)
- **d** When pneumatization of Processus clinoideus ant. is present, operations for Os sphenoidale meningiomas, A. ophthalmica aneurysms, and N. opticus processes may lead to liquor fistulae
- **e** Operations for Dorsum sellae meningiomas, radical transcranial hypophysectomy, with dura extirpation as far as sella entrance, may lead to liquor fistulas, since the typical vascularization may also require extensive electrocoagulation on the Dorsum sellae
- **a + b** Are common localizations of liquor fistulas following skullbrain trauma
- **c to e** Are less frequent and easily accessible through surgery

B Traumatic liquor fistula, schematic sagittal section
- **a** Lamina cribrosa
- **a'** Planum sphenoidale
- **b** Anterior sella wall below Tuberculum sellae
- **f** Posterior wall of Sinus frontalis

Traumatic liquor fistulae occur predominantly near midline; they are easily recognized in the area of **a + a'**. By a direct view of areas **b + f** these fistulae are difficult to see (but they can be seen by using a warmed dental mirror or curved bulb-headed probe)

Frontobasal fracture with liquorhea (Figs. 116 to 134)

Fig. 116. Frontobasal operations.
Frontobasal fracture with liquor fistula. Anatomy. Schematic projection of sinuses onto skull base. Localization possibilities of liquor fistulas
A Projection of nasal sinuses onto skull base in cases of extensive pneumatization. Location of Cellulae

FIG. 116

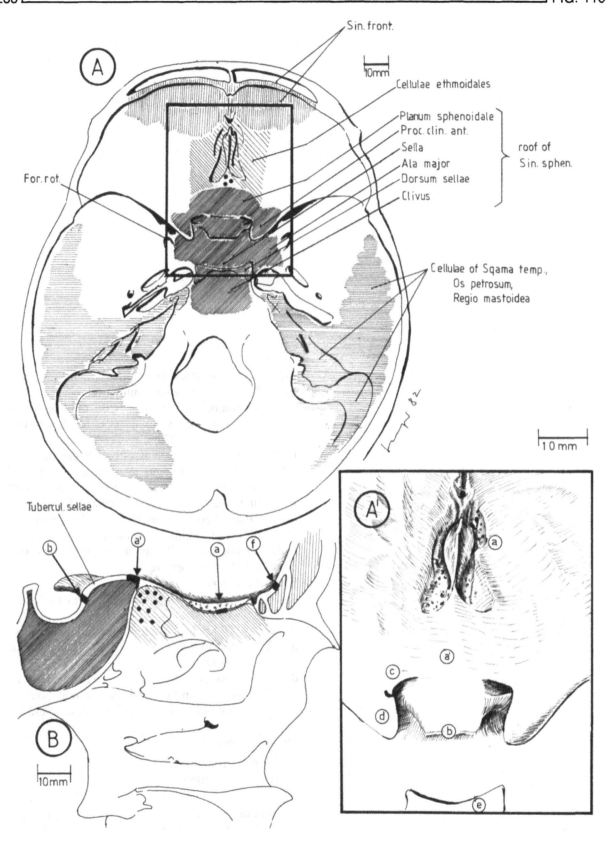

Sin. front.

Cellulae ethmoidales

Planum sphenoidale
Proc. clin. ant.
Sella
Ala major
Dorsum sellae
Clivus

roof of
Sin. sphen.

For. rot.

Cellulae of Sqama temp.,
Os petrosum,
Regio mastoidea

10mm

10 mm

A

Tubercul. sellae

b   a'   a   f

B

10mm

A'

a

a'

c

d   b

e

FIG. 117 ⸤══⸣ 234

Fig. 117. Frontobasal operations.

Frontobasal fracture with liquor fistula

Clinical example of a patient with multiple fronto-basal fractures. Full consciousness for four weeks prior to operation. Then 2 days comatose; after tracheotomy quick regaining of consciousness in outside hospital. Referred to us completely oriented. Bilateral anosmia, decreasing visual acuity on right side, otherwise no neurological findings. Craniotomy, immediately thereafter enucleation of injured right eye ball*. No additional postoperative findings. Quick recuperation. Preoperative psychosyndrome disappeared within few weeks

Clinical findings

A – C   X-ray-studies show multiple fracture zones –x–

D – E   CT findings: multiple fracture zones –x–

A' – B' Postoperative x-ray: bone fragments removed

D'   Postoperative CT: fracture fragment removed; intracranial air accumulation –y– typical finding immediately after operation

Abbreviations:

x   Multiple fracture zone
y   Air accumulation

---

* Enucleation performed by Prof. Dr. H. Wietschel, Universitäts-Augenklinik Freiburg (Director: Prof. Dr. G. Mackensen).

FIG. 117

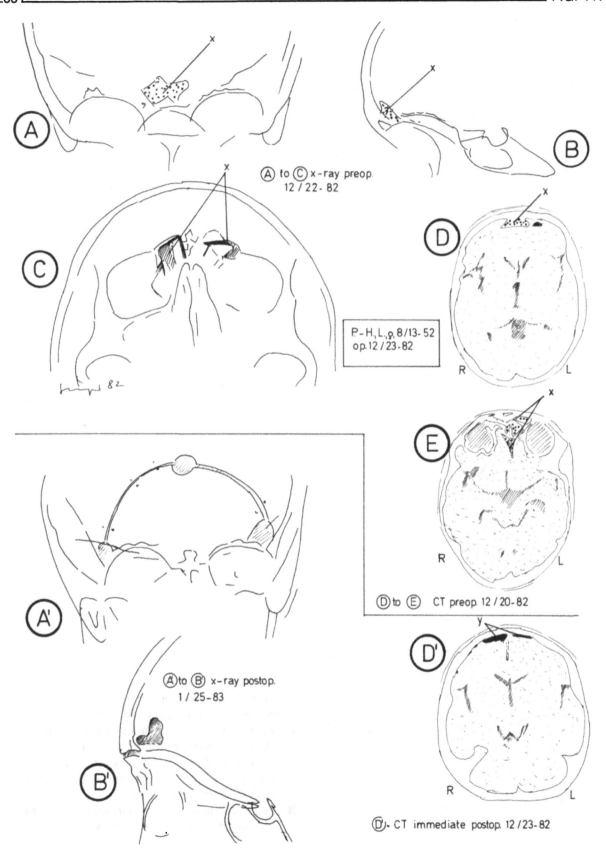

Ⓐ to Ⓒ x-ray preop.
12 / 22 - 82

P - H., L., ♀, 8/13 - 52
op. 12 / 23 - 82

Ⓓ to Ⓔ   CT preop. 12 / 20 - 82

Ⓐ to Ⓑ' x-ray postop.
1 / 25 - 83

Ⓓ'- CT immediate postop. 12 / 23 - 82

FIG. 118 ⊏━━━━━━━━━━━━━━━━━━━━━━━━━⊐ 236

Fig. 118. Frontobasal operations.
Frontobasal fracture with liquor fistula
Anatomical model presentation of clinical case
A   Arrow *1:* Impression fracture of medial portions
    of Squama frontalis and Sinus frontalis
    Arrow *2:* Impression fracture of Os sphenoidale
    with dislocation into skull
B   Arrows as in **A.** Note compression of Falx and of
    anterior portion of Sinus sagittalis sup.

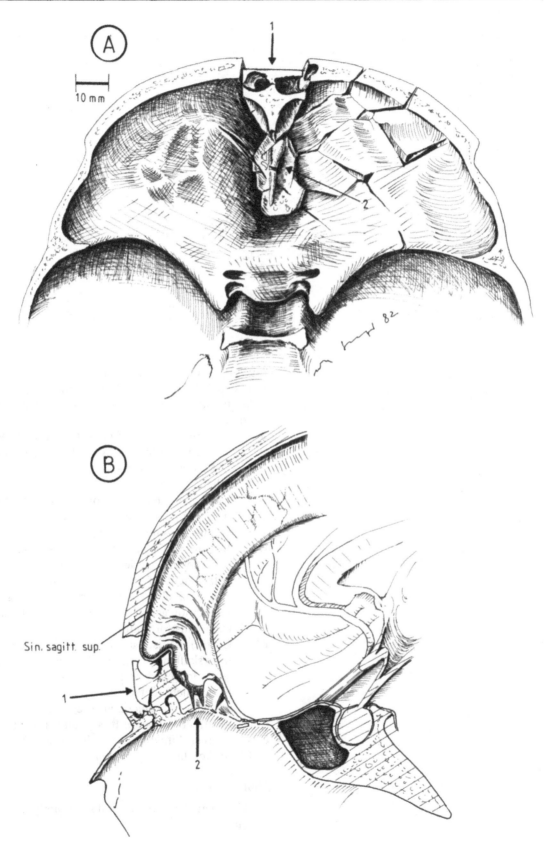

Sin. sagitt. sup.

FIG. 119 ⊏══════════════════════════════════⊐ 238

Fig. 119. Frontobasal operations.

Frontobasal fracture with liquor fistula

Incision and preparation of skin and periosteum. Possible mistakes

A Incorrect incision: frontal branch of N.VII is severed, causing paralysis of anterior portions of M. epicranius –m– (formerly called M. frontalis)

A' Correct incision just before ear. Frontal branch of N.VII preserved, Frontal portion of M. epicranius –m– not paretic

B Incorrect. Galea and cutis detached from periosteum, periosteum left bone. Thus detachment of periosteum from bone is no longer possible without demage to periosteum. In addition galea has been incorrectly detached from cutis for grafting

B' Correct. Cutis, galea and periosteum detached from skull in one piece. As second step, periosteum loosened from galea –arrow–; thus a thickwalled defect-free periosteum-layer is available. M. epicranius preserved

C Incorrect: Situation B, sagittal transection

C' Correct: Situation B', sagittal transection

C, C' Broken line: trepanation

Abbreviation:

m M. epicranius, Pars frontalis (formerly: M. frontalis)

FIG. 119

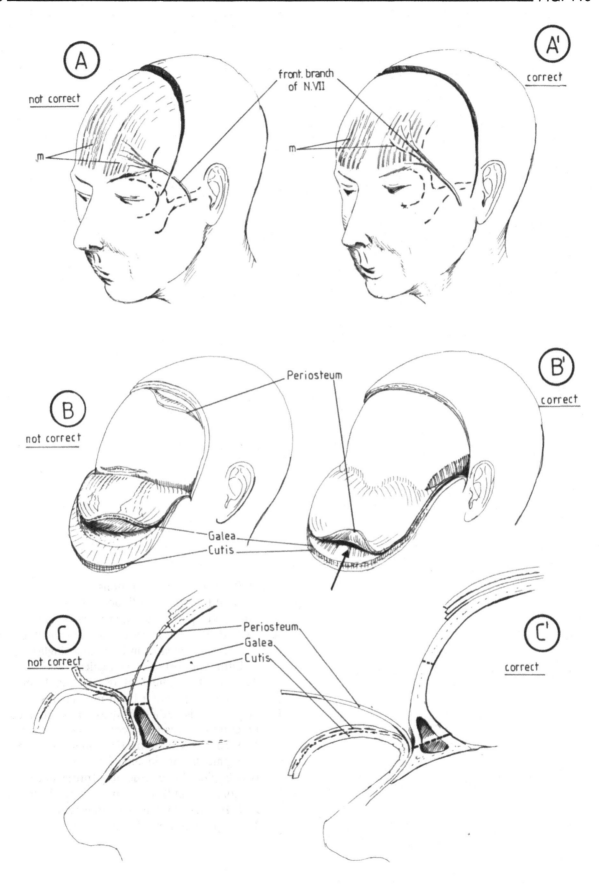

FIG. 120 ⊏━━━━━━━━━━━━━━━━━━━━━━━━━━━━⊐ 240

Fig. 120. Frontobasal operations.
Frontobasal fracture with liquor fistula
Preparation of periosteum and fracture zone

A **1a + 1b** Pushing away periosteum together with
cutis and galea from bone in a **single** layer
2 Lifting periosteum from galea
3a + 3b Detachment of periosteum from galea
using sharp and/or blunt instruments

B Periosteum is pushed away as far as orbita edges.
Fracture zones can be recognized between orbitae
1a + 1b Loosening of scar adhesions between
fragments and Squama frontalis
Broken line: bone structures (projection)

C Sectional detail from **B**, microsurgical site
1a + 1b Blunt loosening of fragments
2 Sharp separation of adhesions

FIG. 120

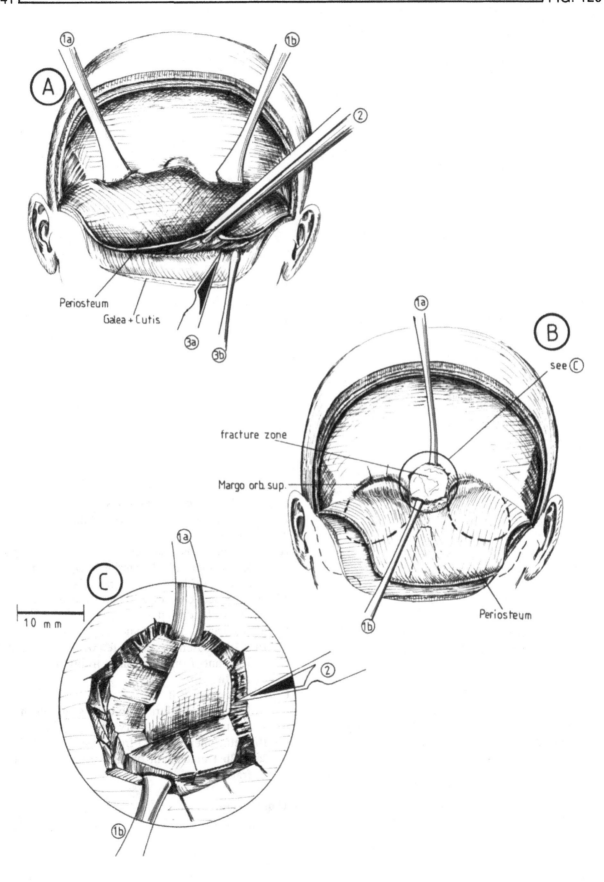

Periosteum

Galea + Cutis

Margo orb. sup.

fracture zone

see C

Periosteum

10 mm

FIG. 121 ⊏──────────────────────────────────────┐ 242

Fig. 121. Frontobasal operations.

Frontobasal fracture with liquor fistula

Trepanation

A Trepanation as small and as far basally as possible. Cosmetically disfiguring burr holes must be
filled with drill shavings at reimplanation

A' **2a – 2d** Sequence of drilling. Midline area is the
last to be drilled

B Microsurgical detail from **A**

  1a – 1d Loosening and removal of mucosa
remnants from right Sinus frontalis

  2a As **1a – 1d**

C Enlargement of **B**

  1a Loosening of dura from bone spur, which had
led to small dura injury –*g*–

  1b Detachment of dura from base

  2a + 2b Detachment of dura from medial bone
fragments

Abbreviation:

g Dura injury

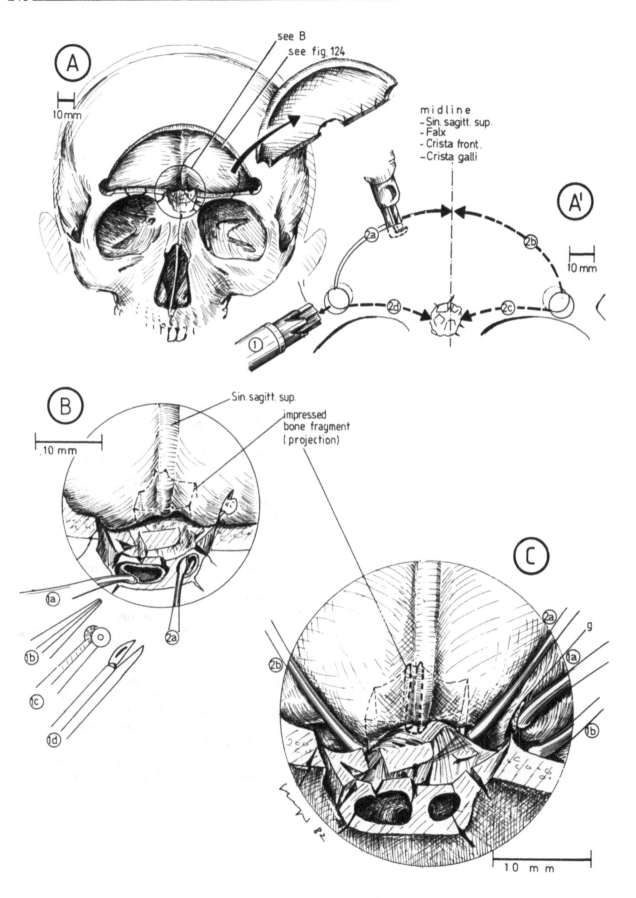

see B
see fig.124

A

10mm

midline
- Sin. sagitt. sup.
- Falx
- Crista front.
- Crista galli

A'

10 mm

1

2a

2b

2c

2d

B

Sin. sagitt. sup.

impressed
bone fragment
(projection)

10 mm

1a

2a

1b

o

1c

1d

C

2a

g

2b

1a

b

10 mm

FIG. 122 ⊏━━━━━━━━━━━━━━━━━━━━━━━━━━━━━⊐ 244

Fig. 122. Frontobasal operations.

Frontobasal fracture with liquor fistula

Closure of both Sinus frontalis remnants by muscle grafting

A Overview, operation site **B** and **F** drawn in

B Incision of fascia temporalis

C **1** Holding back fascia temporalis

    2 Holding incised Aponeurosis temporalis in place

    3 Detachment of Aponeurosis temporalis from M. temporalis

D Removal of muscle piece

D' Corresponding to varying sizes of the small Sinus frontalis remnants, muscle piece is divided in two appropriate-sized portions

E Fascia and Aponeurosis temporalis are sutured

F **1** Muscle piece, soaked with thrombin/calcium, is positioned in Sinus frontalis and squirted from below with fibrinogen concentrate*

    2 Immediately after squirting, muscle piece is pressed firmly into place

G **1** Principle of dura opening and attaching of resulting dura flaps to periosteum at the root of the nose

———————

* Immuno.

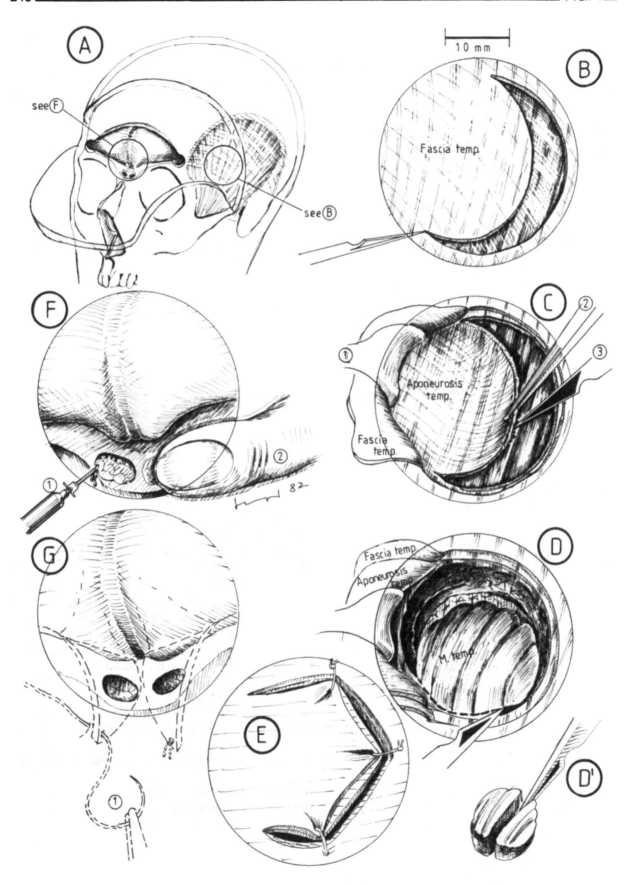

FIG. 123 ⌐━━⌐ 246

Fig. 123. Frontobasal operations.
Frontobasal fracture with liquor fistula
Dura opening and brain retraction; possible mistakes

A   Incorrect

      1 Ligature and separation of Sinus sagittalis sup. and Falx

      2a, 2b Too forceful retraction of both Lobi frontales. During reclination Sinus sagittalis sup. and cerebral veins leading thereinto are simultaneously compressed. Danger of brain edema and encephalomalacia

B   Correct. Sinus sagittalis sup. preserved. In the presence of major cerebrospinal fluid loss it is possible to eliminate use of spatulas; reclination is carried out solely by use of suction device

A' + A''   Anatomical sketch for **B**

B' + B''   Anatomical sketch for **A**

      Arrows: operative approach

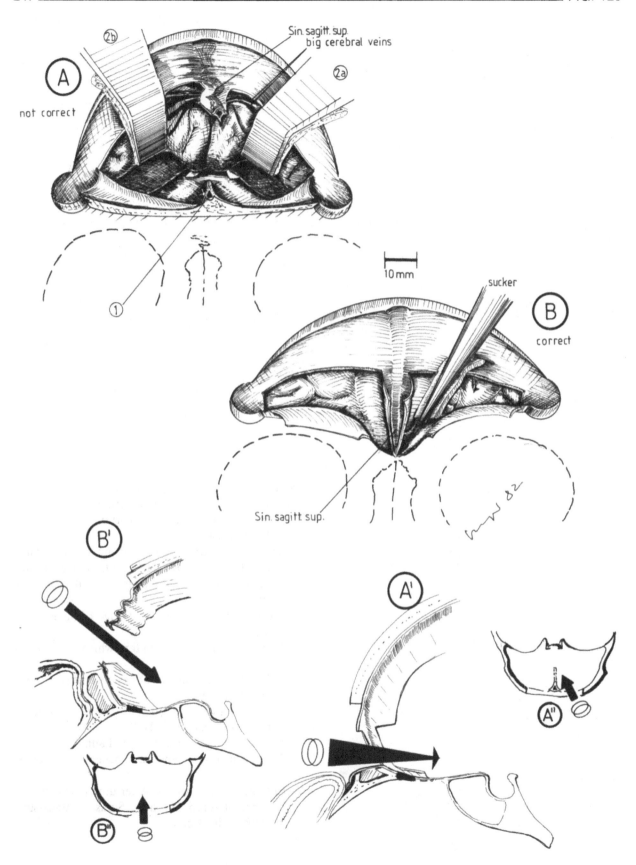

Sin. sagitt. sup.
big cerebral veins

(2b)
(2a)

(A) not correct

①

10 mm

sucker

(B) correct

Sin. sagitt. sup.

(B')

(A')

(A'')

(B'')

FIG. 124 [=================================] 248

Fig. 124. Frontobasal operations.
Frontobasal fracture with liquor fistula
Preparation between dura and cortex

A 1 Dura incision
   2a – 2c Light arrows: folding out of dura flaps.
   Shortly before reaching Sinus a lacuna was
   opened during dura incision, and closed by
   suture

A' Closure of incised lacuna at edge of Sinus sagit-
    talis sup.

B 1 Removal of bone splinters which have pene-
     trated dura
   2 Blunt detachment of adhesions between dura
     and brain surface
   3 As **2,** with forceps (this instrument preferable
     to the one shown in **2**)
   4 Sharp separation of loosened adhesions
   5 Dura incision above and beneath a cerebral
     vein

B' Enlarged detail from **B.** After dura circumcision,
    juncture of cerebral vein to Sinus sagittalis sup.
    remains undisturbed

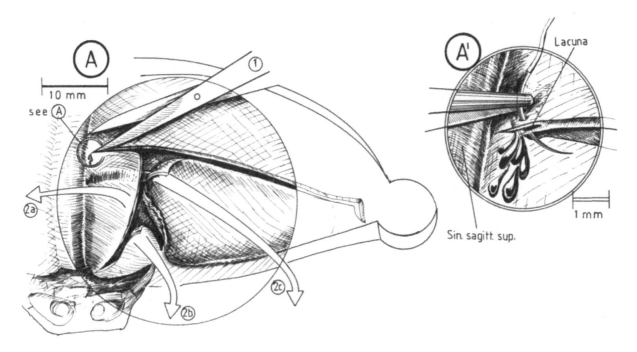

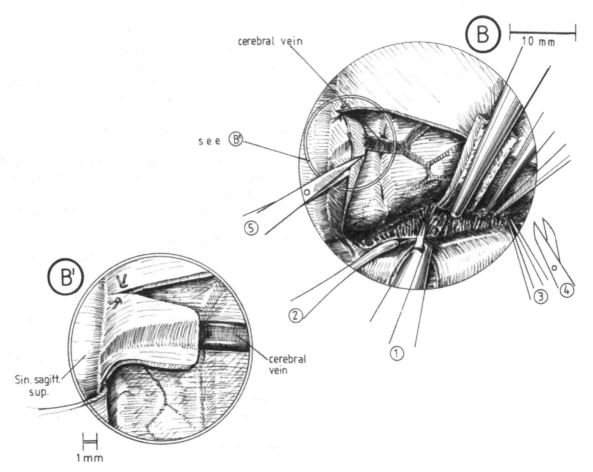

Fig. 125. Frontobasal operations.

Frontobasal fracture with liquor fistula

Removal of basal bone fragments in Sinus sphenoidalis area, particularly in the area of Crista galli and Falx

A Microsurgical site after loosening basal leptomeningeal adhesions. Baso-medial brain reclination amounts to approximately 1 cm. Spatula unnecessary after liquor outflow. Holding back of brain with sucker (with cotton wool beneath it). Nn. olfactorii on both sides are no longer identifiable

B Enlarged detail from A
   1 Reclination of medio-basal frontal brain portions
   2 Reducing impressed bone fragments, after loosening adjoining adhesions
   3a + 3b After falx incision with scalpel, falx resection follows; in case of bleeding, suturing (see clinical example of olfactorius meningioma)

C Resection of impressed bone fragments below incised falx through to the other side

C' Anatomical topographical sketch for C

Abbreviation:

ss Sinus sagittalis sup.

FIG. 125

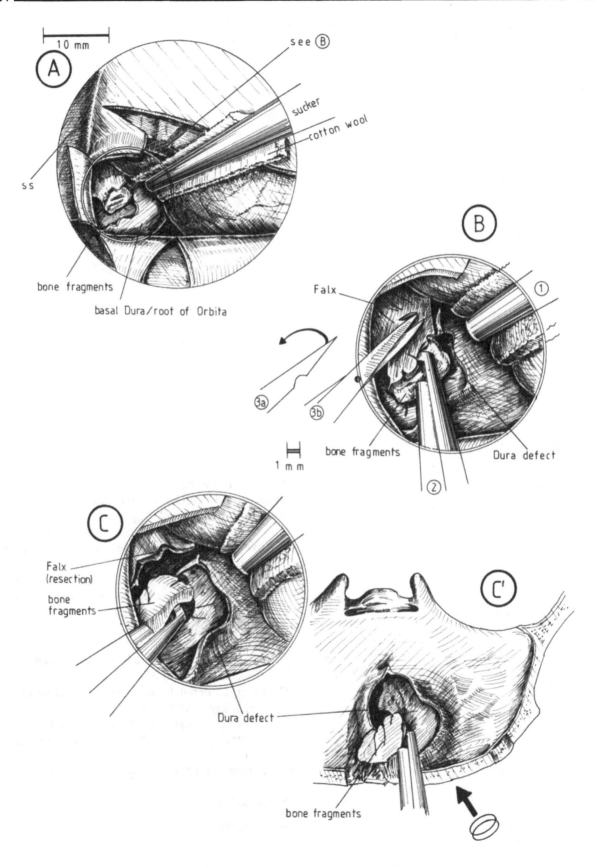

A

10 mm

see Ⓑ

sucker

cotton wool

ss

bone fragments

basal Dura/root of Orbita

Ⓑ

Falx

①

③a

③b

bone fragments

Dura defect

②

1 mm

Ⓒ

Falx
(resection)

bone
fragments

Ⓒ'

Dura defect

bone fragments

FIG. 126 ⊏━━━━━━━━━━━━━━━━━━━━━━━━━━━━━━━━━⊐ 252

Fig. 126. Frontobasal operations.

Frontobasal fracture with liquor fistula

Removal of basal bone fragments

A   Anatomical topographical sketch for **B.** Operative approach on right side. Arrow: microsurgical approach **B**

B   Although fractures are more extensive on right side than on left, only a few leptomeningeal adhesions are found on the right

    1 Dura opening on right side

    2 Pulling back of frontal brain

    3a – 3c Loosening of adhesions between Gyrus rectus and Dura of skull base

C   Enlarged detail from **B.** After loosening of leptomeningeal adhesions

    1a Sucker pushed forward (arrow), and

    1b (arrow) farther pulling back of Gyrus rectus from base

    2 Removal of bone fragments on right side

Abbreviation:

ss   Sin. sagitt. sup.

(A)

see (B)

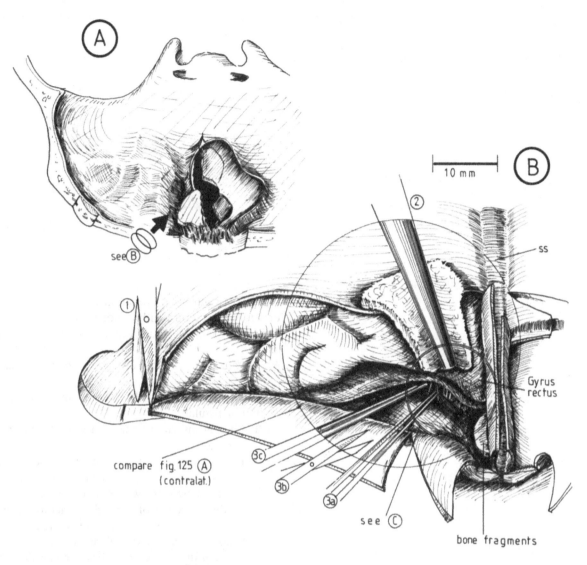

(B)

10 mm

①

②

ss

Gyrus
rectus

③c

③b

③a

compare fig.125 (A)
(contralat.)

see (C)

bone fragments

(C)

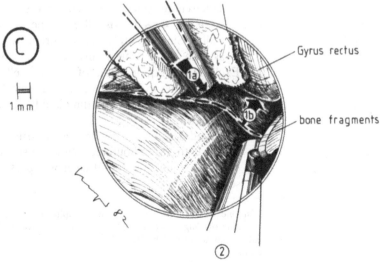

1 mm

Gyrus rectus

1a

1b

bone fragments

②

FIG. 127 ⊏▭▭▭▭▭▭▭▭▭▭▭▭▭▭▭▭▭▭▭▭⊐ 254

Fig. 127. Frontobasal operations.
Frontobasal fracture with liquor fistula
Exposure of liquor fistula and exclusion of additional fistulas

A   Localization of microsurgical approach, skull sketch

B   Microsurgical site with exposure of right medial liquor fistula

   1 Spatula insertion is necessary for frontal base overview

   2 Below torn falx, after removal of bone fragments, dura-bone gap becomes visible. Opening communicates with ethmoid cells

   3 In the presence of extensive fracturing, area between both Nn. optici is examined by bulb headed probe (or dental mirror) to ascertain whether dura cover of anterior sella wall below Tuberculum sellae is intact. **This area cannot often be directly visualized.** Since posterior wall of Sinus frontalis has been removed as far as base, good bilateral inspection is possible.

B' Exclusion of liquor fistula of anterior sella wall, corresponding to **B 3,** shown in anatomical sagittal section sketch. Site of ethmoidal liquor fistula also drawn in

B" Enlarged detail from **B'.** Because instruments lie so close to Infundibulum, there is risk of Diabetes insipidus. Arachnoid layer was preserved *
served *

---

* In one case author observed the complication of Diabetes insipidus of long duration, without additional findings. Liquor fistula was diagnosed by the above method and was closed by grafting.

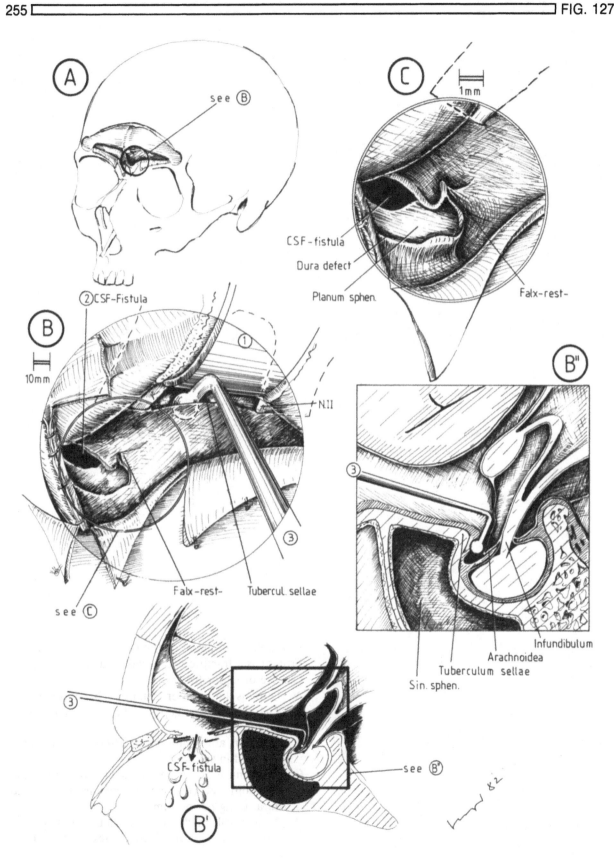

A — see Ⓑ

Ⓑ
10mm

②CSF-Fistula
①
N.II
③

see Ⓒ

Falx-rest-
Tubercul. sellae

Ⓒ
1mm

CSF-fistula
Dura defect
Planum sphen.
Falx-rest-

Ⓑ″
③
Infundibulum
Arachnoidea
Tuberculum sellae
Sin. sphen.

Ⓑ′
③
CSF-fistula
see Ⓑ′

FIG. 128 ⊏══════════════════════════════════⊐ 256

Fig. 128. Frontobasal operations.
Frontobasal fracture with liquor fistula
Closure of liquor fistula

A   Dura is loose after extensive bone fracturing. Therefore, dura gap can be made smaller by suture

B   Situation after dura suture. Small falx remnant included in suture

C   Anatomical sketch for **B.** Light arrow: principle of additional covering of incompletely closed dura, using periosteum

D   Anatomical model of periosteum graft. Light arrows: direction in which sutures are pulled

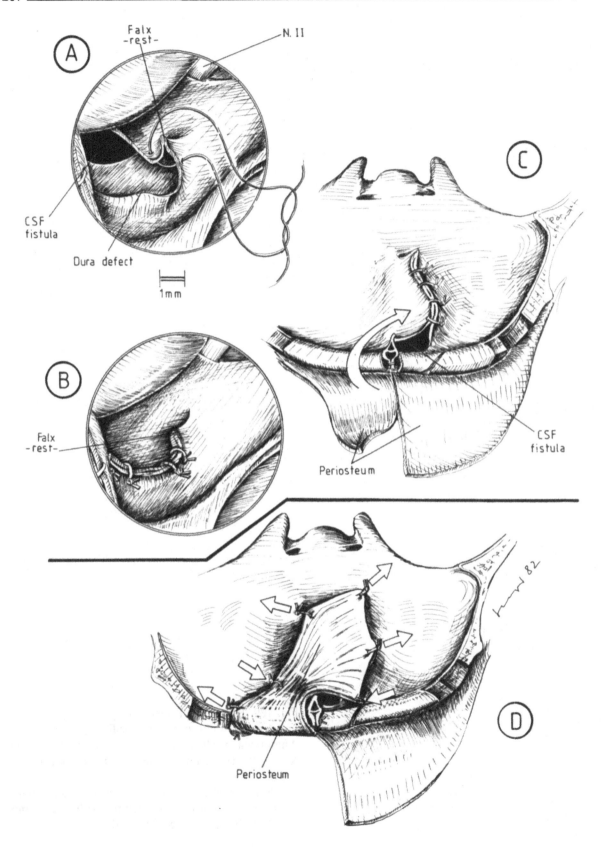

FIG. 129 ⊏══════════════════════════════════════⊐ 258

Fig. 129. Frontobasal operations.
Frontobasal fracture with liquor fistula
Anatomical model of liquor fistula closure by grafting

A   Light arrow: positioning of left periosteum flap
    onto base

B   Situation after fixation of both periosteum flaps.
    Liquor fistula is covered from both sides, Sinus
    sagittalis sup. not compressed

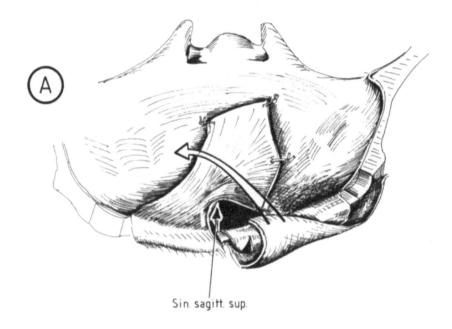

Sin. sagitt. sup.

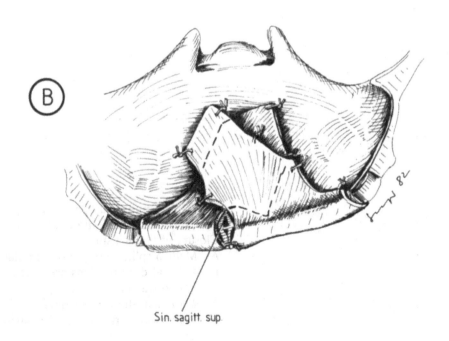

Sin. sagitt. sup.

FIG. 130 ⊏━━━━━━━━━━━━━━━━━━━━━━━━━⊐ 260

Fig. 130. Frontobasal operations.
Frontobasal fracture with liquor fistula
Closure of liquor fistula
A   Median splitting of periosteum flap
B   1 Basal dura portions are fastened by suture to
       periosteum
    2 Medial dura portions from both sides are
       joined together over Sinus sagittalis sup.

FIG. 130

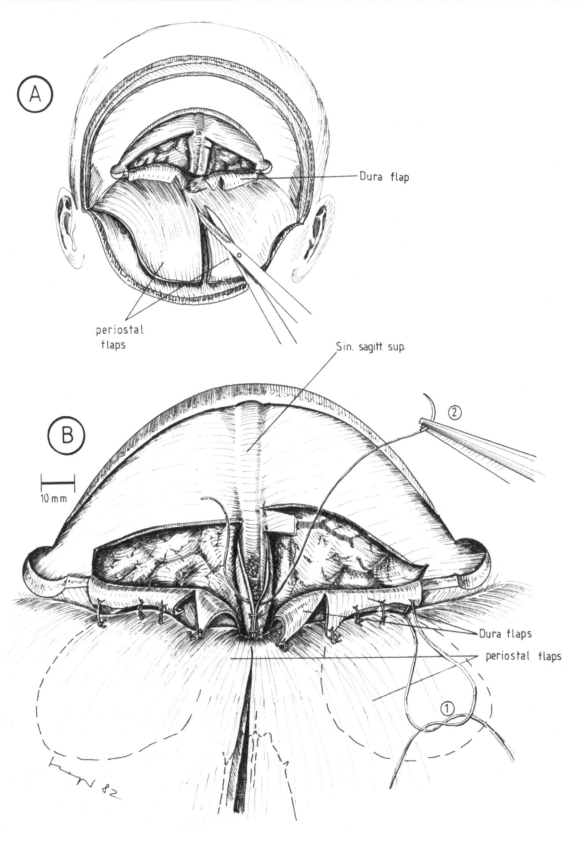

Dura flap

periostal
flaps

Sin. sagitt. sup.

②

10 mm

Dura flaps

periostal flaps

①

FIG. 131 262

Fig. 131. Frontobasal operations.
Frontobasal fracture with liquor fistula
Closure of liquor fistula

A Position sketch of microsurgical operation site **A'**
– left side –

A' Periosteum graft is pushed in from the right, then
from left microsurgical site it is fastened to base
by suture

B As **A,** contralateral – right side – approach

B' Microsurgical site, right side. Right periosteum
graft, already fastened contralaterally (see **A'**),
now is fastened to the base on the right by suture,
using moderate tension

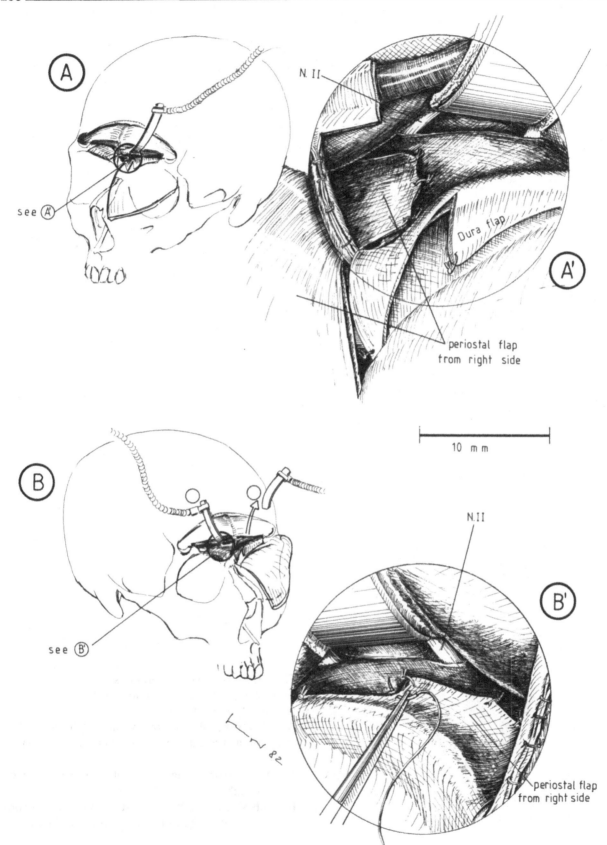

A

see Ⓐ

A'

N. II

Dura flap

periostal flap
from right side

10 mm

B

see Ⓑ'

B'

N. II

periostal flap
from right side

FIG. 132 ⸤══⸣264

Fig. 132. Frontobasal operations.
Frontobasal fracture with liquor fistula
Closure of liquor fistula

A Microsurgical site, overview sketch. Operative approach is changed once again to left side (see **A'**)

B As **A,** again changing side of operative approach – to right –

B' Left sided periosteum graft is now fastened contralaterally – right – by suture, using slight tension

FIG. 132

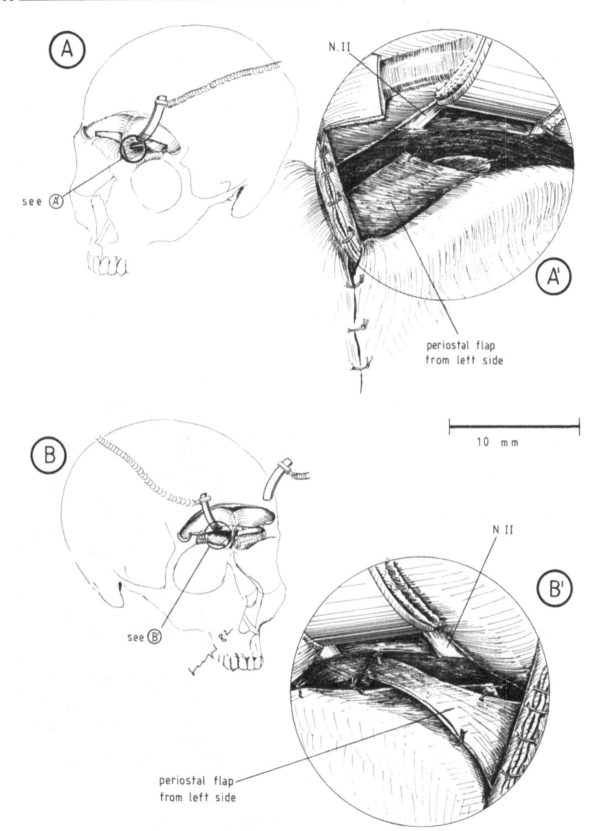

N. II

see Ⓐ'

Ⓐ'

periostal flap
from left side

10 mm

N. II

see Ⓑ

Ⓑ'

periostal flap
from left side

FIG. 133 ⊏▭▭▭▭▭▭▭▭▭▭▭▭▭▭⊐ 266

Fig. 133. Frontobasal operations.
Frontobasal fracture with liquor fistula
Closure of liquor fistula

A   Anatomical topographical sketch, after fastening of both periosteal grafts by suture. Sinus sagittalis sup. preserved. Additional securing by tissue glue *

    1a + 1b The grafts are squirted from beneath on both sides with thrombin/calcium solution and then with fibrinogen concentrate

    2 Immediately after injection of fibrin glue, grafts are pressed against skull base using sponge (in case of ample space and good overview, use of finger also possible).

    The closer the contact surfaces lie to one another and the thinner the glue film is, the more reliable is the result because a thin fibrin layer is more quickly grown through by connective tissue than a thick fibrin layer

A' + A'' Sketch of anatomical longitudinal section for A

B   Dura suture

---

* Fibrinogen concentrate Immuno.

FIG. 133

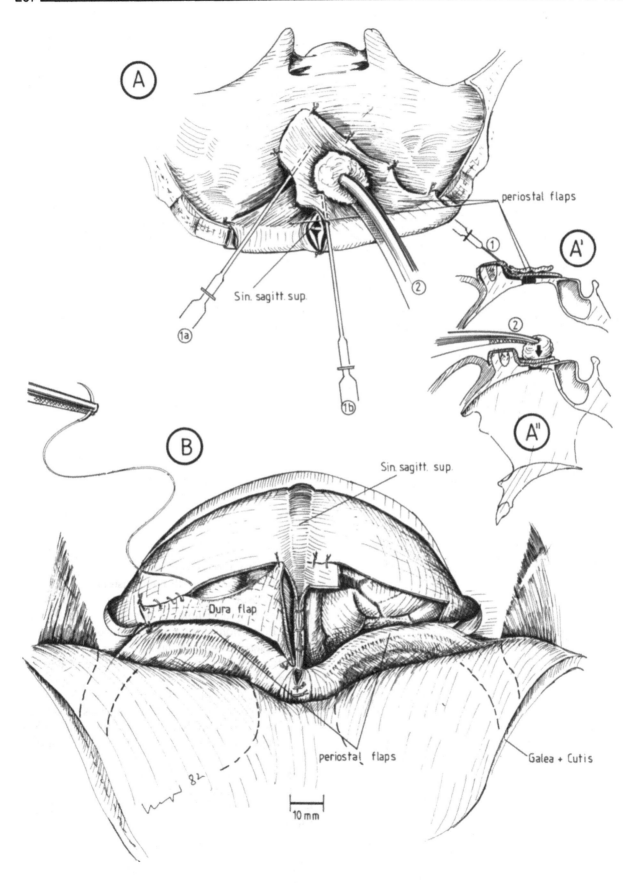

A

A'

A"

B

periostal flaps

Sin. sagitt. sup.

1a

1b

1

2

Sin. sagitt. sup.

Dura flap

periostal flaps

Galea + Cutis

82

10 mm

FIG. 134 ⊏ ⊐ 268

Fig. 134. Frontobasal operations.
Frontobasal fracture with liquor fistula
Wound closure

A **1a** Making burr holes at bone edge
    1b Protection of dura and brain from drill
    2 Insertion of bone flap
A' After creating small burr holes along edge of bone flap, follows:
    3 Fastening of bone flap by sutura
A" **4** For cosmetic reason bone shavings, preserved from operation's beginning, are put in bone gaps (and soaked with fibrinogen concentrate) *
    5 Insertion of drain
    6 Galea- and skin suture

---

* Immuno.

FIG. 134

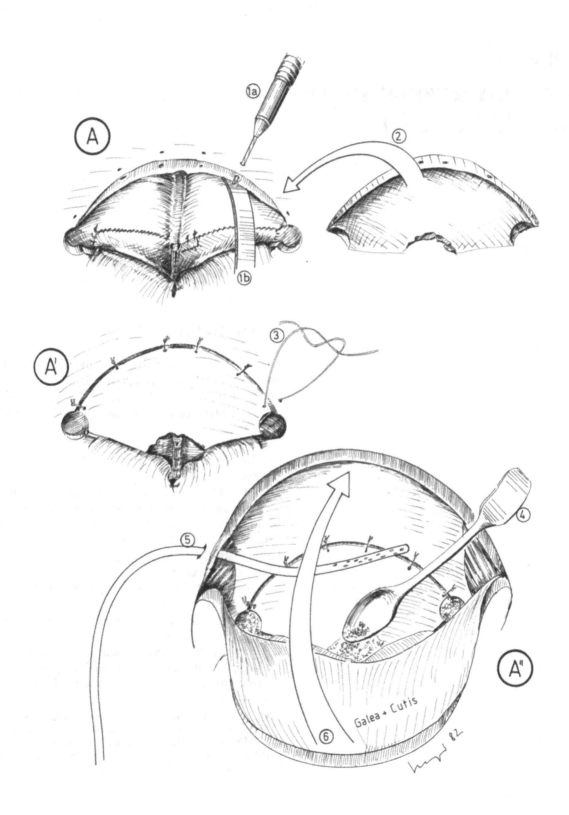

Galea + Cutis

FIG. 135 [==] 270

Chapter 4
Extra-intracranial Bypass
(Figs. 135 to 167)

"STAMCA" (Figs. 135 to 156)

Figs. 135–156. Extra-intracranial bypass supratentorial: bypass between Ramus parietalis of A. temporalis superficialis and branch of A. cerebri media (superficial temporal artery – middle cerebral artery – "STAMCA")

Fig. 135. Extra-intracranial bypass "STAMCA"
Clinical example of total occlusion of left A. carotis int. with TIA's. Additionally, stenosis of Truncus brachiocephalicus with vertebral steal syndrome. For months, progressive stenosis of right A. carotis int. also, without clinical findings*.
Postoperatively, no neurological deficits.
Diagnostic procedures
A Arrow: left sided angiogram shows occlusion of A. carotis int. at its origin
B Right A. carotis int. supplies Aa. carot. intt. areas on both sides
C X-ray confirms trepanation site. Because the Doppler sonogram** showed clearly patency of anastomosis, angiography was superfluous

---

* Operation performed by Dr. W. Hassler, author's coworker.
** Microvascular Doppler MF 20, Fa. EME medical electronic, D-7770-Überlingen, Christophstrasse 36, Federal Republic of Germany. The clinical application was developed by Dr. J. Gilsbach, author's coworker. See Fig. 113–154.

FIG. 135

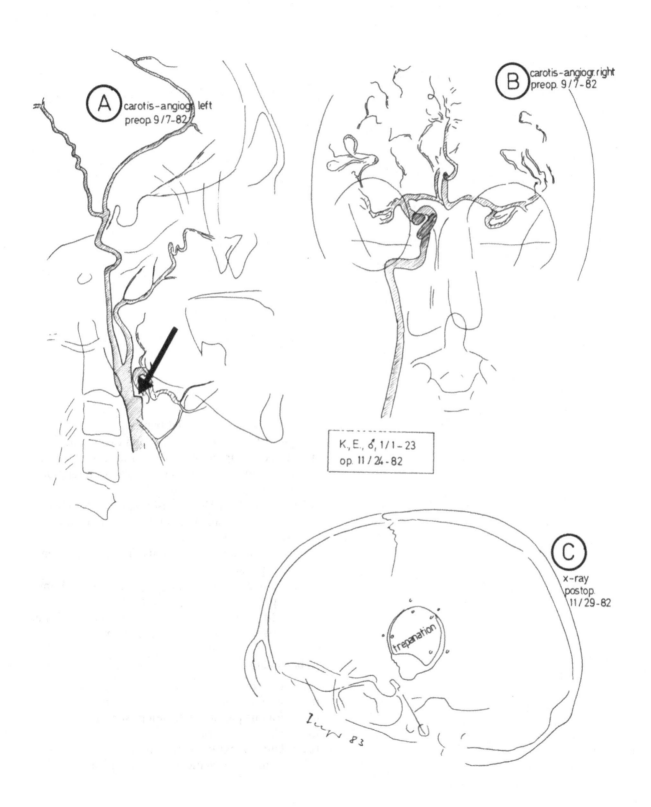

A carotis-angiogr. left preop. 9/7-82

B carotis-angiogr. right preop. 9/7-82

K., E., ♂, 1/1-23
op. 11/24-82

C x-ray postop. 11/29-82

trepanation

FIG. 136 ⊏═══⊐ 272

Fig. 136. Extra-intracranial bypass "STAMCA"

Mapping of A. temp. superfic. and Fissura lat. Sylvii

A Projection upon external skull surface of Fiss. lat. Sylvii and its anatomical topographical relation to A. temp. superfic. and its branches

B Sketch of Doppler ultrasonographic localization of A. temp. superfic. and of its branches upon external skull surface

   1a Localization of Ramus front. of A. temp. superfic.

   1b Doppler sonographic localization of Ramus pariet. of A. temp. superfic.

   1c, 1d Further localization points of Ramus pariet. using Doppler sonograph

Abbreviations:

(fl) Fissura lat. Sylvii (projection)
rf Ramus front. of A. temp. superfic.
rp Ramus pariet. of A. temp. superfic.
US Ultrasonograph
(US) Ultrasonograph (projection)
zo Ramus zygomaticus of A. temp. superfic.

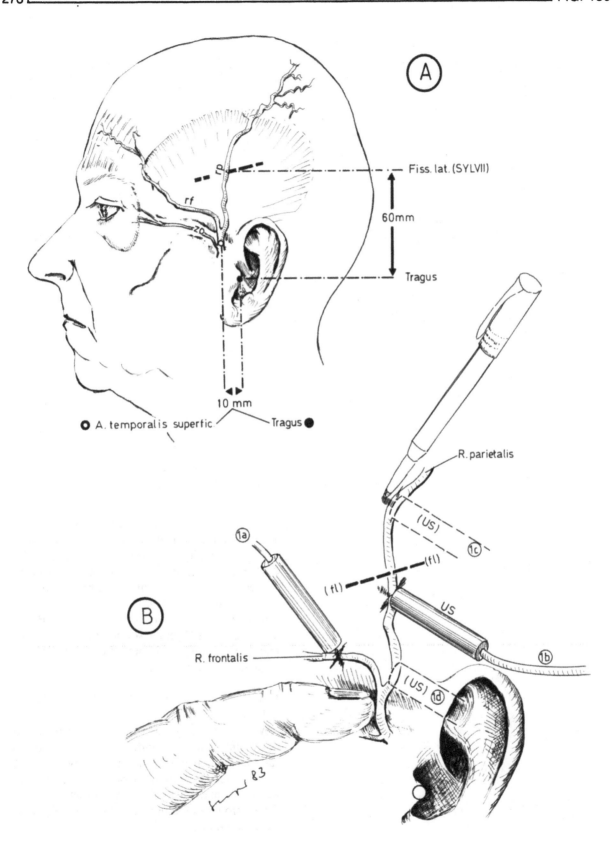

Ⓐ

Fiss. lat. (SYLVII)

60mm

Tragus

10 mm

Tragus ●

○ A. temporalis superfic.

rf

zo

Ⓑ

R. parietalis

1a

(US)

1c

(fl)

(fl)

US

1b

R. frontalis

(US)

1d

FIG. 137 274

Fig. 137. Extra-intracranial bypass "STAMCA"

A 1 Localization of main trunk of A. temp. superfic. by Doppler sonograph
   2 Path of arteries drawn upon external skull surface by felt tip pen, corresponding to Doppler sonographic markings
B Examination of Ramus front. and Ramus angularis using Doppler sonograph. Result: normal blood flow in Ramus front. and Ramus angularis-"external type"

   1 + 2 Normal direction of blood flow in Ramus front.
B' Reversed in the direction of carotis siphon, so-called "internal type"; indications of cerebro-vascular insufficiency with blood flow reversal in A. ophthalmica. Examination of Ramus front. and Ramus angularis using Doppler sonograph.
   Open arrows: blood flow direction. Black graphs: ultrasonograms

FIG. 137

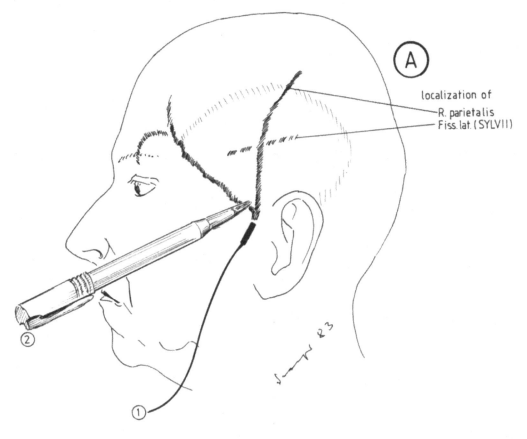

A) localization of
R. parietalis
Fiss. lat. (SYLVII)

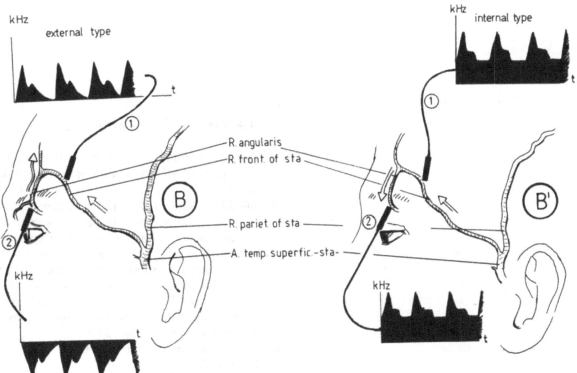

external type

kHz

internal type

kHz

R. angularis
R. front. of sta
R. pariet of sta
A. temp. superfic.-sta-

B

B'

kHz

kHz

FIG. 138 ⊏━━━━━━━━━━━━━━━━━━━━━━━━━━━⊐ 276

Fig. 138. Extra-intracranial bypass "STAMCA"
Skin incision

A Position of skin incision – approx. 100 mm long –
corresponding to Doppler ultrasonic localization of
artery

B **1a – 1d** Incision of skin and subcutaneous fatty
tissue is carried out in several consecutive
steps, whereby only skin and subcutaneous
fatty tissue, but not Galea, is incised

C **1** Detachment of subcutis from galea. One sees
that Ramus pariet. and Ramus front. of A.
temp. superfic. run partly above and partly
beneath galea, thereby contacting subcutis

2 Insertion of wound spreader

C' Anatomical section sketch for **C**

1 As in **C**

FIG. 138

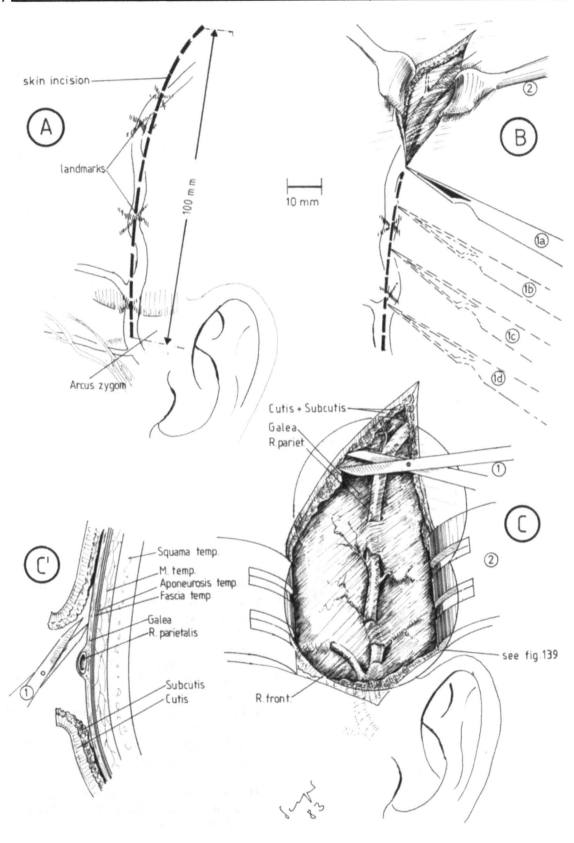

A

skin incision

landmarks

100 mm

Arcus zygom

10 mm

B

1a

1b

1c

1d

Cutis + Subcutis

Galea
R.pariet

1

C

2

see fig.139

R.front.

C'

Squama temp.
M. temp.
Aponeurosis temp.
Fascia temp

Galea
R. parietalis

Subcutis
Cutis

1

83

FIG. 139 ◻▭▭▭▭▭▭▭▭▭▭▭▭▭▭▭◻ 278

Fig. 139. Extra-intracranial bypass "STAMCA"
Preparation of Ramus par. of A. temp. superf.
A 1 Coagulation of small branches of the artery,
   but not too close to arterial trunk
   2 Cutting of coagulated small branches
   3 Incision of galea parallel to arterial path
A' Anatomical section sketch, corresponding to A,
   indications as in A
B 1 Lengthening of incision started in A 3, after
   interruption of small side branches
   2 + 3 Coagulation and interruption of small
   arteries alternating with further galea incision
   –1–
   4a + 4b Further insertion of wound spreader
B' Anatomical section sketch, corresponding to B,
   indications as in B

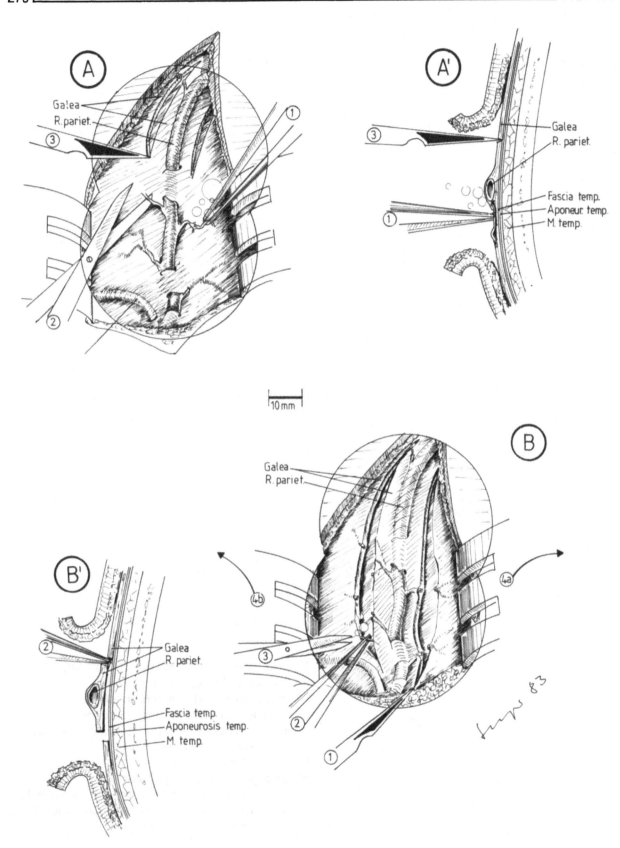

Galea
R. pariet.
③
Ⓐ
①
②

Ⓐ'
③
Galea
R. pariet.
Fascia temp.
Aponeur. temp.
M. temp.
①

10 mm

Galea
R. pariet.
Ⓑ
④b
④a
③
②
①

Ⓑ'
②
Galea
R. pariet.
Fascia temp.
Aponeurosis temp.
M. temp.

FIG. 140

Fig. 140. Extra-intracranial bypass "STAMCA"

A Incision of M. temporalis

A' Preparation of M. temporalis, anatomical model. Anterior muscle portion –x–, together with Ramus parietalis is folded forward, the muscle thus covering this artery

B Detachment of muscle

B' Spreader holds back portions of M. temporalis. Anterior muscle portions cover Ramus parietalis of A. temporalis superficialis. Broken line: Fissura lateralis –(fl)– (projection)

FIG. 140

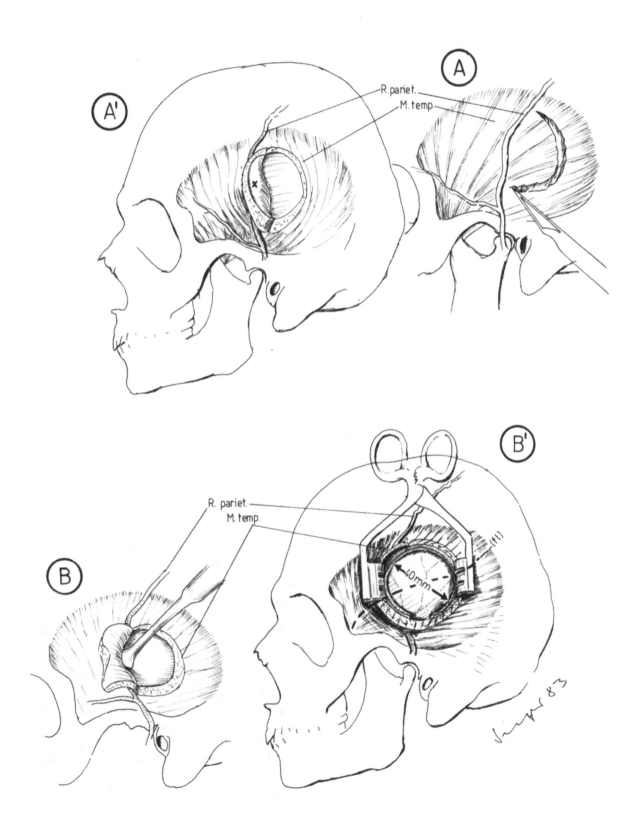

FIG. 141 ⊏━━━━━━━━━━━━━━━━━━━━━━━━━━━━━━━⊐ 282

Fig. 141. Extra-intracranial bypass "STAMCA"
Preparation of M. temporalis, microsurgical prepara-
tion
A   1a Holding back posterior M. temporalis portion
        with spatula
      1b + 1c Holding back Ramus parietalis and the
        Galea strip containing artery
      2 Curved incision of M. temporalis
      3 Detachment of muscle and periosteum from
        Squama temporalis
A' Anatomical section sketch, corresponding to A
B   1a – 1c Removal of spatula
      2a, 2b Insertion of spreader. Ramus parietalis of
        A. temporalis superficialis is protected from
        spreader by M. temporalis
B' Anatomical section sketch, corresponding B

FIG. 141

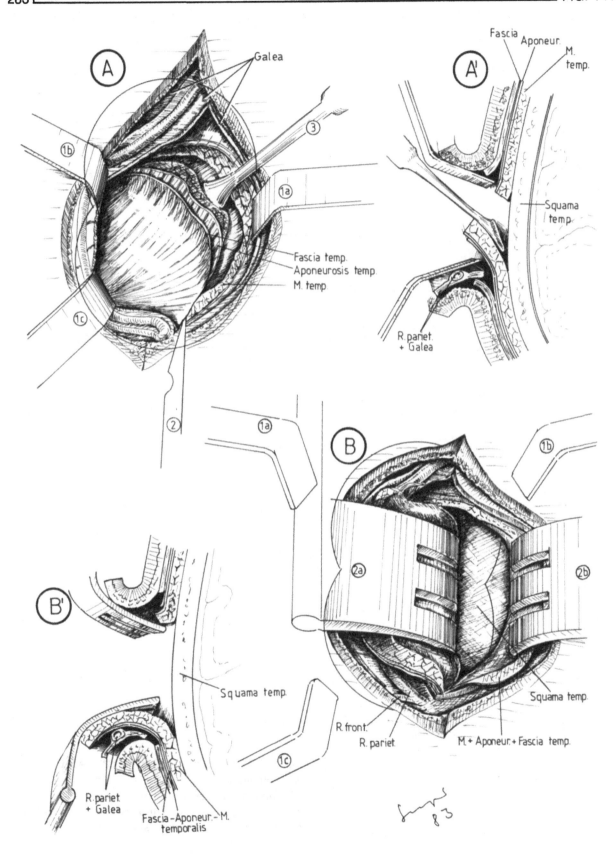

Ⓐ

Galea

③

①b

①a

①c

②

Fascia temp.
Aponeurosis temp.
M. temp.

Ⓐ'

Fascia Aponeur. M.
temp.

Squama
temp.

R. pariet.
+ Galea

①a

Ⓑ

①b

②a

②b

Ⓑ'

Squama temp.

Squama temp.

R. front.

R. pariet.

M. + Aponeur. + Fascia temp.

①c

R. pariet.
+ Galea

Fascia – Aponeur. – M.
temporalis

83

FIG. 142 ⊏━━━━━━━━━━━━━━━━━━━━━━━━━━⊐ 284

Fig. 142. Extra-intracranial bypass "STAMCA"
A   Trepanation
A' Anatomical transection sketch for A
B   Bone flap removed. Dura incision (broken line)
B' Anatomical transection sketch for B

FIG. 142

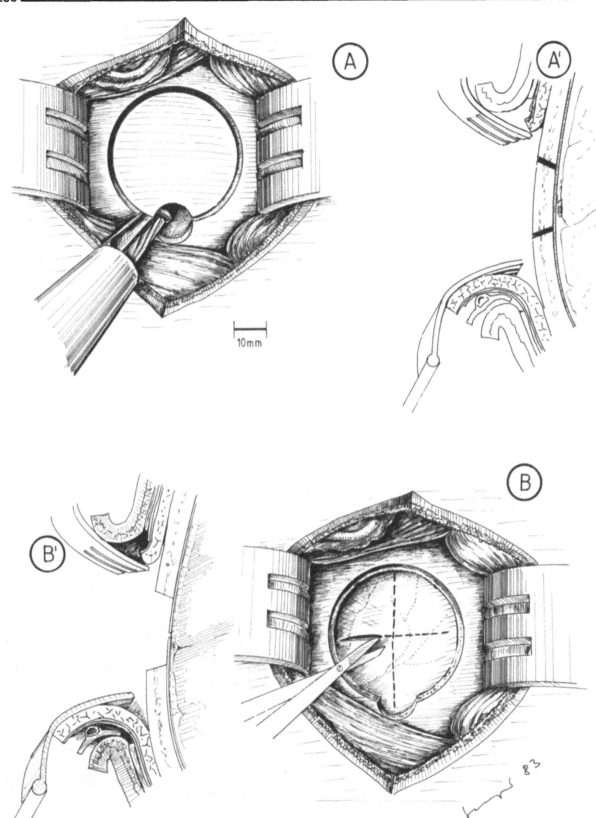

10mm

FIG. 143 ⊏━━━━━━━━━━━━━━━━━━━━━━━━━━━━⊐ 286

Fig. 143. Extra-intracranial bypass "STAMCA"
Site after dura opening
A Fissura lateralis Sylvii with temporal branch of A. cerebri media is exposed
A' Anatomical transection sketch for **A**
B Enlarged detail from **A**
   1 Doppler ultrasonographic check* of various exposed arteries, in this case, a parietal branch of A. cerebri media
   2 The same check of A. cerebri media branch shown in **A** and **A'**
   3 Having verified that temporal branch of artery has the best blood flow (which is usually the case), arachnoidea is opened over this vessel. Light arrow: flow direction verified by Doppler sonograph

* Method of Dr. J. Gilsbach, author's coworker.

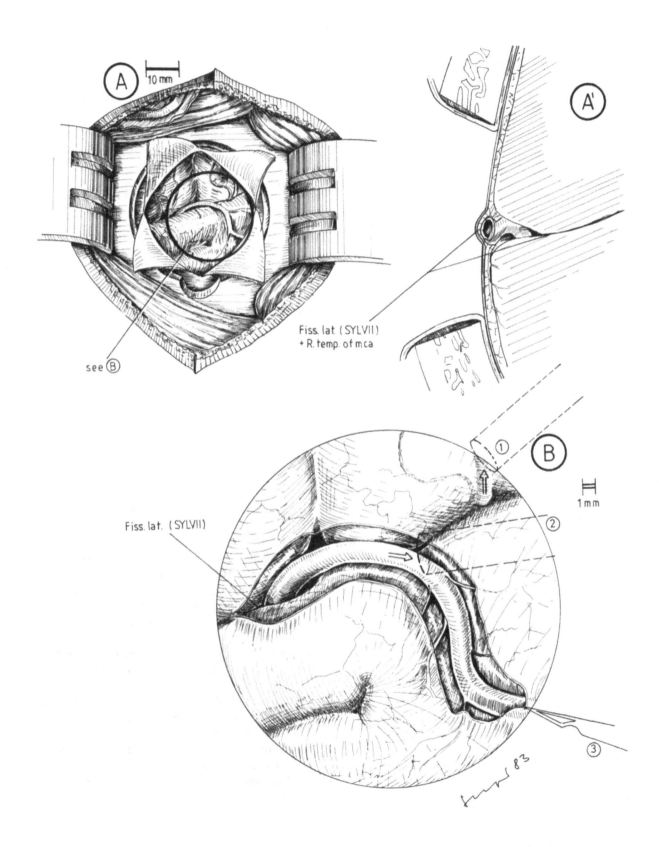

Ⓐ 10 mm

see Ⓑ

Fiss. lat (SYLVII)
+ R. temp. of m.ca

Ⓐ'

Ⓑ

1 mm

Fiss. lat. (SYLVII)

① ② ③

FIG. 144 ⊏══⊐ 288

Fig. 144. Extra-intracranial bypass "STAMCA"
Preparation of Ramus temporalis of A. cerebri media
1   Detachment of arachnoidea
2a Coagulation of smallest cerebral arterial branches
2b Cutting of these branches
3   Check by Doppler sonograph, to see whether manipulation caused spasms
A' Anatomical transection sketch for **A,** Indications as in **A**
B   **1a + 1b** Introduction of small piece of rubber foil between Ramus temporalis of A. cerebri media and cortex
    2   Check of blood flow by Doppler sonograph
        Light arrow: flow direction, verified by Doppler sonograph.
        Light arrow: flow direction, verified by Doppler sonograph
B' Anatomical transection sketch, corresponding to **B**

FIG. 144

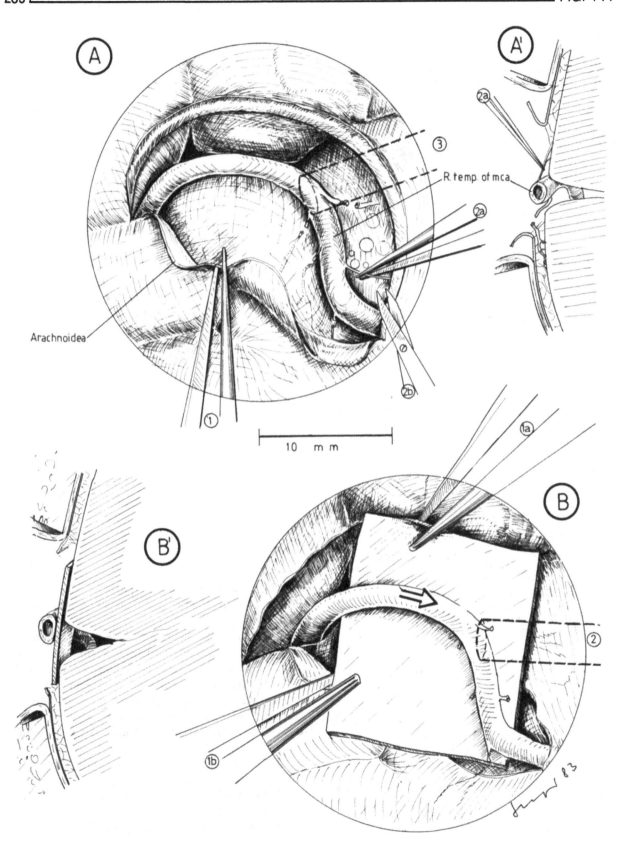

Ⓐ

③

R. temp. of mca.

②a

Ⓐ'

②a

Arachnoidea

①

⓪

②b

10   m m

Ⓑ'

①a

Ⓑ

②

①b

FIG. 145 ⊏══════════════════════════════════════⊐ 290

Fig. 145. Extra-intracranial bypass "STAMCA"
Preparation of Ramus parietalis of A. temporalis
superficialis

A **1a + 1b** After removal and reinsertion of
spreader, freed Ramus parietalis of A. temporalis superficialis slides over and beyond M.
temporalis and now lies over trepanation area

A' As **A.** Arrow shows dislocation of Ramus
parietalis corresponding to **A**

B Galea resection along distal path of Ramus
parietalis

B' **1** Distal ligation of Ramus parietalis of A. temporalis superficialis

2 Proximal temporary clipping of Ramus
parietalis

3 Distal cutting of Ramus parietalis

FIG. 145

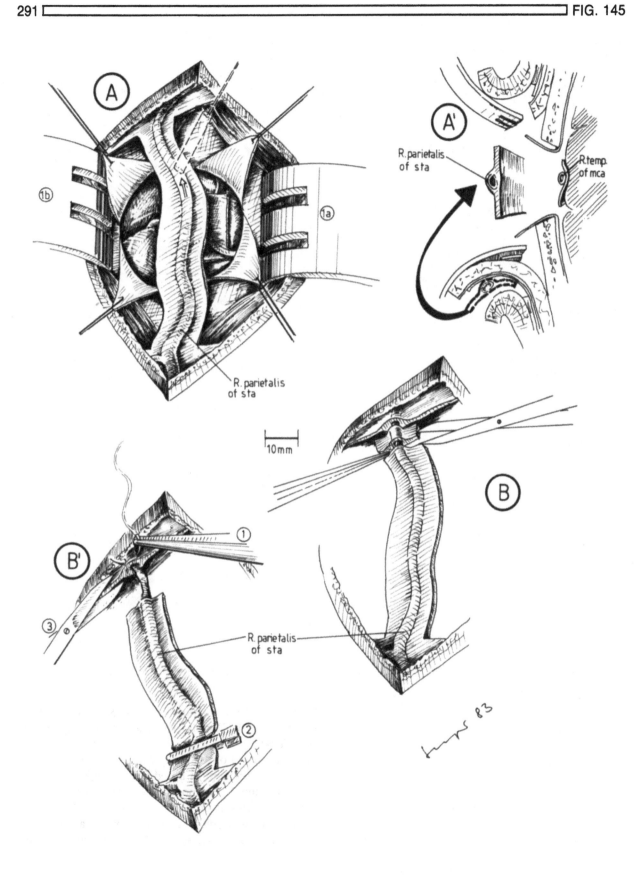

R. parietalis of sta

R. parietalis of sta

R. temp. of mca

R. parietalis of sta

10mm

FIG. 146 ⊏━━━━━━━━━━━━━━━━━━━━━━━━━━━━⊐ 292

Fig. 146. Extra-intracranial bypass "STAMCA"
Preparation of Ramus parietalis of A. temporalis
superficialis
A 1 Removal of temporay clip
   2 Measurement of blood flow per/min.
B 1 Proximal temporary clipping of Ramus
      parietalis again
   2 Remaining blood is washed out of artery with
      saline solution. Abocat plastic cannula is used

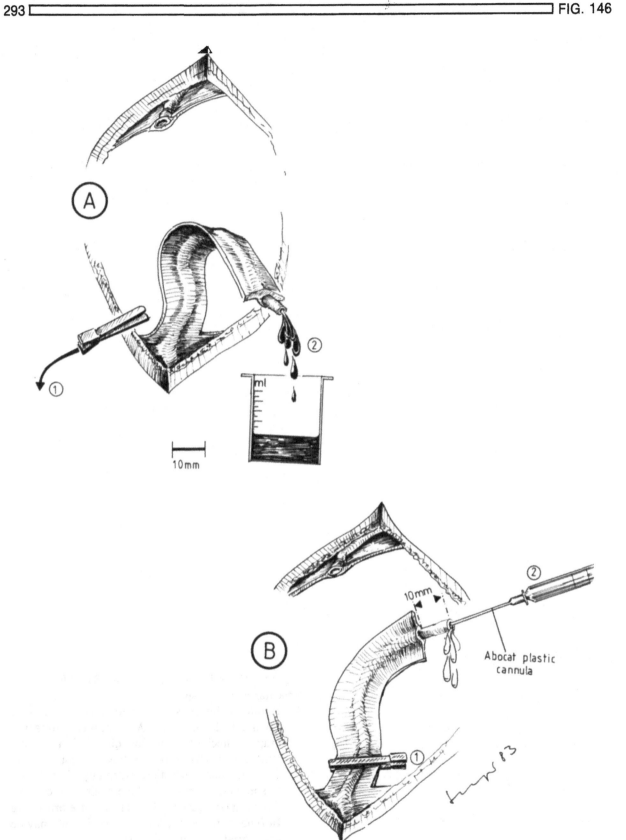

FIG. 147 ⸤━━━━━━━━━━━━━━━━━⸥ 294

Fig. 147. Extra-intracranial bypass "STAMCA"
Vascular anastomosis
A Ramus parietalis is positioned on cortical surface
B Enlarged detail from **A.** Doppler ultrasonographic check of blood flow direction in cerebral
vessels (arrows). Blood is flowing from Fissura
Sylvii in a distal direction. Normally, Doppler ultrasonographic check is done against blood flow
direction (see curve at **1b**). The reverse procedure
1a (check in the direction of blood flow) may be
appropriate, given limited space

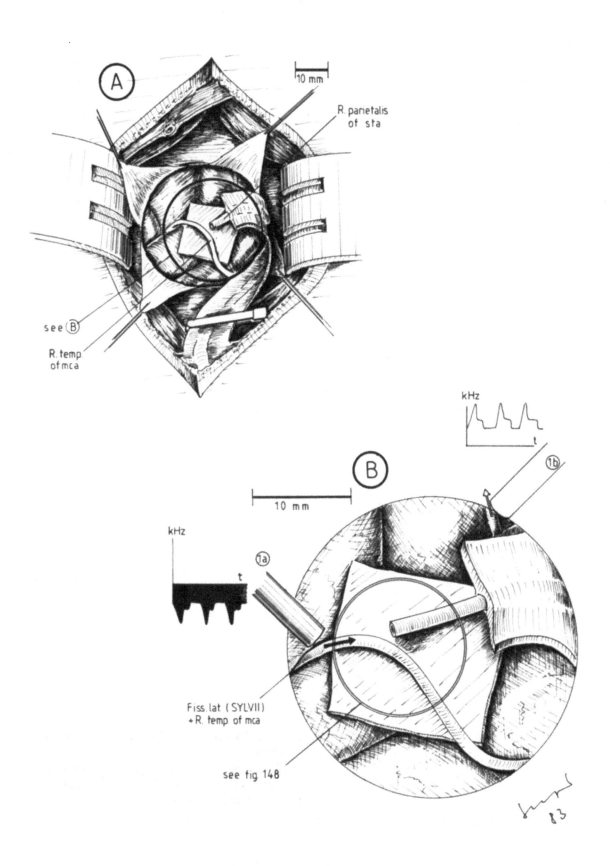

A

10 mm

R. parietalis
of sta

see B

R. temp.
of mca

kHz

t

1b

B

10 mm

kHz

1a

t

Fiss. lat (SYLVII)
+ R. temp of mca

see fig 148

FIG. 148 ⊏━━━━━━━━━━━━━━━━━━━━━━━━━━━━━━━━⊐ 296

Fig. 148. Extra-intracranial bypass "STAMCA"
Vascular anastomosis
A Enlarged detail from Fig. 147 B. End of donor
  vessel (Ramus parietalis) is cut obliquely
B Additionally, this vessel is incised lengthwise –1–

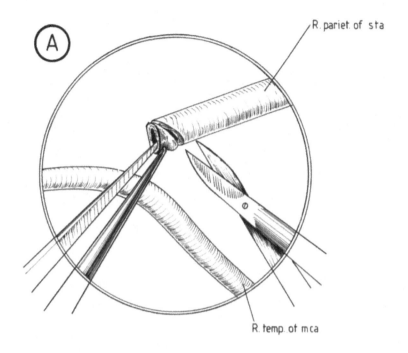

A

R. pariet. of sta

R. temp. of mca

1mm

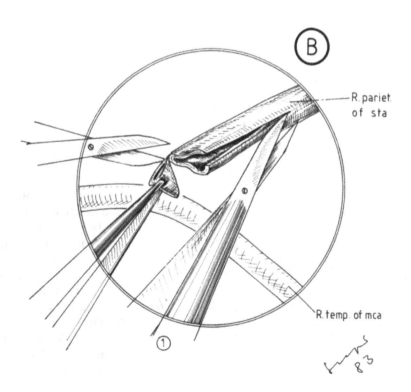

B

R. pariet. of sta

R. temp. of mca

FIG. 149 ⊏━━━━━━━━━━━━━━━━━━━━━━━━━━━━⊐ 298

Fig. 149. Extra-intracranial bypass "STAMCA"
Continuation from Fig. 148. Vascular anastomosis

A **1a + 1b** Temporary clipping of Ramus temporalis
of A. cerebri media

   2 Incision of Ramus temporalis of A. cerebri
   media. Incisions –a– of Ramus parietalis and
   –a'– of Ramus temporalis of A. cerebri media
   are of equal length

B Donor vessel – Ramus parietalis – is positioned
along the receiver vessel – light arrow – against
receiver's blood flow direction. First suture is
applied

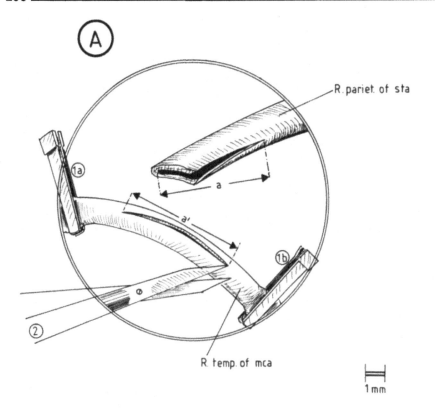

Ⓐ

R. pariet. of sta

a

a'

1a

1b

②

R. temp. of mca

1 mm

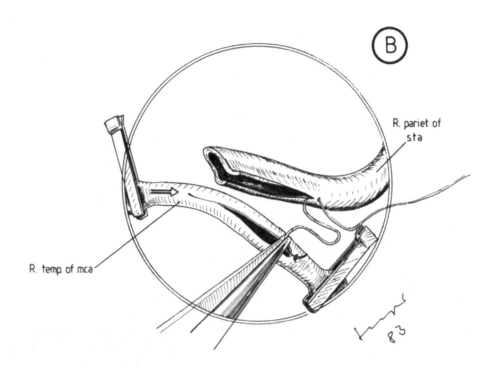

Ⓑ

R. pariet of
sta

R. temp. of mca

FIG. 150 ⊏ ⊐ 300

Fig. 150. Extra-intracranial bypass "STAMCA"
A Application of second suture
B 1 Donor vessel – Ramus parietalis – is folded
      downwards (light arrow)
   2 First row of stitches is applied at back side of
      vessels

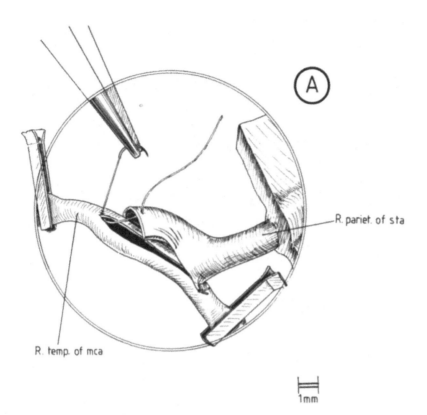

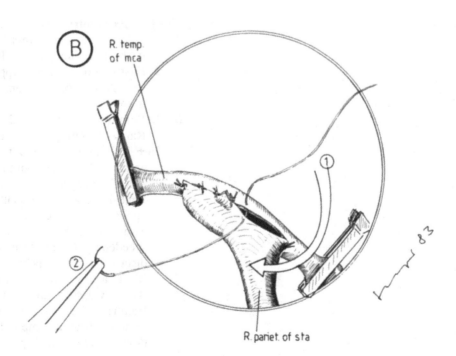

R. pariet. of sta

R. temp. of mca

1mm

R. temp.
of mca

R. pariet. of sta

FIG. 151 ⬚⬚⬚⬚⬚⬚⬚⬚⬚⬚⬚⬚⬚⬚⬚⬚⬚⬚⬚⬚⬚⬚ 302

Fig. 151. Extra-intracranial bypass "STAMCA"

A **1** Folding of donor vessel (Ramus parietalis) back to original position (light arrow)

2 First row of stitches is applied at vessel's front side. A total of approximately 15 sutures 0-00- is applied

B **1a** Removal of temporary clip from donor artery – Ramus parietalis – (light arrow)

1b + 1c Removal of temporary clip from receiver artery – Ramus temporalis – (light arrows)

2a – 2c Doppler ultrasonographic check of anastomosis. Even if visually inspected suture appears to be correct, stenosis should be assumed, if blood flow is shown to have speeded up. Greatest stenosis risk occurs at the distal anastomosis portion – sonography **2d** –. Black arrows: correct flow direction; blood flow divides in the area of donor vessel – Ramus parietalis – anastomosis; the receiving vessels – Ramus temporalis – shows reversed flow at measurement point **2c**

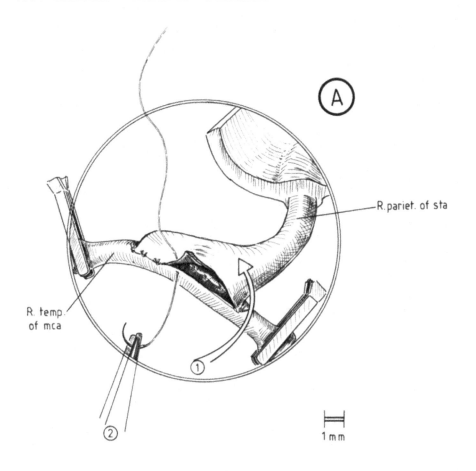

R.pariet. of sta

R. temp. of mca

1 mm

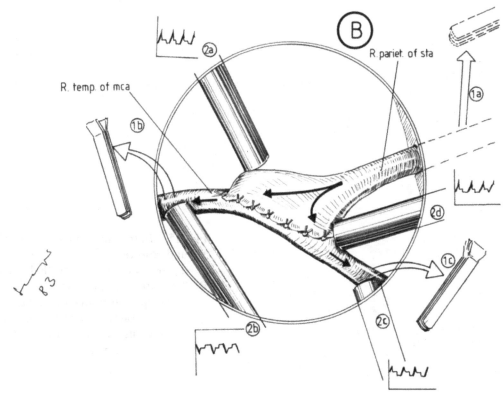

R. temp. of mca

R.pariet. of sta

FIG. 152 ⊏━━━━━━━━━━━━━━━━━━━━━━━━━━⊐ 304

Fig. 152. Extra-intracranial bypass "STAMCA"
Wound closure

A Removal of rubber foil (light arrow)

B Operation site, overview

    1 Doppler ultrasonographic check of donor vessel – Ramus parietalis – especially at point of previous clipping, to verify that clip caused no flow disturbance

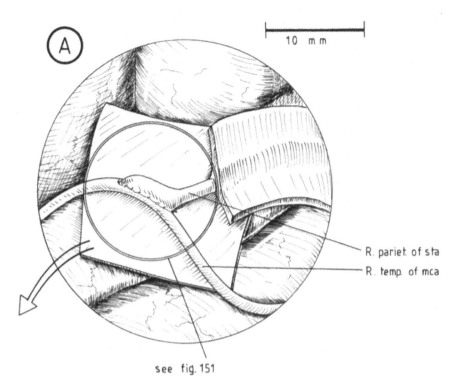

Ⓐ

10 mm

R. pariet. of sta
R. temp. of mca

see fig. 151

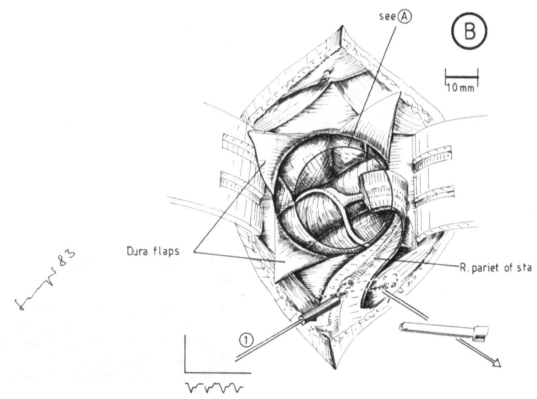

see Ⓐ

Ⓑ

10 mm

Dura flaps

R. pariet of sta

①

83

FIG. 153 □―――――――――――――――――――――――――――――□ 306

Fig. 153. Extra-intracranial bypass "STAMCA"
Wound closure
A Dura suture
B 1 Widening of trepanation at penetration point
      of Ramus parietalis of A. temporalis super-
      ficialis, in order to avoid pinching of vessel
    2 Doppler ultrasonographic check of vessel for
      free passage after dura closure and bone resec-
      tion

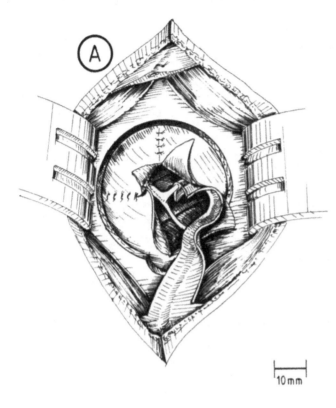

10 mm

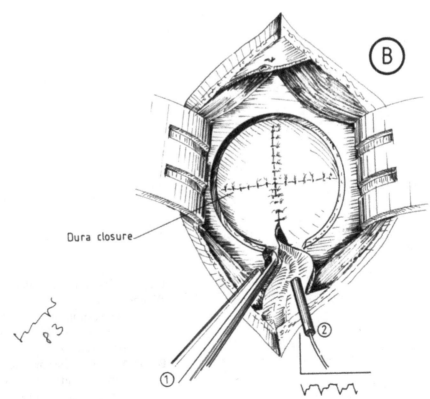

Dura closure

① ②

FIG. 154 ⊏━━━━━━━━━━━━━━━━━━━━━━━━━━━━━━━━━━━━⊐ 308

Fig. 154. Extra-intracranial bypass "STAMCA"
Wound closure
A 1 Reinsertion of bone flap
   2 Ultrasonographic check of Ramus parietalis
      for free flow
B 1 After suturing muscle, fascia, gaela and skin,
      Ramus parietalis is checked again by
      ultrasonograph, this time through closed skin

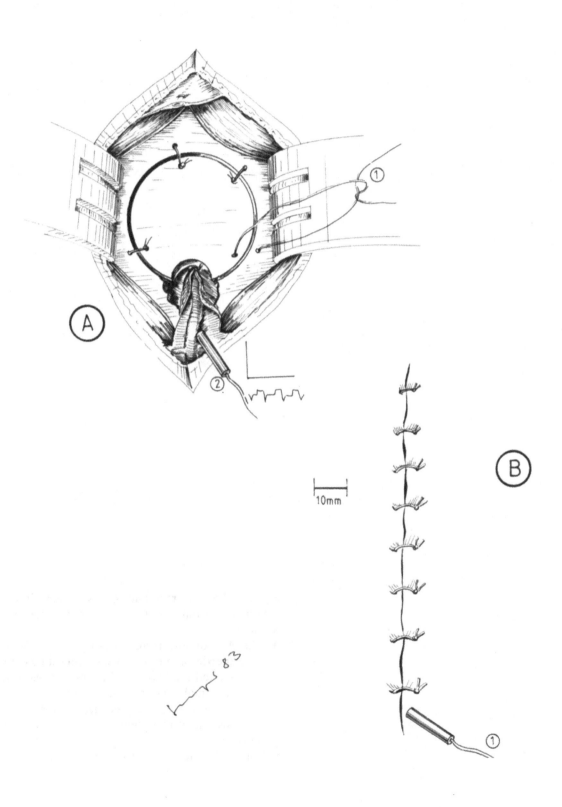

FIG. 155 ⊏══════════════════════⊐310

Fig. 155. Extra-intracranial bypass "STAMCA"
Appendix. Comparison of various anastomosis techniques

A + B Anastomosis technique according to Yaşargil, Spetzler and others. Classic, most commonly applied method, which, however, as proven in animal experiments, is not ideal*

B' Using this classic technique, stenoses are possible at two points

---

* J. Gilsbach, Thesis, Freiburg 1983.

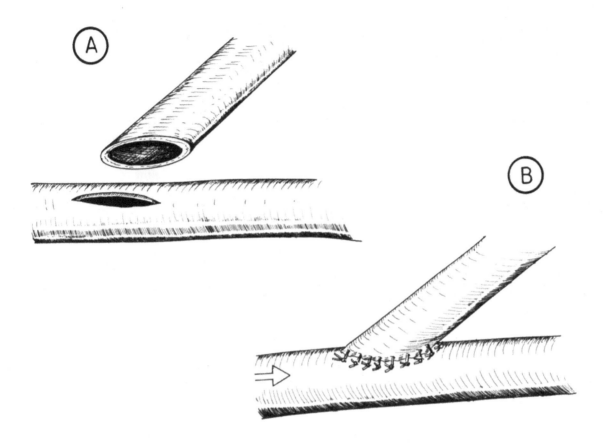

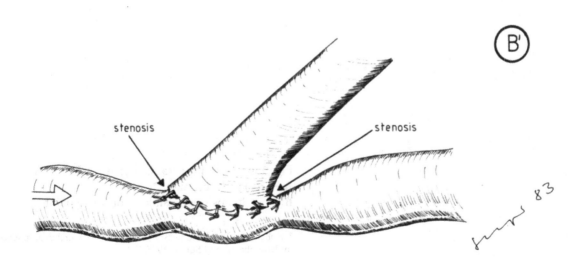

stenosis

stenosis

FIG. 156 ⌐━━━━━━━━━━━━━━━━━━━━━━━━━━━━━━━━⌐ 312

Fig. 156. Extra-intracranial bypass "STAMCA"

A + B Patch technique*

B' Stenosis is possible at only **one** point

---

* Robertson, J. H., Robertson, J. T., 1978, Animal experiments by Rosenbaum and Sundt, 1977.

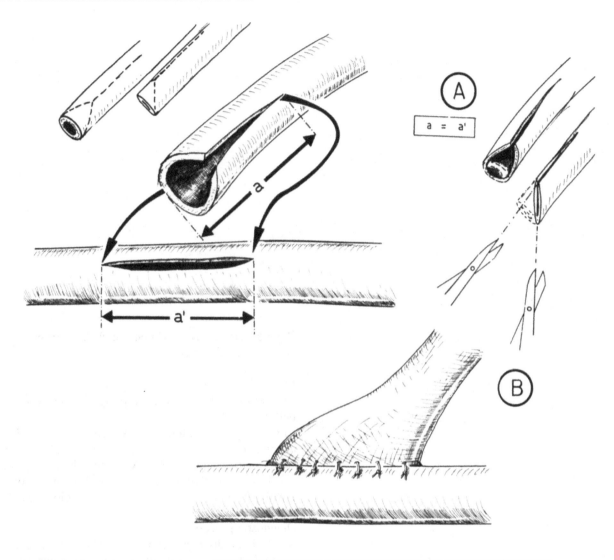

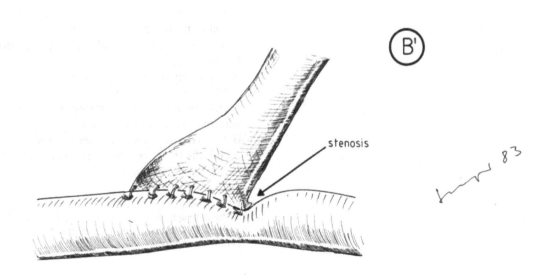

stenosis

FIG. 157 ⬚─────────────────────────⬚ 314

Bypass between A. occipitalis and A. cerebelli inf. post. (Figs. 157 to 167)

Fig. 157. Extra-intracranial bypass
Infratentorial: bypass from A. occipitalis and A. cerebelli inf. post.
Clinical example of left sided A. vertebralis occlusion in congenital hypoplasia of right A. vertebralis, which supplies only the right A. cerebelli inf. post. –"PICA"–. Increasing daily attacks of dizziness for 3 months. No pre- and postoperative * neurological deficits**.
Diagnostic procedures
A   A. cubitalis angiography, left side: black arrow indicates A. vertebralis occlusion in upper cervical area.
Light arrow: faint contrast appearance of left A. vertebralis above occlusion point.
X: contrast-medium-uptake into A. vertebralis in the nape muscles
B   Aortography shows hypoplastic right A. vertebralis continuing directly as A. cerebralis inf. post.-"PICA", without showing intracranial A. vertebralis-basilaris circulation
C   Black arrow: operative anastomosis from A. occipitalis to A. cerebelli inf. post. –"PICA"–
D   X-ray shows trepanation

---

* Since anastomosis cannot be ascertained through thick nape muscles by Doppler sonograph – in contrast to "STAMCA" – postoperative angiography must be carried out.
** Operation performed by Dr. W. Hassler, author's coworker.

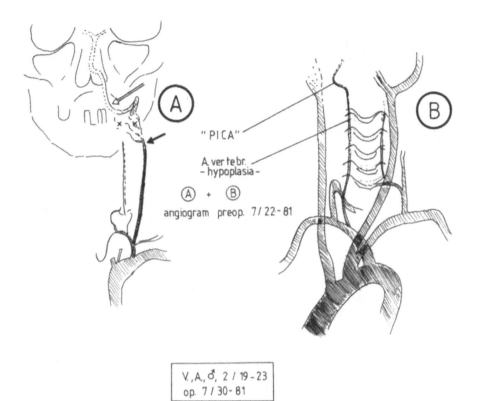

"PICA"

A.vertebr.
- hypoplasia -

Ⓐ + Ⓑ

angiogram preop. 7/22-81

V.,A., ♂, 2/19-23
op. 7/30-81

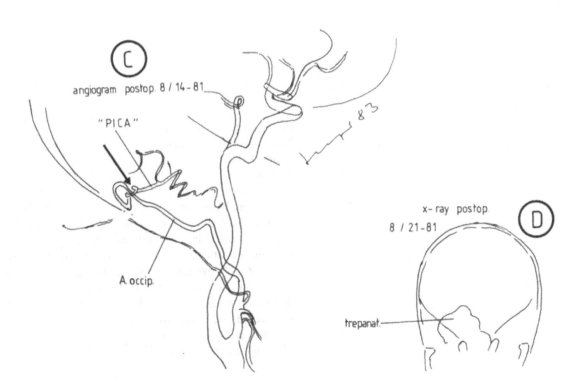

angiogram postop. 8/14-81

"PICA"

A.occip.

x-ray postop.
8/21-81

trepanat.

FIG. 158 ⊏━━━━━━━━━━━━━━━━━━━━━━━━━━━⊐ 316

Fig. 158. Extra-intracranial bypass
Infratentorial: bypass from A. occipitalis and A. cere-
belli inf. post.
Anatomy
A   Anatomical topographical relation between N.
    occipitalis major and A. occipitalis, overview
A' Enlarged detail from A. A. occipitalis penetrates
    Fascia nuchalis approximately 40 mm lateral from
    midline and there N. occipitalis major crosses
    over it. Nerve must be saved during artery prepa-
    ration because of danger of neuralgia
B   Anatomical topographical relation of A.
    occipitalis, Processus mastoideus and middle
    muscle layer
B' Enlarged detail from B

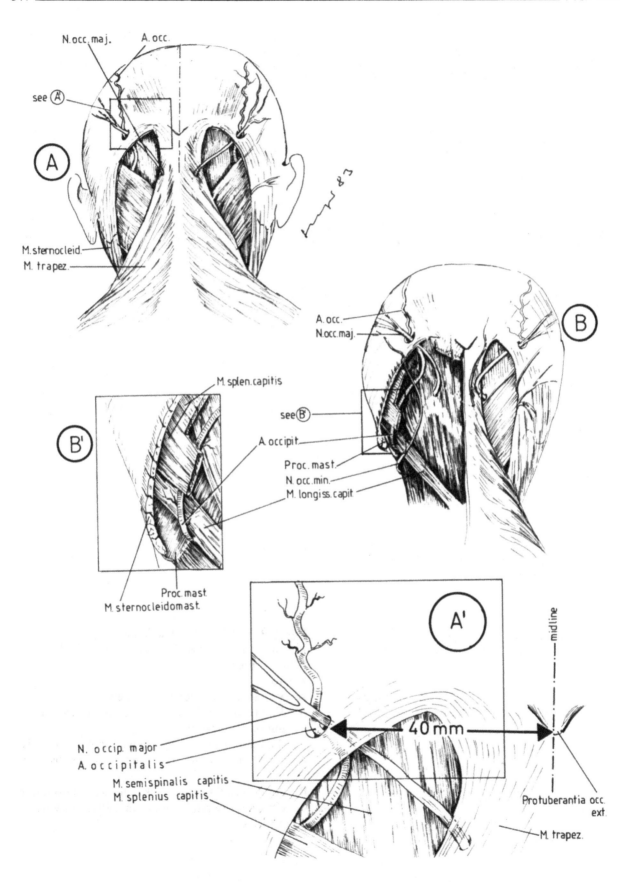

FIG. 159 ⬛══════════════════════════════════════⬛318

Fig. 159. Extra-intracranial bypass
Infratentorial: bypass from A. occipitalis and A. cerebelli inf. post.
Anatomy
A   Processus mastoideus, overview
A' Enlarged detail from A. Incisura mastoidea: origin of M. digastricus.
    Sulcus a. occip.: bony groove for A. occipitalis
A" As A', deep muscle layer and A. occipitalis drawn in
B   Anatomical overview sketch, with position of both Aa. occipitales drawn in, between deep nape muscles

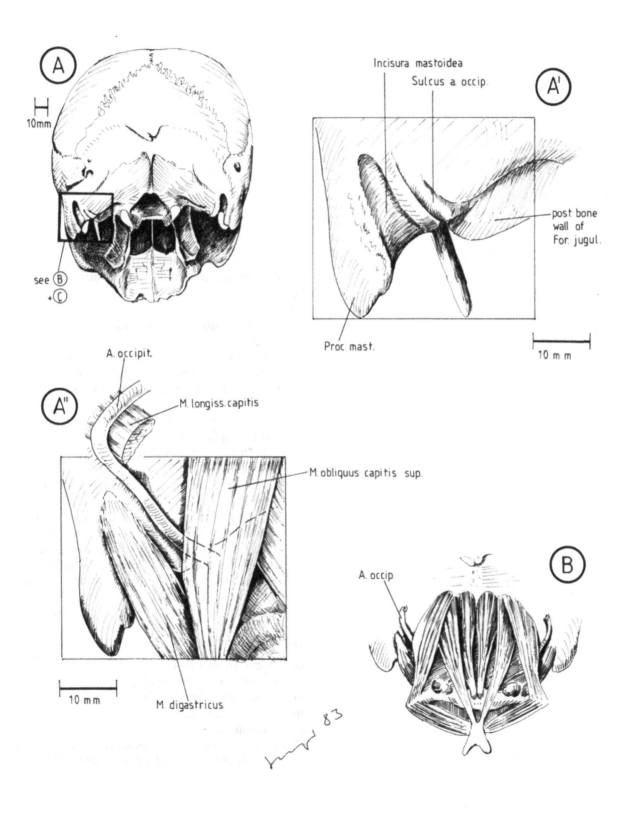

(A)

10mm

see (B)
+(C)

(A')

Incisura mastoidea
Sulcus a. occip.

post. bone
wall of
For. jugul.

Proc. mast.

10 m m

(A")

A. occipit.

M. longiss. capitis

M. obliquus capitis sup.

10 mm

M. digastricus

(B)

A. occip.

83

FIG. 160 ⊏━━━━━━━━━━━━━━━━━━━━━━━━━━━━━⊐ 320

Fig. 160. Extra-intracranial bypass

Infratentorial: bypass from A. occipitalis and A. cerebelli inf. post.

Operation

A **1 + 2** Localization of midline on the sitting patient

    1 Palpation of Processus spinosus axis

    2 Palpation of Protub. occipitalis ext.

    3 Palpation of Processus mastoideus on both sides

    4a – 4c Defining of A. occipitalis path by Doppler sonography

    5a + 5b Skin incision drawn in

    5a Portion of skin incision in the midline between Protuberantia occip. ext. and Processus spinosus axis

    5b Lateral portion of skin incision nearly parallel to and above path of A. occipitalis (broken lines), defined by Doppler ultrasonogram

B At first, median skin incision only, splitting of Lig. nuchae, exposure of Arcus atlantis post. –*aa*– and exposure of Planum nuchae –*pn*–

C Enlarged detail from **B,** microsurgical site

Abbreviations:

aa Arcus atlantis post.

fo Foramen occipitale (edge)

map Membrana atlanto-occipitalis post.

nm Neck musculature

pn Planum nuchae

vl A. vertebralis over Sulcus a. vertebralis of Arcus atlantis post. (palpable; pulsations visible)

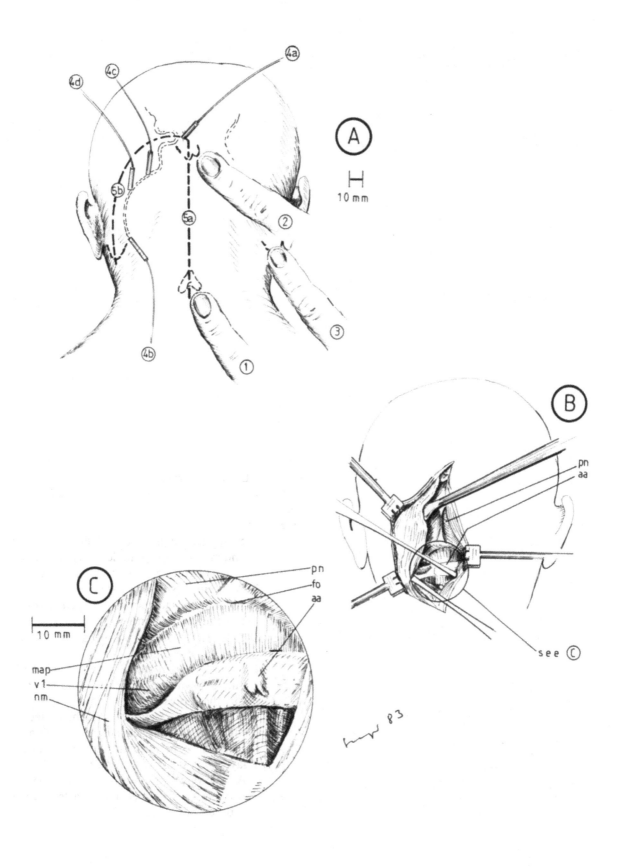

FIG. 161 ⊏━━━━━━━━━━━━━━━━━━━━━━━━━━⊐ 322

Fig. 161. Extra-intracranial bypass
Infratentorial: bypass from A. occipitalis and A. cerebelli inf. post.
Operation

A   **1** Skin incision is extended laterally. Skin and muscle flap are folded outwards. Ligation and cutting of A. occipitalis, see **A'**

A'   **2a** A. occipitalis ligated distally

      2b A. occipitalis temporarily clipped proximal to penetration point

      3 After ligation and clipping of A. occipitalis, it is cut

      4 (arrow) clipped stump of A. occipitalis is pulled downwards under N. occipitalis major; then, preserving N. occipitalis major, musculature is sectioned to the bone (see **A**)

B + C Composite microsurgical site presentation

      1 Incision of periosteum and deep muscle layer almost to A. occipitalis.
Arrow: direction of artery preparation.
Broken lines: projection of artery upon exposed periosteum

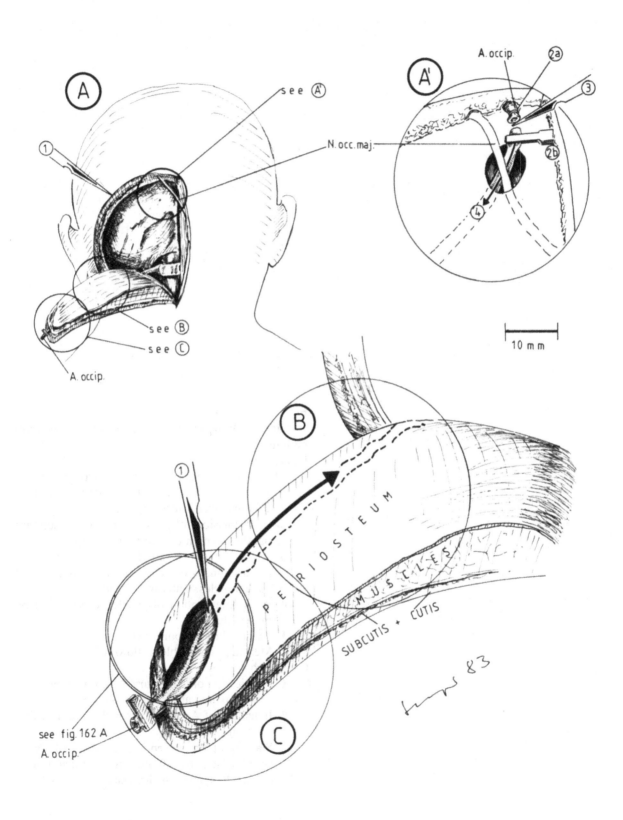

FIG. 162 ⊏━━━━━━━━━━━━━━━━━━━━━━━━━━━━━⊐ 324

Fig. 162. Extra-intracranial bypass

Infratentorial: bypass from A. occipitalis and A. cerebelli inf. post.

Operation

A   Microsurgical site. Enlarged detail from Fig. 161 C

    1 Extension of incision of periosteum and musculature over artery path (arrow)

    2a + 2b Incisions of periosteum and musculature parallel to path of artery, and deeper

    3 Artery, with surrounding musculature and periosteum, is detached from periosteum and nape muscles. Cutis and subcutis are preserved

    4a + 4b Interruption of smaller vessels in nape musculature

B   **1** Removal of temporary clip

    2 Measurement of blood flow/min.

C   Sketch

    1 Application of temporary clip to A. occipitalis, very proximal and close to skull base

    2 Irrigation of A. occipitalis with isotonic saline solution.

    Starting at the cut end of A. occipitalis for a length of approx. 20 mm the periosteum muscle envelope must be detached from vessel

FIG. 162

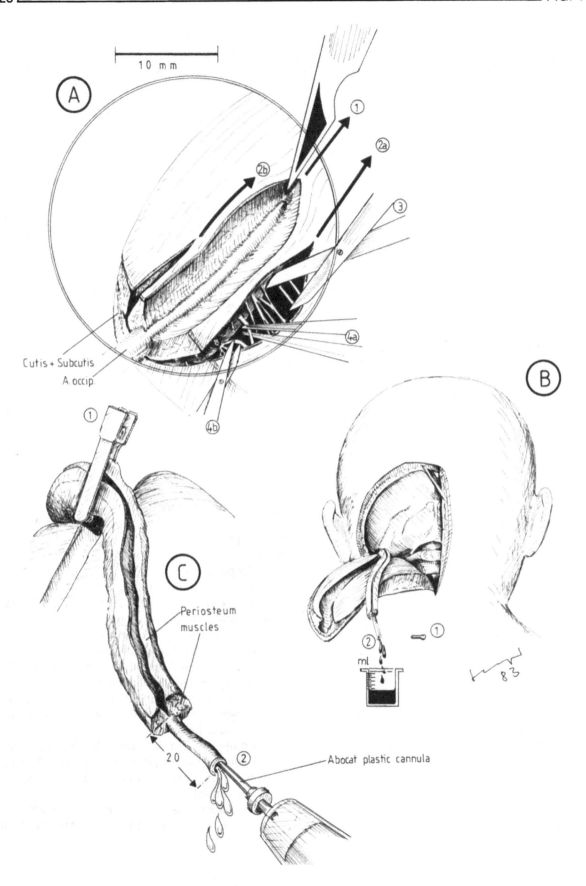

10 mm

Ⓐ

①

②a

②b

③

④a

Cutis + Subcutis

A. occip.

④b

①

Ⓒ

Ⓑ

Periosteum
muscles

②

①

ml

②

Abocat plastic cannula

2 0

83

FIG. 163 ══ 326

Fig. 163. Extra-intracranial bypass
Infratentorial: bypass from A. occipitalis and A. cere-
belli inf. post.
Operation
A   1 Trepanation
    2 Localization of dura incision
B   Microsurgical site, detail from **A.** Dura and
    arachnoidea are opened up
    1 Detachment of arachnoidea from Tonsilla
    cerebelli and medial Lobulus biventer portions
    2a + 2b Lifting Tonsilla cerebelli off Medulla
    oblongata; cutting of adhesions
    3a + 3b Lifting Tonsilla cerebelli and medial
    Lobulus biventer portions off basal dura; cut-
    ting of adhesions
C   1 Lifting of Tonsilla cerebelli and adjoining
    Lobulus biventer portions by spatula. A. cere-
    belli inf. post. –"PICA"– and N.XI become
    recognizable.
    For anastomosis, trunk of A. cerebelli inf.
    post. –"PICA"– is used, not the lateral branch

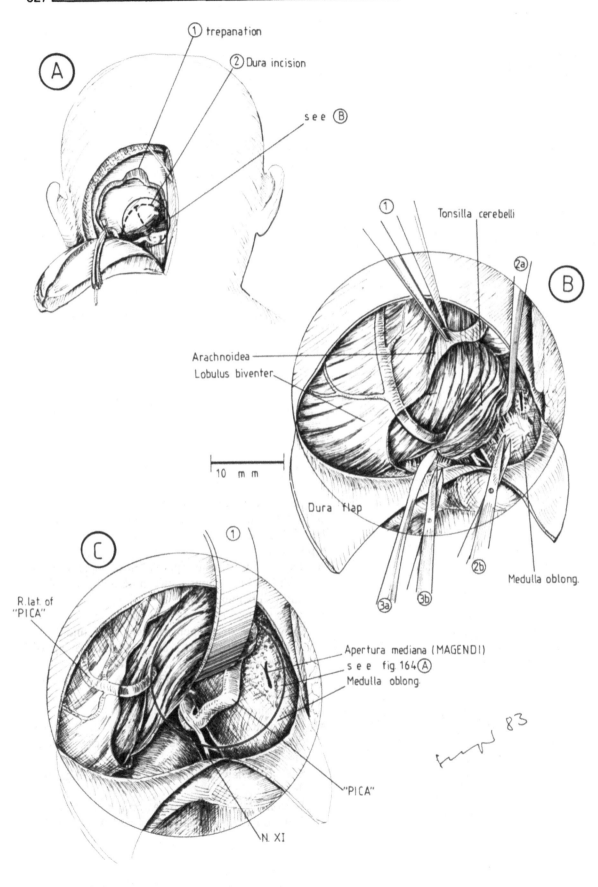

A
① trepanation
② Dura incision
see Ⓑ

B
① Tonsilla cerebelli
②a
Arachnoidea
Lobulus biventer
10 m m
Dura flap
②b
③a ③b
Medulla oblong.

C
R.lat. of "PICA"
①
Apertura mediana (MAGENDI)
see fig 164Ⓐ
Medulla oblong.
"PICA"
N. XI

FIG. 164

Fig. 164. Extra-intracranial bypass

Infratentorial: bypass from A. occipitalis and A. cerebelli inf. post.

Operation

A Deeper insertion of spatula, after separation of
  additional adhesions between Medulla oblongata
  and cerebellum

  1 Retraction of cerebellum

  2 A piece of rubber foil is placed under A.
  cerebelli inf. post., after careful freeing of
  artery from Medulla oblongata

  3a + 3b Temporary clipping of A. cerebelli inf.
  post.

  4 Incision of A. cerebelli inf. post.

A' Anatomical topographical sketch of Medulla
  oblongata and A. cerebelli inf. post., corresponding to A

B Site, overview. Microsurgical site of Fig. 165
  drawn in

C 1 Oblique transection of A. occipitalis

C' Situation after extended incision of A. occipitalis

FIG. 164

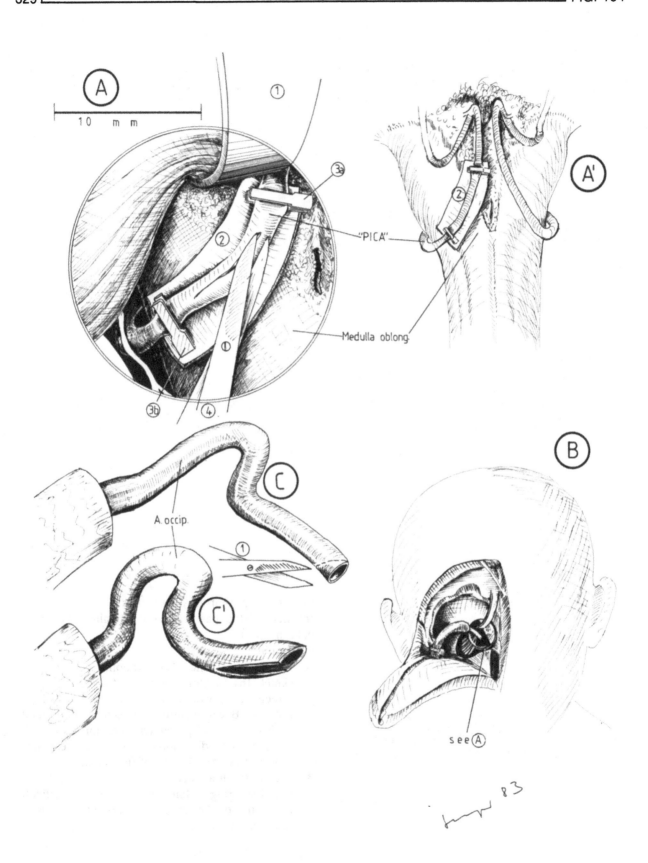

A

10 m m

① 3a ② "PICA" ③b ④ Medulla oblong.

A'

②

B

C A. occip. ① C'

see Ⓐ

83

FIG. 165 ⊏━━━━━━━━━━━━━━━━━━━━━━━━━━━━━━━━━━⊐ 330

Fig. 165. Extra-intracranial bypass
Infratentorial: bypass from A. occipitalis and A. cerebelli inf. post.
Operation
A Microsurgical site. Localization, see overview sketch 164 **B.** Donor vessel – A. occipitalis – is directed in flow direction of receiver vessel – light arrow –. Because suturing is technically difficult in this deep area, placement of donor vessel with or against flow direction depends on the technical possibilities. Application of first stitch
B Second stitch applied
C Initial suturing is done on the side most difficult to reach. For that purpose A. occipitalis is dislocated upwards

FIG. 165

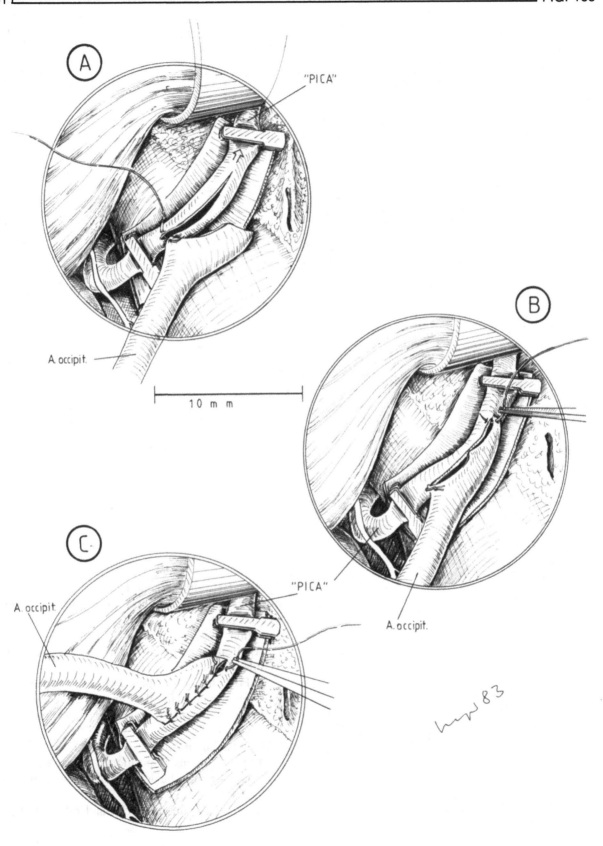

"PICA"

A. occipit.

10 m m

"PICA"

A. occipit.

A. occipit.

wp 83

FIG. 166 ⸤▭⸥ 332

Fig. 166. Extra-intracranial bypass
Infratentorial: bypass from A. occipitalis and A. cerebelli inf. post.
Operation
A   Application of suture on more easily accessible side of vessel
   1   First, lumen of opened vessel is inspected, to see if contralateral sutures lie correctly
   2   First stitch on the more easily accessible side of vessel
B   1   Finishing of sutures
   2   A. occipitalis is positioned upwards, so that later it may be led through dura gap (light arrow)
C   Removal of temporary clip and rubber foil (arrows)

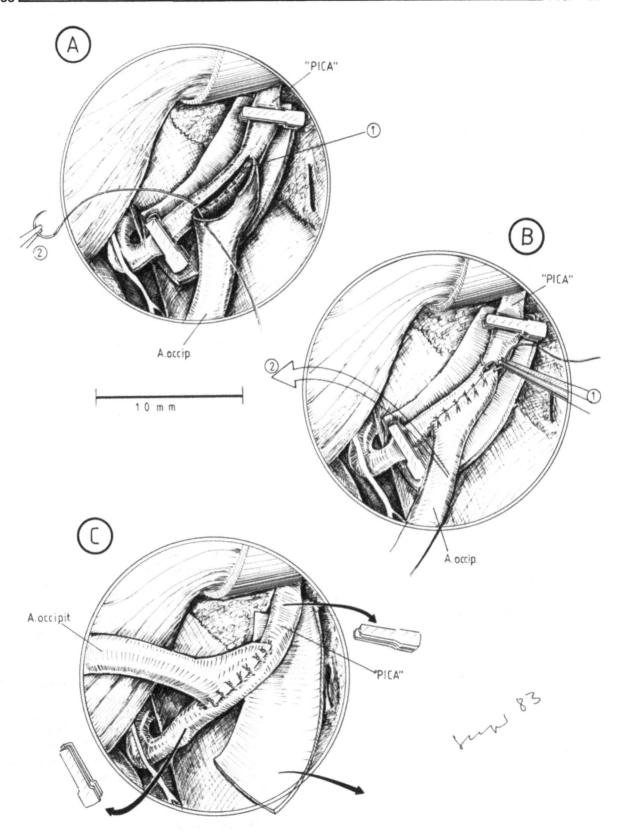

A "PICA"

① ②

A.occip.

10 mm

B "PICA"

② ①

A.occip.

C A.occipit.

"PICA"

ハル 83

FIG. 167 ☐───────────────────────────☐ 334

Fig. 167. Extra-intracranial bypass
Infratentorial: bypass from A. occipitalis and A. cerebelli inf. post.
Operation
A 1 Removal of temporary clip from A. occipitalis
   2 Doppler sonographic check of blood flow in A.
      occipitalis
A' Microsurgical site
   3a Doppler sonographic check of anastomosis at
   point where danger of stenosis is greatest
   3b Doppler sonographic check of anastomosis at
      point where there is less danger of stenosis
B 1 Doppler sonographic check of A. occipitalis
      after dura closure in order to exclude stenosis
      at dura penetration point, overview
B' Microsurgical site for **B**
   1 As in **B.**
      Wound closure

FIG. 167

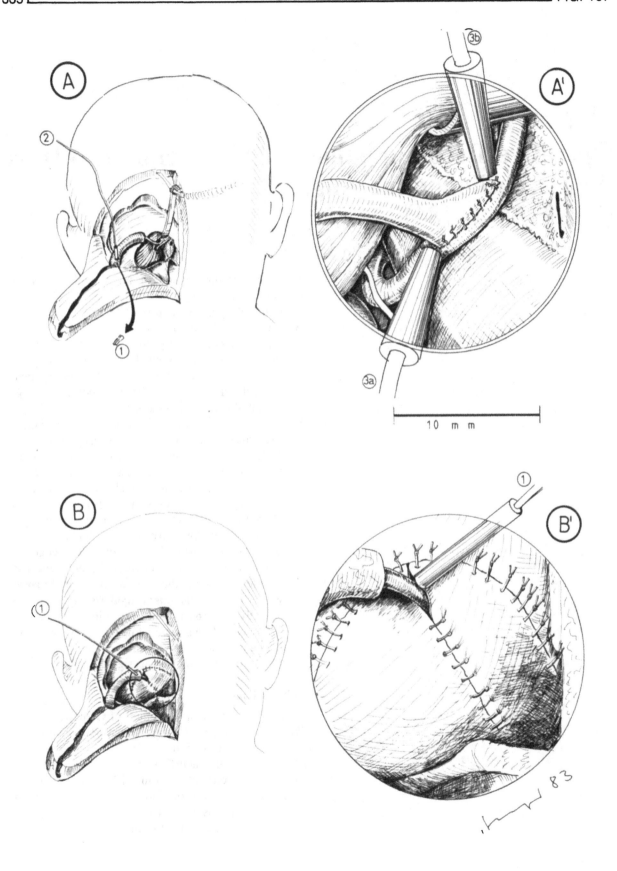

10 m m

FIG. 168 🖵 ▬▬▬▬▬▬▬▬▬▬▬▬▬▬▬▬▬▬▬▬▬▬▬▬▬▬▬▬▬▬▬▬▬▬ 336

Chapter 5

Operative Decompressions of N. V and N. VII in the Cerebellopontine Angle
(Figs. 168 to 184)

Fig. 168. Decompression of N. V and N. VII in cerebello-pontine angle.

Anatomy of operative approach (arrows)

A Dura gap, through which N. trigeminus leaves liquor space, directly adjoins edge of Lobulus quadrangularis cerebelli. Dura penetration point of N. VII and VIII (= Porus and Meatus acusticus int.) adjoins Flocculus, Brachium pontis and edge of Lobulus quadrangularis.

B Sketch of a portion of skull base showing Sulcus petrosus sup. which surrounds Sinus petrosus sup. Note their adjoining relationships to Porus acusticus int. –pa– and to Impressio trigemini –it–

C Planum nuchae, through which Sinus transversus, Sinus sigmoideus, Sinus knee –(k)– and exit of N. V to N. VIII show translucently. Sulcus petrosus sup. of Os petrosum with Sinus petrosus sup. within tentorial insertion, and edge of Lobulus quadrangularis cerebelli adjoin and run parallel to each other. **Between Sinus petrosus sup. and Lobulus quadrangularis cerebelli lies operative approach.** Starting point of operative approach is Sinus knee (juncture Sinus transversus/sigmoideus and entrance of Sinus petrosus sup. into Sinus transversus/sigmoideus)

Abbreviations:

it	Impressio trigemini of Os petrosum
(k)	Knee of Sinus transversus/sigmoideus (projection)
pa	Porus acusticus int.
pV	Penetration point of N. V at Tentorium
pVII/VIII	Penetration point of N. VII/VIII = Porus acusticus int.
te	Edge of Tentorium

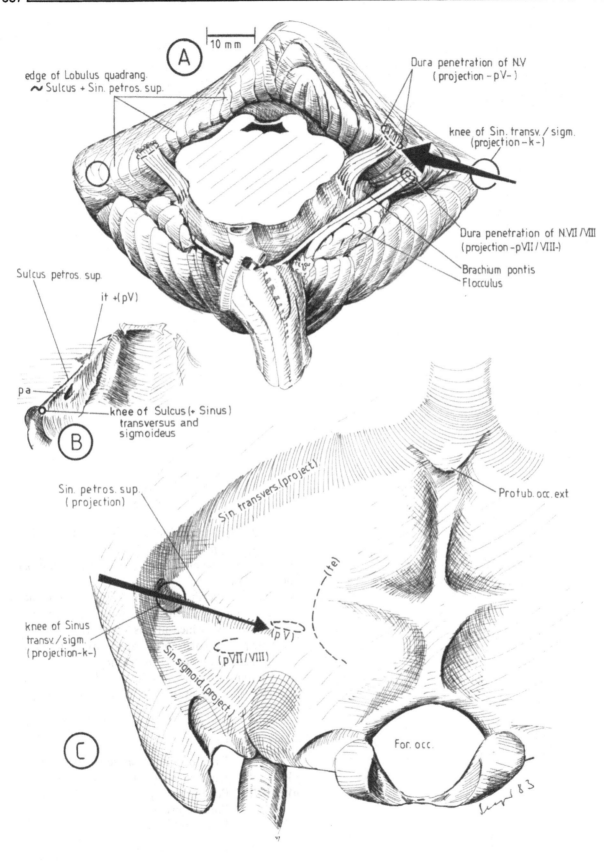

10 mm

(A)

edge of Lobulus quadrang.
∼ Sulcus + Sin. petros. sup.

Dura penetration of N.V
(projection –pV–)

knee of Sin. transv. / sigm.
(projection–k–)

Dura penetration of N.VII /VIII
(projection –pVII / VIII–)

Brachium pontis
Flocculus

Sulcus petros. sup.

it +(pV)

pa

knee of Sulcus (+ Sinus)
transversus and
sigmoideus

(B)

Sin. petros. sup.
(projection)

Sin. transvers (project)

Protub. occ. ext

(te)

(p V)

knee of Sinus
transv. / sigm.
(projection–k–)

(pVII / VIII)

Sin. sigmoid (project)

For. occ.

(C)

FIG. 169 ⌐‗‗‗‗‗‗‗‗‗‗‗‗‗‗‗‗‗‗‗‗‗‗‗‗‗‗‗‗‗‗‗‗‗‗⌐338

Fig. 169. Decompression of N. V and N. VII in cerebello-pontine angle.

Anatomical schematic sketches of operative approach (black arrows)

A Schematic reclination of Lobulus quadrangularis and Pons (double arrows), in order to show position of N.V, which in this sketch is cut through. Note position of Sinus petrosus sup. to the adjoining Tentorium and Os petrosum

B Anatomical sketch of duraclad skull base, detail view, showing arterial loops at N.V and N.VII/ VIII

Abbreviations:

k	Knee of Sinus transversus/sigmoideus
pV	Dura penetration point of N.V
pVII/VIII	Penetration point of N.VII/VIII = Porus acusticus int.
VP	V. petrosa sup.

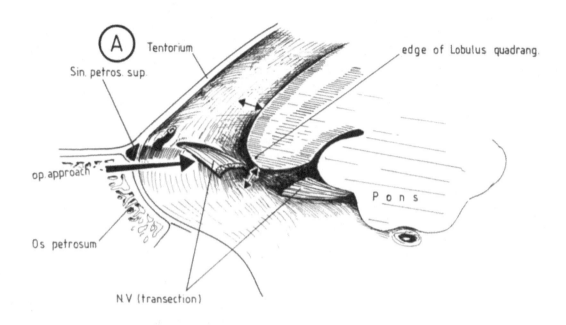

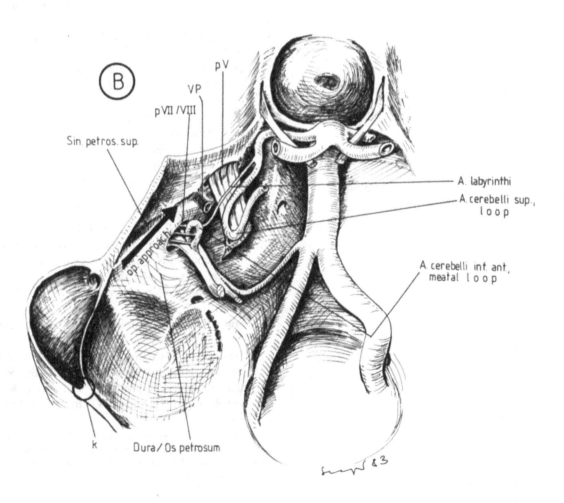

FIG. 170 ⌐━━━⌐ 340

Fig. 170. Decompression of N. V and N. VII in cerebello-pontine angle.

Possibilities of vascularly-induced compression of N.V. and N.VII

A Lower brainstem region, left lateral view, with vessels.

Leptomeningeal structures omitted

a1 – a4 Compression of N. trigeminus by arteries:

a1 by A. cerebelli sup.

a2 A. basilaris

a3 A. vertebralis

a4 A. cerebelli inf. ant. –"AICA"–

b1 – b3 Compression of N. facialis

b1 by meatal loop of "AICA"

b2 A. vertebralis

b3 A. cerebelli inf. post. –"PICA"–

Arrows: Enlargements of arterial loops in the direction of N. trigeminus exit from Pons and near Porus acust. int.

B Typical compression points on N. V. Nomenclature **a1 – a4**

C Typical compression points on N. VII. Nomenclature **b1 – b3** see **A**

Every artery of the posterior fossa may lead to a compression of N. V as well as N. VII (also VIII); most common compressions are: N. V by A. cerebelli sup. (a1), and N. VII by "AICA" b1 *

---

* One also speaks of compressions of other basal cranial nerves such as Nn. IX to XI; however, they are not discussed in this book, since author has not experienced them, and therefore he cannot evaluate them.

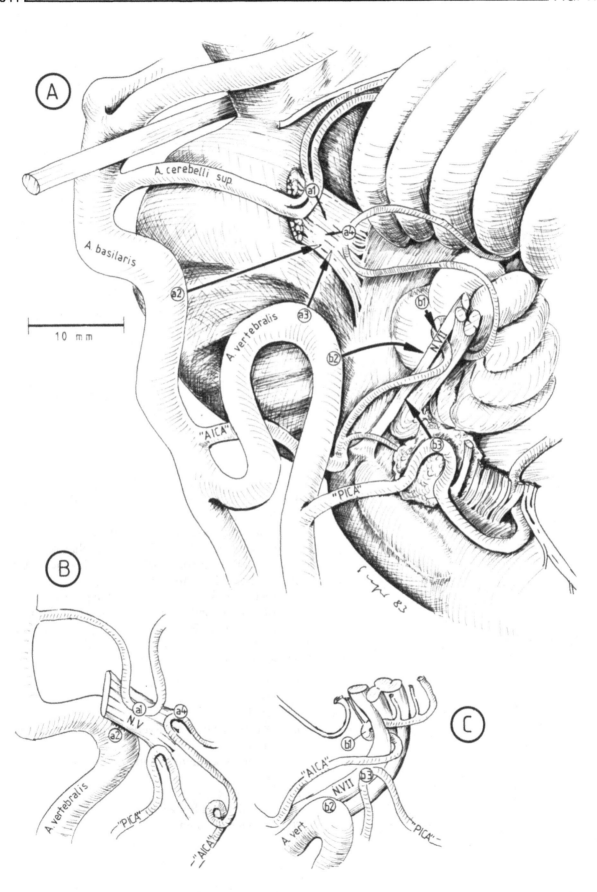

FIG. 171 ⊏==⊐ 342

Fig. 171. Decompression of N. V and N. VII in cerebello-pontine angle.

A   Anatomical sketch, normal finding
B   Compression of N. V by A. cerebelli sup. This is the most common cause of trigeminal neuralgia
B' Enlarged detail from **B.**
    Light arrows: artery shown compressing N. V, Brachium pontis –*bp*– and Pons –*p*– at exit point of N. V from Pons

Abbreviations:

bi   Lobulus biventer
bp   Brachium pontis
bl   A. basilaris
k   Knee of Sinus transversus/sigmoideus (projection)
lss Lobulus semilunaris sup.
p   Pons
pl   A. cerebri post.
qu   Lobulus quadrangularis
si   Lobulus semilunaris inf.

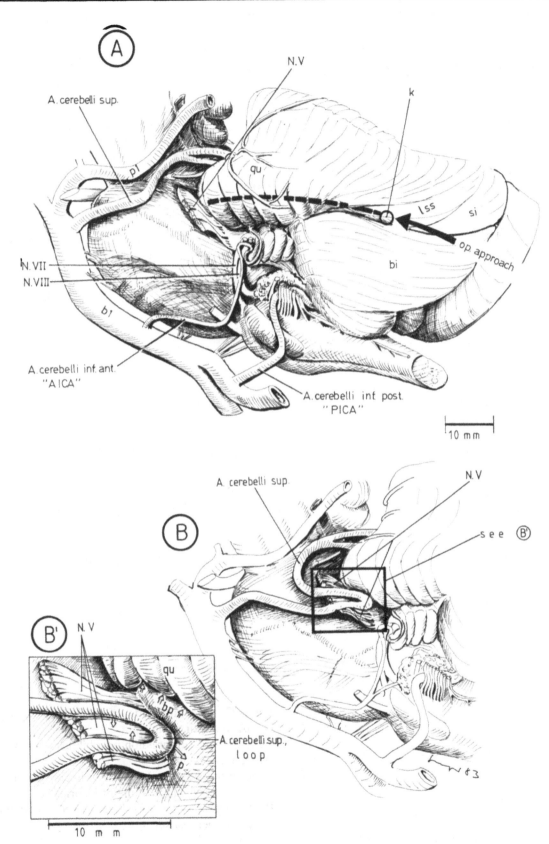

FIG. 172 ⊏──────────────────────────────────⊐ 344

Fig. 172. Decompression of N. V and N. VII in
cerebello-pontine angle.
Less frequent compression possibilities of N. V
Anatomical sketches
A Compression of N. V by circular looping of
   A. cerebelli sup. or one of its branches
B Compression by veins, i. e. by lateral pontine vein
   (or V. petrosa sup.)

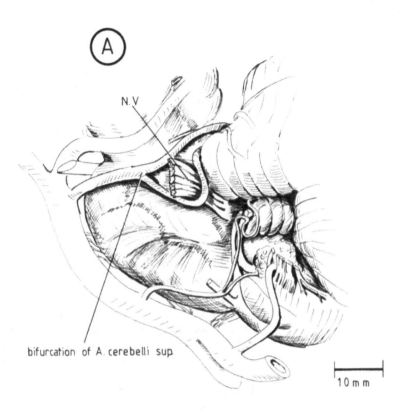

N.V

bifurcation of A. cerebelli sup.

10 mm

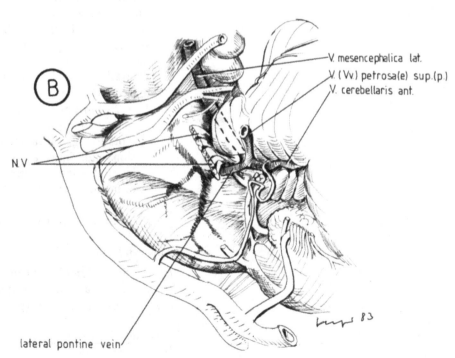

V. mesencephalica lat.
V. (Vv.) petrosa(e) sup.(p.)
V. cerebellaris ant.

N.V

lateral pontine vein

FIG. 173 346

Fig. 173. Decompression of N. V and N. VII in cerebello-pontine angle.

Operation

A Localization of skin incision drawn in (broken line). Condition after skin incision and pushing back of muscles. Processus mastoideus exposed. Sinus transversus/sigmoideus drawn in (broken lines)

B Trepanation, anatomical sketch. Burr hole **a** lies above Sinus transversus in order to permit upward view unobstructed by protruding bone structures*. Burr hole **b** lies medial to Sinus sigmoideus, to prevent injury to thin Sinus sigmoideus wall

C Operation site after cutting of skin, fascias and musculature

    1 + 2 Further preparation of musculature, periosteum pushed away from Planum nuchae. Note topographical relation between skin incision and Sinus transversus/sigmoideus (skin incision – heavy broken lines – lies just medial of medial Sinus sigmoideus wall – light broken line –)

    3 Control of retractor position

Abbreviations:

(ss) Sinus sigmoideus (projection)
(sss) Sinus sagittalis sup. (projection)
(st) Sinus transversus (projection)

---

* Indication from Prof. Dr. G. Yaşargil, Neurosurgical Clinic, University of Zürich.

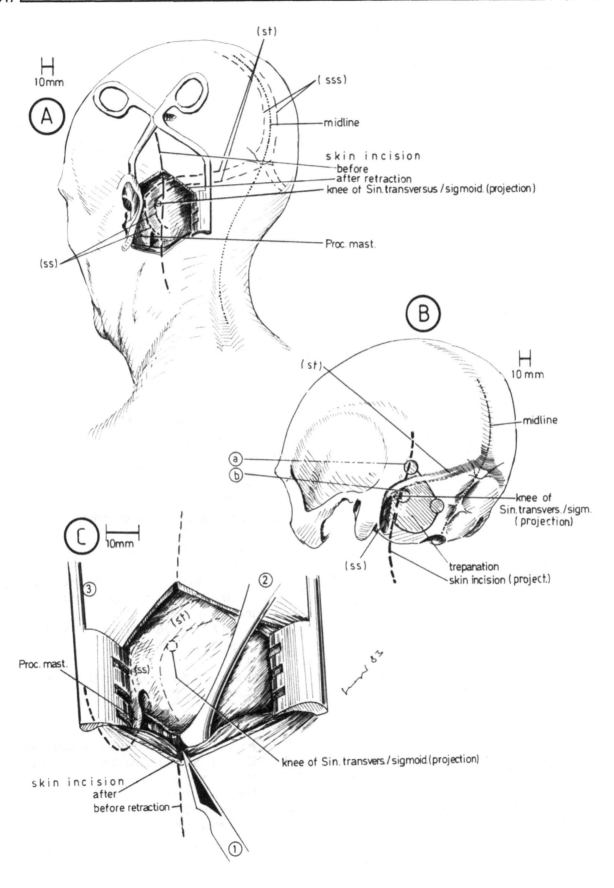

A
H 10mm

(st)

(sss)

midline

skin incision
before
after retraction
knee of Sin. transversus / sigmoid. (projection)

Proc. mast.

(ss)

B
H 10 mm

(st)

midline

(a)
(b)

knee of
Sin. transvers./sigm.
(projection)

(ss)

trepanation
skin incision (project.)

C
10mm

③

②

(st)

(ss)

Proc. mast.

knee of Sin. transvers./sigmoid.(projection)

skin incision
after
before retraction

①

FIG. 174 ⬚ 348

Fig. 174. Decompression of N. V and N. VII in cerebello-pontine angle.

Operation

A 1 Wider opening of wound spreader, after drilling burr holes (light arrow)

2 Continuation of craniotomy

B 1 Loosening of dura from Sinus transversus as far as Sinus knee –(k)–

2 Loosening on dura from bone medial to Os mastoideum

3a + 3b Cautious bone resection over Sinus sigmoideus (projection) –(ss)– as far as Processus mastoideus

C Edges of Sinus transversus and Sinus sigmoideus are exposed

Arrows: Especially endangered are Sinus sigmoideus edges (projection –(ss)–)

Abbreviations:

k Knee of Sinus transversus/Sinus sigmoideus

(k) Knee of Sinus transversus/Sinus sigmoideus (projection)

(ss) Sinus sigmoideus (projection)

st Sinus transversus

(st) Sinus transversus (projection)

FIG. 174

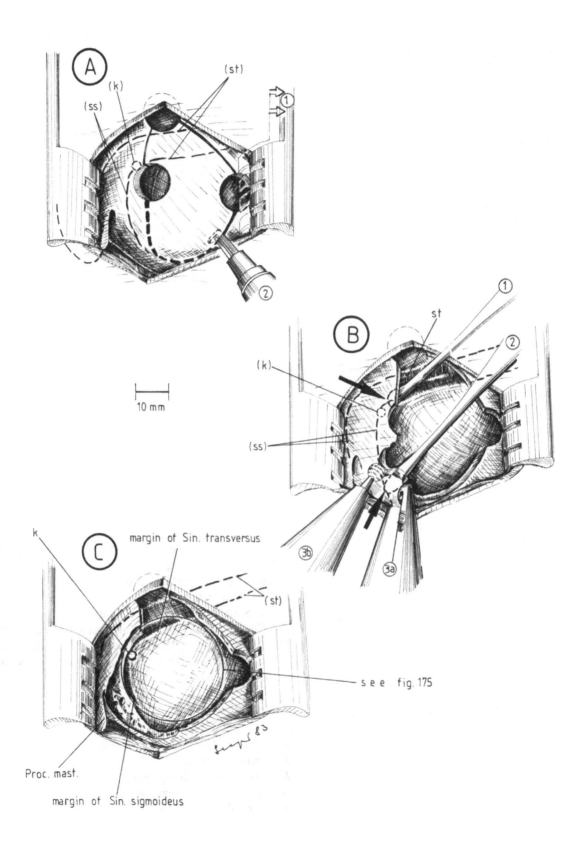

FIG. 175 ⊏━━━━━━━━━━━━━━━━━━━━━⊐ 350

Fig. 175. Decompression of N. V and N. VII in cerebello-pontine angle.
Microsurgical operation. Dura opening
A 1 Dura incision
    2 Suture of Lacuna near sinus
B Cerebellar surface after folding back of dura flaps
C Anatomical sketch of microsurgical site **B**; dorsal view of cerebellum, not dorso-lateral view, as during operation

Abbreviations:

bi Lobulus biventer cerebelli
fh Fissura horizontalis cerebelli
k   Knee of sinus
lq Lobulus quadrangularis
si Lobulus semilunaris inf.
ss Lobulus semilunaris sup.

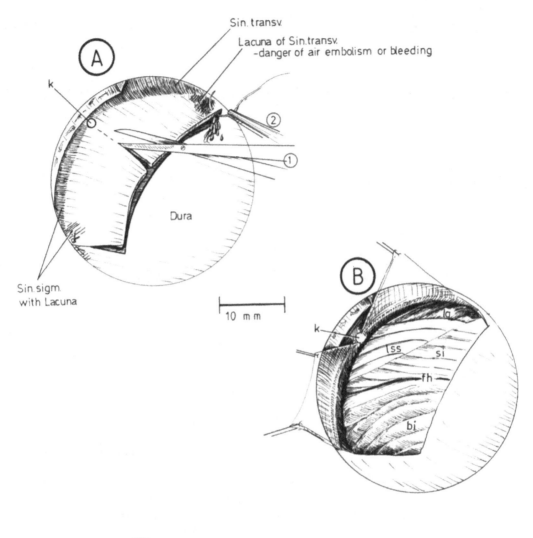

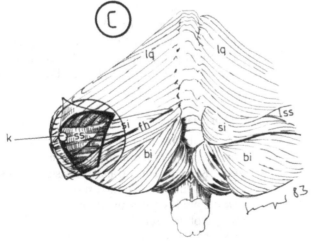

10 mm

FIG. 176 ⊏━━━━━━━━━━━━━━━━━━━━━━━━━━━━━━━━⊐ 352

Fig. 176. Decompression of N. V and N. VII in cerebello-pontine angle.
Microsurgical operation. Reclination of cerebellum

A Insertion of spatula

A' Anatomical sketch for microsurgical site **A.**
Arrow: view as in **A**

B After separation of slight adhesions, spatula is inserted more deeply

B' Anatomical sketch for microsurgical site **B**

C Enlarged detail from **B.** Separation of adhesions in the area of N. VII/VIII, Flocculus, V. petrosa sup. and N. V

Abbreviations:

bi Lobulus biventer
fh Fissura horizontalis cerebelli
k Knee of Sinus transversus/sigmoideus
lss Lobulus semilunaris sup.
qu Lobulus quadrangularis
si Lobulus semilunaris inf.
PS V. petrosa sup.

FIG. 176

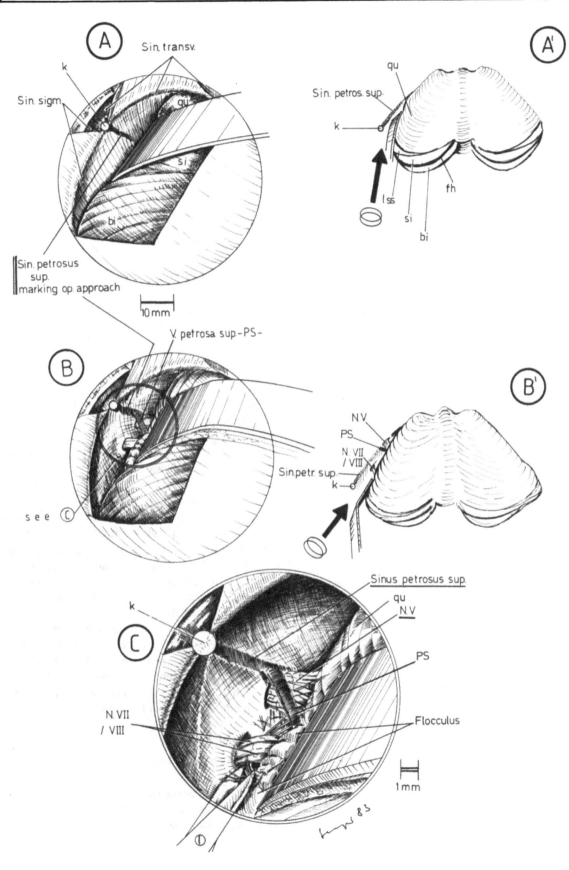

A

Sin. transv.

k

Sin. sigm.

qu

si

bi

Sin. petrosus
sup.
marking op. approach

10 mm

A'

qu

Sin. petros. sup.

k

lss

si

bi

fh

B

V. petrosa sup.-PS-

see C

B'

N V

PS

N. VII
/ VIII

Sin. petr. sup.

k

C

k

Sinus petrosus sup.

qu

N. V

PS

N. VII
/ VIII

Flocculus

1 mm

FIG. 177 ⊏━━━━━━━━━━━━━━━━━━━━━━━━━━━━━━━━━━⊐ 354

Fig. 177. Decompression of N. V and N. VII in cerebello-pontine angle.

Microsurgical operation

A **1** Separation of adhesions between Flocculus *–fl–* and V. petrosa sup. *–PS–*

    2 Separation of arachnoidal adhesions of N. V., A. cerebelli sup. and Lobulus quadrangularis *–qu–*. Further reclination of cerebellum by changing spatula position (light arrows)

A' Anatomical transection sketch of microsurgical site **A.** Anatomical topographical relation of loop of A. cerebelli sup., to N. V. and Pons

B **1** Separation of arachnoidal adhesions near A. cerebelli sup. loop

    2 Reclination of deeper lying cerebellar structures over N. V (structures close to surface can be reclined over N. V 5 to 10 mm, but deeper structures not more than 5 mm)

B' Anatomical topographical sketch for **B.** Section plane **A'** drawn in (broken line)

Abbreviations:

bp   Brachium pontis
fl   Flocculus
k   Knee of Sinus transversus/sigmoideus
qu   Lobulus quadrangularis
PS   V. petrosa sup.

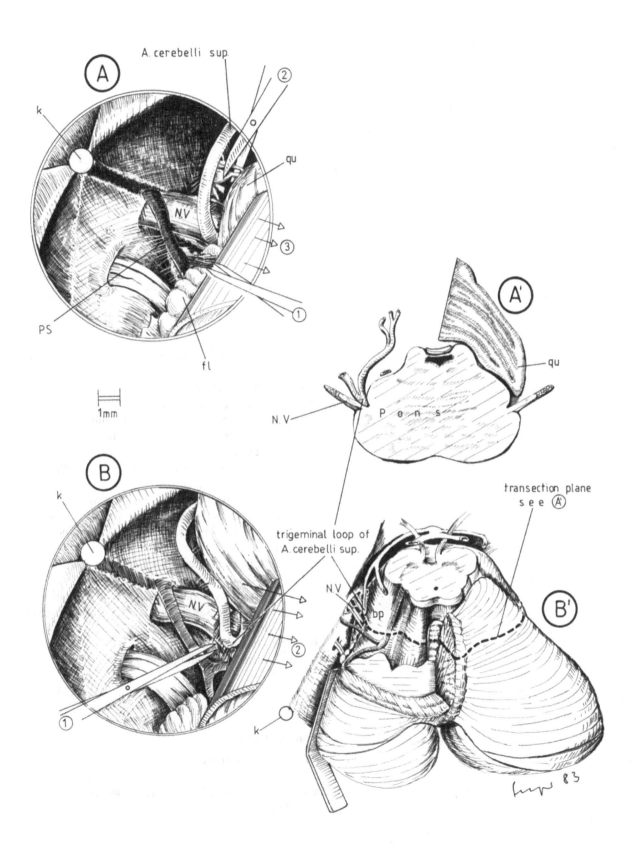

A. cerebelli sup.

k

qu

N.V

PS

fl

1mm

trigeminal loop of
A.cerebelli sup.

N.V

bp

transection plane
see Ⓐ'

k

Pons

qu

N.V

FIG. 178 ⌐⎯⎯⎯⎯⎯⎯⎯⎯⎯⎯⎯⎯⎯⎯⎯⎯⎯⎯⎯⎯⎯⌐ 356

Fig. 178. Decompression of N. V and N. VII in cerebello-pontine angle.

Microsurgical operation

A **1** Loosening and cutting of remaining adhesions between N. VII/VIII and Flocculus *–fl–*

2 Loosening of remaining adhesions at dura penetration point of N. V

3 Separation of remaining arachnoidal adhesions on A. cerebelli sup. loop

4 Again, slight forward positioning of spatula (light arrows), until the juncture Pons – Brachium pontis can be seen, at pontine N. V exit

B **1** Lifting of A. cerebelli sup. loop from N. V. and Brachium pontis *–bp–*.

Light arrow: small muscle piece is positioned between dorsal surface of N. V and A. cerebelli sup. loop

B' Operation site, overview

2 Excision of small muscle piece from nape muscles

3 Positioning of muscle piece between N. V. and A. cerebelli sup. loop, see **B**

Abbreviations:

bp   Brachium pontis
fl   Flocculus
k   Knee of Sinus transversus/sigmoideus
p   Pons

FIG. 178

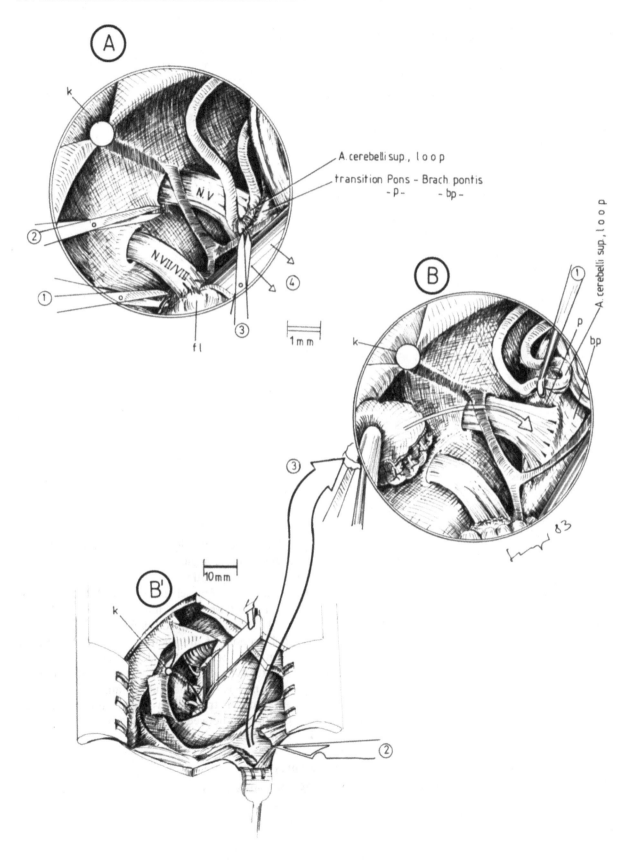

A

k

N V

② ②

① ①

N.VII/VIII

③

f l

④

A. cerebelli sup., l o o p

transition Pons – Brach. pontis
– p –   – bp –

1 mm

B

k

①

p

bp

A. cerebelli sup., l o o p

③

83

B'

10 mm

k

②

FIG. 179 ⬜━━━━━━━━━━━━━━━━━━━━━━━━━━━━━━━━━⬜ 358

Fig. 179. Decompression of N. V and N. VII in cerebello-pontine angle.

Microsurgical operation

A   **1** Insertion of muscle piece under V. petrosa sup. –*PS*–. Fascia and muscle are soaked with thrombin-calcium-solution*

      2 Injection of fibrogen concentrate* beneath muscle (between muscle and N. V)

      3 Attachment of A. cerebelli sup. loop to fascia by means of tissue glue*, similar to **2**

A' Anatomical transection sketch for **A.** Muscle positioning between artery and nerve

B   Dura suture, wound closure

Abbreviation:

PS   V. petrosa sup.

—————

* Immuno.

FIG. 179

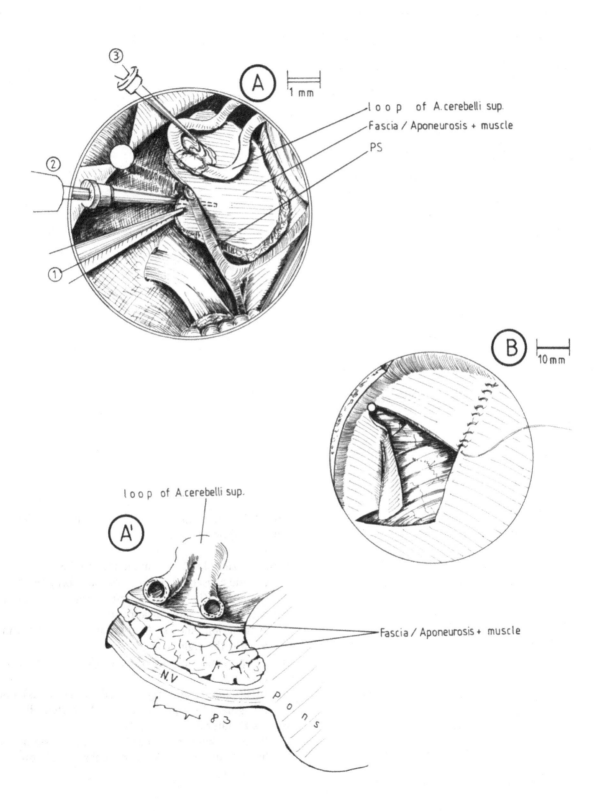

loop of A.cerebelli sup.
Fascia / Aponeurosis + muscle
PS

loop of A.cerebelli sup.

Fascia / Aponeurosis + muscle

N.V

Pons

FIG. 180 ⊏━━━━━━━━━━━━━━━━━━━━━━━━━━━━━━━━━⊐ 360

Fig. 180. Decompression of N. V and N. VII in cerebello-pontine angle.

Microsurgical operation

Clinical example of trigeminal neuralgia with facial tic on left side caused by A. basilaris loop compression of N. V and N. VII. After operation trigeminal neuralgia and facial tic have disappeared

A Angiogram shows A. basilaris loop, pointing toward the right side

A' Loop is not only pointing to the right side, but also dorsally

B In ap-angiogram (right sided A. cubitalis) one recognizes hypoplasia of right A. vertebralis

B' As B, lateral view

C Position sketch of A. basilaris and brain stem with hypoplastic right A. vertebralis based on angiogram

FIG. 180

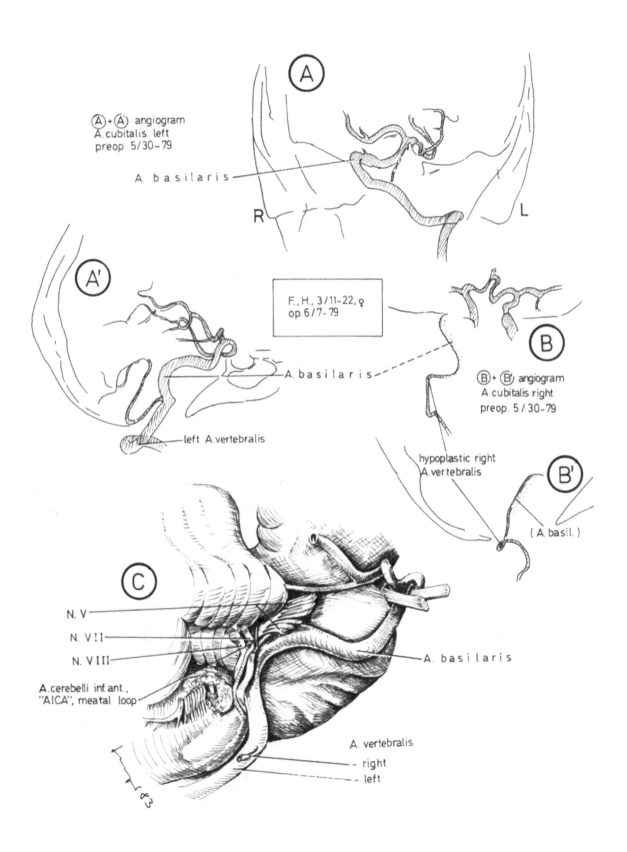

Ⓐ + Ⓐ́ angiogram
A.cubitalis left
preop. 5/30–79

A. basilaris

R   L

Ⓐ́

F., H., 3/11–22, ♀
op. 6/7– 79

A. basilaris

Ⓑ

Ⓑ + Ⓑ́ angiogram
A.cubitalis right
preop. 5/30–79

left A.vertebralis

hypoplastic right
A.vertebralis

Ⓑ́

(A. basil.)

Ⓒ

N. V

N. VII

N. VIII

A. basilaris

A.cerebelli inf.ant.,
"AICA", meatal loop

A. vertebralis

– right

– left

FIG. 181 ⊏══⊐ 362

Fig. 181. Decompression of N. V and N. VII in cerebello-pontine angle.

Microsurgical operation

A Microsurgical site. For teaching purposes, reclination of cerebellum between spatula and Porus acusticus int. is drawn approx. 2 cm wide. This site constitutes a combination of several microsurgical sites where, each time, reclination amounted to only 0,5 cm (repeated repositioning of spatula). One recognizes the close topographical relation of A. basilaris to N. V, VII and VIII

A' Anatomical sketch of cerebellum and lower brain stem, corresponding to microsurgical site **A**

B Cerebellum and lower brain stem, view from right sided dorsobasal direction. The drawn-in right cerebellum-pontine angle is deformed, corresponding to deformation caused by the atypical path of A. basilaris. Broken lines: projection of A. basilaris upon brain stem.

Arrows: **I** Operative approach to N. VII
II Operative approach to N. V

Abbreviations:

fl   Flocculus
(k) Knee of Sinus transversus/sigmoideus (projection)
pch Plexus chorioideus
sp Sinus petrosus sup.
te Tentorium
PS V. petrosa sup.

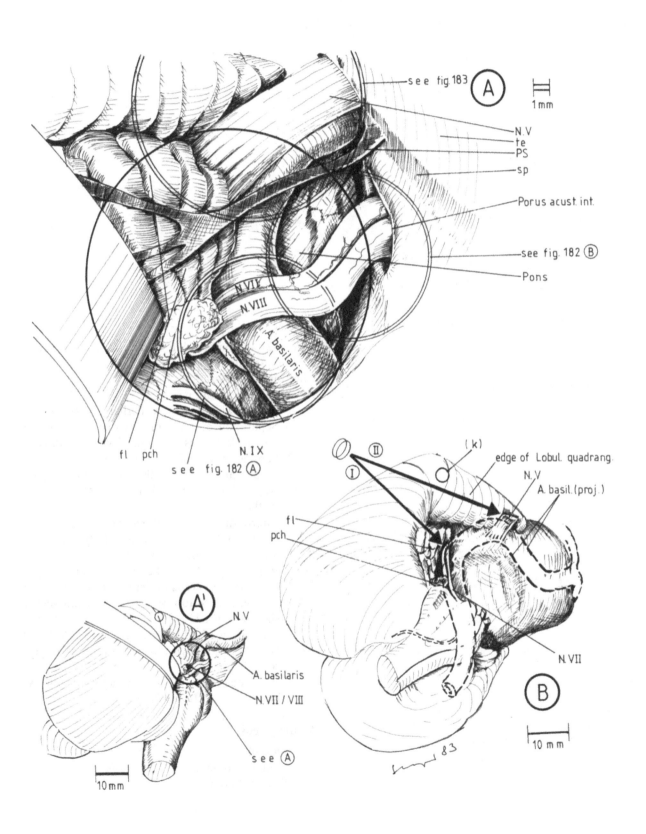

see fig.183 Ⓐ

1mm

N.V
te
PS
sp

Porus acust. int.

see fig. 182 Ⓑ

Pons

N.VII
N.VIII

A.basilaris

fl pch   N.IX

see fig. 182 Ⓐ

Ⓘ Ⓘ Ⓘ Ⓘ (k)   edge of Lobul. quadrang.

N.V
A. basil.(proj.)

fl
pch

N.VII

Ⓑ

10 mm

Ⓐ'

N.V
A. basilaris
N.VII / VIII

see Ⓐ

10 mm

FIG. 182

Fig. 182. Decompression of N. V and N. VII in cerebello-pontine angle.

Microsurgical operation

A Medial preparation

    1 **Slight** reclination of A. basilaris by sucker

    2 Separation of adhesions between A. basilaris and N. VII at its exit from Fossa supraolivaris

    3 Separation of adhesions between N. VII and A. basilaris at the middle portion of nerve path

    4 Repositioning of sucker, to check whether further adhesions must be separated

    5 Interposition of a muscle piece taken from nape muscles (with remnants of fibrous tissue)

B Lateral preparation at Porus acusticus int.

    1 Repositioning of sucker (during all preparations in the cerebello-pontine angle, minimal suction and cotton wool layer beneath sucker should be used)

    2 Separation of adhesions between N. VII and N. VIII. A. labyrinthi with branches is preserved

    3 + 4 Separation of further adhesions of A. basilaris, N. VII and N. VIII

Abbreviations:

fl   Flocculus
obl Medulla oblongata
pch Plexus chorioideus

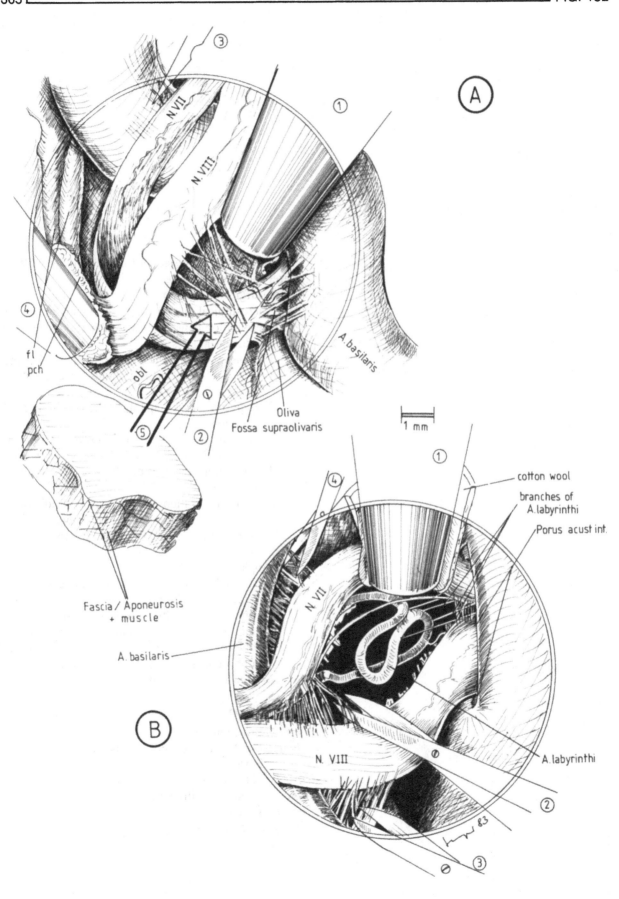

N. VII

③

N. VIII

①

④

fl
pch

obl

A. basilaris

①

⑤

②

Oliva
Fossa supraolivaris

1 mm

Fascia / Aponeurosis
+ muscle

A. basilaris

④

N. VII

N. VIII

B

①

cotton wool

branches of
A. labyrinthi

Porus acust. inf.

A. labyrinthi

②

③

FIG. 183 366

Fig. 183. Decompression of N. V and N. VII in cerebello-pontine angle.

Microsurgical operation

A Microsurgical site of N. V. As in Fig. 181, this presentation constitutes a combination of several microsurgical sites

  1 Separation of adhesions between N. V. and Pons –p–, as well as Lobulus quadrangularis –qu–

  2 Repositioning of spatula, after separation of adhesions

  3 Separation of adhesions between Tentorium –tc– and N. V

  4 Separation of adhesions between A. basilaris and N. V

  5a + 5b Preparation and separation of adhesions of N. V, Brachium pontis/Pons –bp/p–, as well as Flocculus. Note: V. petrosa sup. –PS– is hypoplastic

B Supplement to A

  2 Normally, Lobulus quadrangularis covers exit point of N. V from Brachium pontis/pons area –bp/p–. Only after preparation of Lobulus quadrangularis with separation of arachnoidal adhesions between Lobulus quadrangularis, brain stem and N. V., can reclination – as in 2 – be carried out, arrow

Abbreviations:

bp	Brachium pontis
bp/p	Brachium pontis/pons transition area
f	Flocculus
p	Pons
qu	Lobulus quadrangularis
te	Tentorium
PS	V. petrosa sup.

FIG. 183

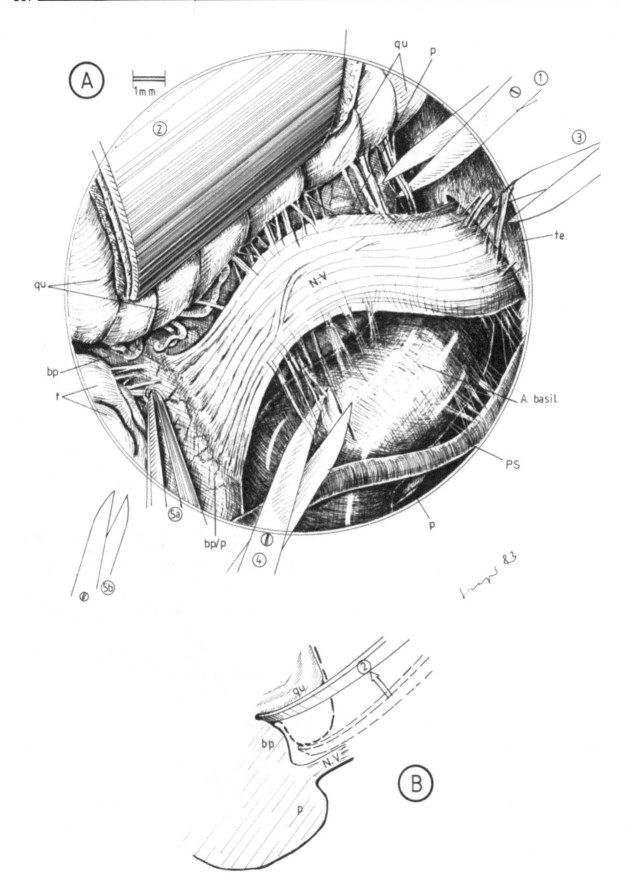

FIG. 184 ⊏ ⊐ 368

Fig. 184. Decompression of N. V and N. VII in cerebello-pontine angle.

Microsurgical operation

A   Microsurgical site. Muscle piece taken from nape muscles (with connective tissue) was inserted between N. V, VII and VIII and A. basilaris

    1 Muscle piece, soaked with thrombin/calcium solution, is squirted with fibrinogen concentrate*, in order to attach to A. basilaris

    2 Pressing of muscle piece against A. basilaris. **The thinner the fibrin film, the more reliable is the gluing**

B + B' Brain stem transections of mid-Pons and upper Medulla oblongata

B   Positioning of muscle between A. basilaris and N. V. Light arrow: Pushing A. basilaris away from N. V

B'   Positioning of muscle between A. basilaris and N. VII. Light arrow: Pushing A. basilaris from N. VII.

Wound closure

Abbreviations:

fl   Flocculus
pch Plexus chorioideus
qu   Lobulus quadrangularis
PS   V. petrosa sup.

---

* Immuno.

FIG. 184

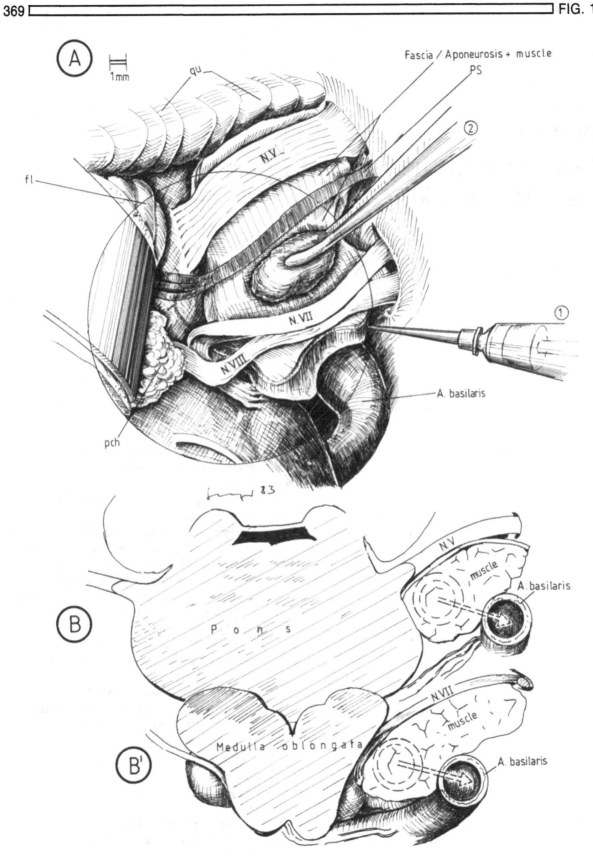

A

1mm

qu

Fascia / Aponeurosis + muscle

PS

2

N.V.

fl

N.VII

1

N.VIII

A. basilaris

pch

B

Pons

N.V

muscle

A. basilaris

Medulla oblongata

B'

N.VII

muscle

A. basilaris

FIG. 185   370

Chapter 6
Operations at the Base of Fossa cranii post.
(Figs. 185 to 200)

Epidermoid, pre- and paramedullary (Figs. 185 to 194)

Fig. 185. Basal tumors of posterior Fossa.
Clinical example of epidermoid: pre- and paramedullary, pre- and parapontine, pre- and paramesencephalic; no pre- or postoperative neurological deficits.
Diagnostic procedures

A   Premedullary tumor between Clivus and Medulla oblongata, extending to the right

B   Pre- and parapontine tumor portion. Beyond Tentorium temporomedially –x– a tumor portion is seen which expanded from Cisterna ambiens, beneath parahippocampal area, into supratentorial space

C   Tumor lies in front of and alongside Mesencephalon and widens Cisterna ambiens irregularly

A' – C'   Postoperative findings: no tumor remnant can be recognized; supratentorial temporomedial portion –x– is removed also

Abbreviations:

m   Mesencephalon
o   Medulla oblongata
p   Pons
p-m Ponto-mesencephalic transition
x   Temporo-medialy tumor portion

FIG. 185

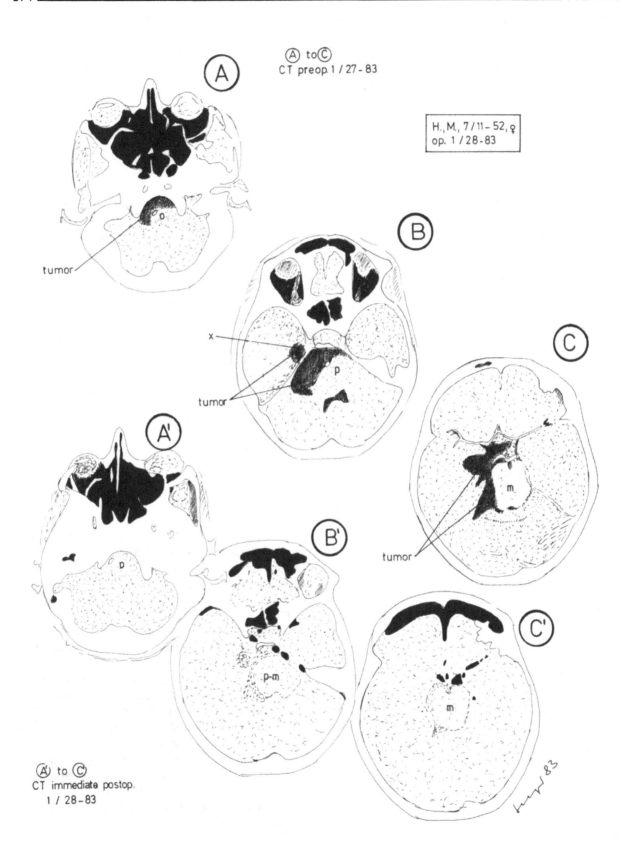

(A) to (C)
CT preop. 1 / 27 - 83

H., M., 7 / 11 – 52, ♀
op. 1 / 28 - 83

A

tumor

B

x

tumor

p

C

m

tumor

A'

p

B'

p-m

C'

m

(A) to (C)
CT immediate postop.
1 / 28 - 83

FIG. 186 ⬒━━━━━━━━━━━━━━━━━━━━━━━━━━━━━━━━━━━━━⬓372

Fig. 186. Basal tumors of posterior Fossa.
Operation of an epidermoid.
Microsurgical operation

A Anatomical sketch corresponding to Fig. 185 CTs.
Anatomical section planes lie transverse to brain stem axis, and thus lie in a different plane than that of CTs Fig. 185 **A – C**

B Anatomical section sketch, section planes see **A.**
Tumor displaced Medulla oblongata and expanded within several cisterns

C Anatomical section sketch, section plane see **A.**
Pons is compressed and displaced

D Anatomical section sketch, section plane see **A.**
Tumor reaches from Corpora quadrigemina area to N. oculomotorius, surrounding it.
(x): temporo-medial portion, projection on Tentorium undersurface

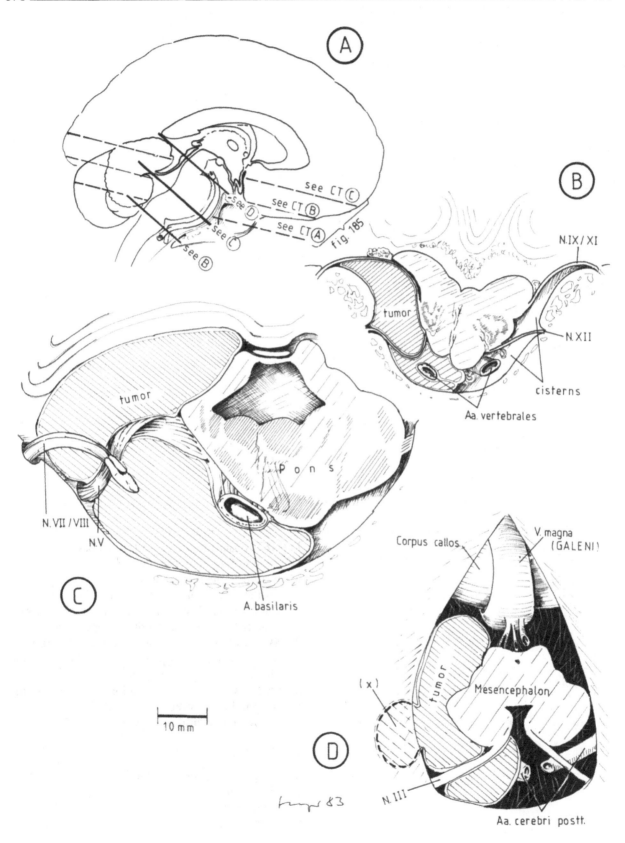

A

B

N.IX / XI

tumor

N.XII

cisterns

Aa. vertebrales

tumor

P o n s

N. VII / VIII

N.V

A. basilaris

C

10 mm

Corpus callos.

V. magna (GALENI)

(x)

tumor

Mesencephalon

D

N. III

Aa. cerebri postt.

FIG. 187 ⊏━━━━━━━━━━━━━━━━━━━━━━━━━━━⊐ 374

Fig. 187. Basal tumors of posterior Fossa.
Operation of an epidermoid.
Microsurgical operation

A Position of trepanation and dura incision, indicated on skull sketch. Position of skull corresponds to head position during operation

A' Sketch of skull base, view from above, trepanation sketched in, supplement to **A.** Arrow: initial direction of operative approach

B Operative site after trepanation and dura opening

C Reclination of cerebellum using spatula.
Arrow: microsurgical view for Fig. 188

Abbreviations:

fo Edge of Foramen occipitale
pm Processus mastoideus
ss Sinus sigmoideus
st Sinus transversus

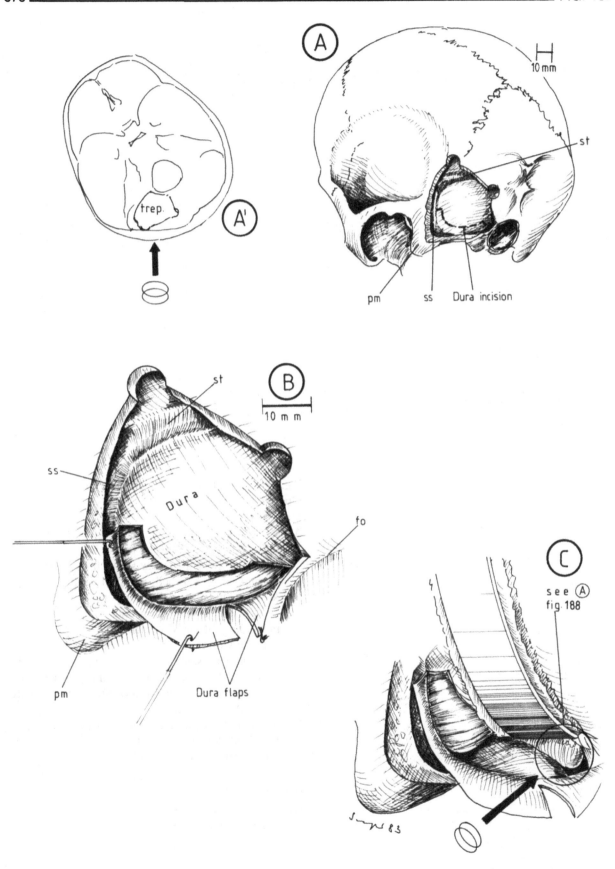

A

st
10 mm

A'

trep.

pm   ss   Dura incision

B
st
10 mm

ss

Dura

fo

pm   Dura flaps

C
see Ⓐ
fig. 188

FIG. 188 ⬚───────────────────────────────⬚ 376

Fig. 188. Basal tumors of posterior Fossa.
Operation of an epidermoid.
Microsurgical operation

A Microsurgical site. Continuation of Fig. 187
    1 Reclination of ·Tonsilla cerebelli
    2 Pulling away an artery (branch or hypoplastic trunk of A. cerebelli inf. post. -PICA-)
    3a + 3b Opening and pulling away arachnoidea lying over lower tumor end

B 1a Holding tumor with sucker
    1b Hollowing tumor with curette
    2a + 2b The same procedure as in 1a + 1b applied to a medial tumor lump in a second cistern chamber, in front of Medulla oblongata and A. vertebralis

C Anatomical position of tumor portions shown in A + B; posterior view, not lateral inferior view as microsurgical site

Abbreviations:

pch Plexus chorioideus
tj Tuberculum jugulare

FIG. 188

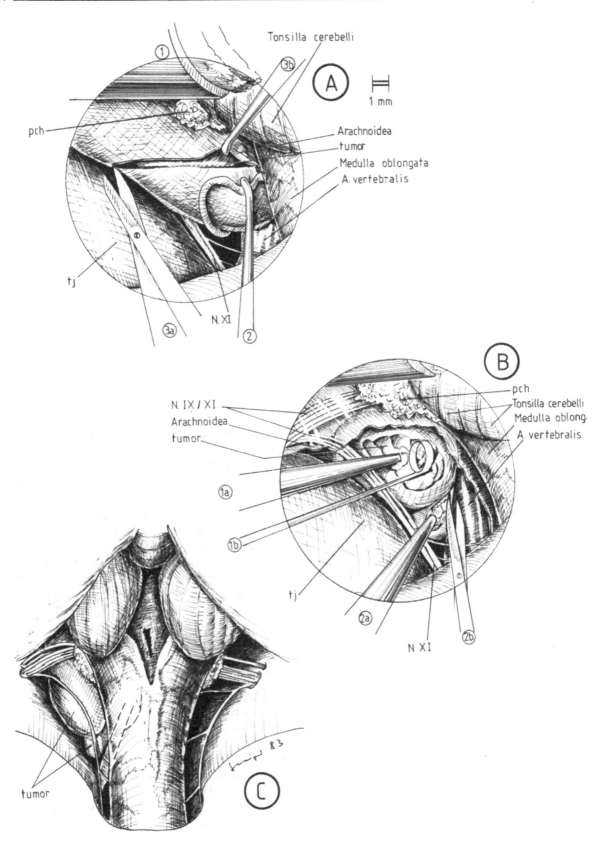

Tonsilla cerebelli

(A)

⊢⊣
1 mm

pch

Arachnoidea
tumor
Medulla oblongata
A. vertebralis

tj

N. XI

(B)

N. IX / XI
Arachnoidea
tumor

pch
Tonsilla cerebelli
Medulla oblong.
A. vertebralis

tj

N. XI

(C)

tumor

FIG. 189 ▭ 378

Fig. 189. Basal tumors of posterior Fossa.
Operation of an epidermoid.
Microsurgical operation

A Topographical relation after removal of lower tumor portions

B **1** Spatula placed farther laterally
2 Change of microsurgical approach (arrow)

C Microsurgical site, enlargement from **B**
1 Preparation and incision of arachnoidea and tumor (broken line), corresponding to **D** –x–. Microsurgical preparation corresponding to this sketch is presented in Fig. 190

D Anatomical sketch showing caudal tumor portion removed as far as hatched zone –x–

Abbreviations:

df   Dura flap
fl   Flocculus
mo Medulla oblongata
pch Plexus chorioideus
tj   Tuberculum jugulare
to   Tonsilla cerebelli
vl   A. vertebralis
x   Tumor resection surface (broken line in C)
PS V. petrosa sup.

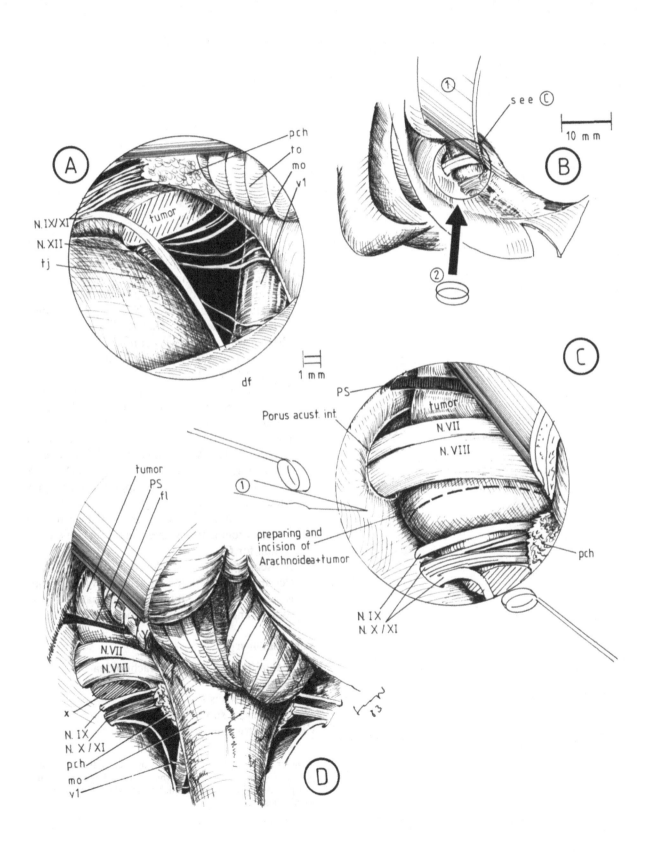

FIG. 190 ☐══════════════════════════════════════☐ 380

Fig. 190. Basal tumors of posterior Fossa.
Operation of an epidermoid.
Microsurgical operation

A **1a** Holding (and removal by suction) of tumor portion beneath N. IX to XI

    1b Hollowing tumor with curette

    2a + 2b The same procedure as in **1a + 1b** beneath N. VII and VIII

    3 Arachnoidea preparation and tumor incision as in Fig. 188 **A + B,** here between V. petrosa sup. –*PS*– and N. VII

B Loosening of tumor from undersurface of N. VII and N. VIII. Arachnoidal layer –*a*– covering tumor is left on undersurface of N. VII and N. VIII. Tumor shell can be separated from thickened arachnoidea in a single piece *

    2 + 3 Examination of arachnoidal niches for tumor remnents. Arrow: Change of view direction for **C**

C Loosening of tumor-enclosed N. V. Nerve fascicles are held together by arachnoidal layer, which is saved. In the meantime V. petrosa sup. –*PS*–, solitary and grossly hypoplastic, was interrupted

Abbreviations:

a   Membranous cisternal arachnoidea
fl   Flocculus
sp Sinus petrosus sup.
PS V. petrosa sup. (After ligation)
VP V. petrosa sup. (before Ligation)

---

* Tumor was completely enveloped by greatly thickened membranous cisternal arachnoidea (which here faciliated preparation and particularly protected cranial nerves sheathed by cisternal membranes).

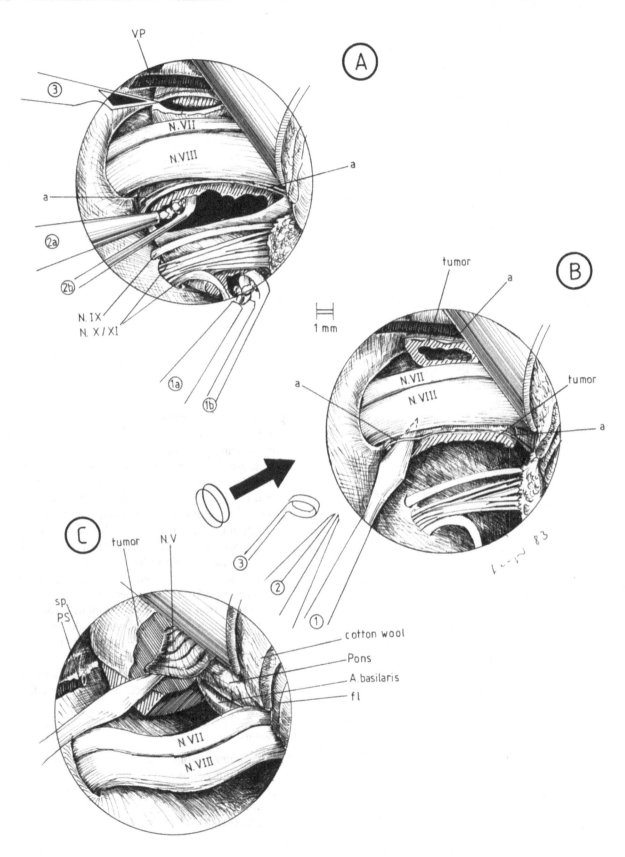

FIG. 191 ⊏══════════════════════════════════════⊐ 382

Fig. 191. Basal tumors of posterior Fossa.
Operation of an epidermoid.
Microsurgical operation

A Microsurgical site. Tumor loosened from N. V on all sides, however, tumor portions crowd rostrally and displace trigeminal fibers downwards.

B Site after removal of additional tumor portions

C Anatomical sketch of cerebellar and brain stem preparation, dura structures drawn in. Arrows: **A – C**: operative approaches for Figs. 192–194

  a Preparation in the direction of prepontine cistern and Cisterna interpeduncularis

  b Preparation in Fissura horizontalis cerebelli as far as Corpora quadrigemina region

  c Preparation in Cisterna ambiens as far as base of parahippocampus region

Trigonum lemnisci at lateral mesencephalon wall is, because of rich vascularization, specifically designated

Abbreviations:

bc Brachium conjunctivum
bp Brachium pontis
fl Flocculus
sp Sinus petrosus sup.
PS V. petrosa sup. (remnant)

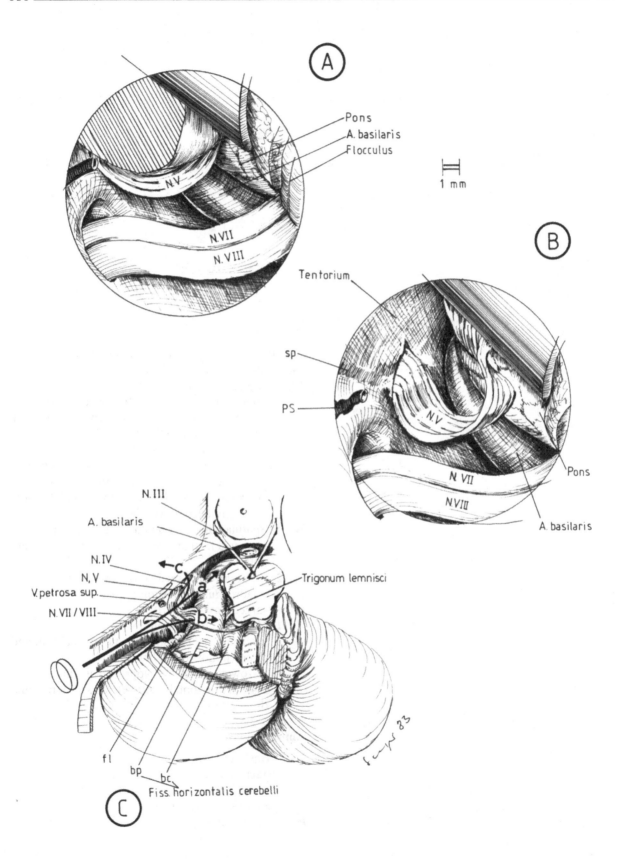

A

Pons
A. basilaris
Flocculus

N.V

N.VII
N.VIII

1 mm

B

Tentorium

sp

PS

N.V

Pons

N VII

N VIII

A. basilaris

N.III
A. basilaris
N.IV
N, V
V. petrosa sup.
N. VII / VIII

c
a
b

Trigonum lemnisci

fl
bp   bc
Fiss. horizontalis cerebelli

C

FIG. 192 384

Fig. 192. Basal tumors of posterior Fossa.
Operation of an epidermoid.
Microsurgical operation.
Microsurgical preparation **a** + **b** from Fig. 191 **C**

A **1** Further insertion of spatula and pulling back Lobulus quadrangularis *-qu-*. Brachium pontis *-bp-* becomes visible

2a + **2b** Arachnoidea preparation and opening of tumor as before. During tumor hollowing, A. cerebri post., N. IV and Crus cerebri *-cc-* gradually become visible

B **1** Spatula lying on Lobulus quadrangularis *-qu-*, is moved farther rostrally on Lobulus quadrangularis

2 Light arrows: reclination of rostral Lobulus quadrangularis portions *-qu-*

C Enlarged detail from **B**
1 New spatula position
2 Arachnoidea preparation, tumor incision, and tumor hollowing as before.
Arrow **b**: operative approach in direction of Fissura horizontalis cerebelli and Cisterna quadrangularis

Abbreviations:

a   Arachnoidea
bp Brach. pontis
cc Crus cerebri
qu Lobulus quadrangularis
te Tentorium

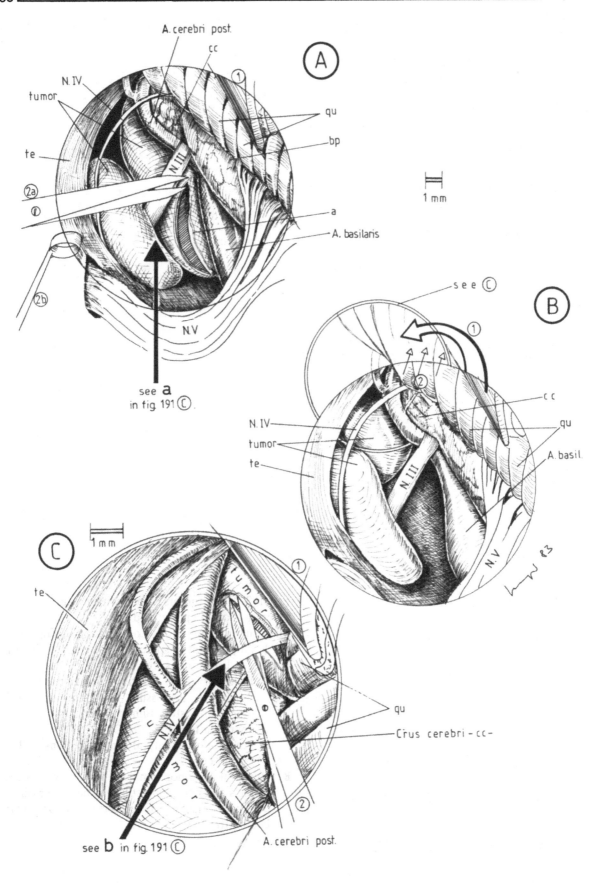

A

A. cerebri post.
cc
N. IV
tumor
te
①
qu
bp
N. III
②a
①
a
A. basilaris
②b
N V

see **a**
in fig. 191 ⓒ.

1 mm

B

see ⓒ
①
②
cc
N. IV
qu
tumor
te
A. basil.
N. III
N. V

C

1 mm
te
tumor
①
N. IV
②
qu
Crus cerebri – cc –
A. cerebri post.

see **b** in fig. 191 ⓒ

FIG. 193 □━━━━━━━━━━━━━━━━━━━━━━━━━━━━━━━━━□386

Fig. 193. Basal tumors of posterior Fossa.
Operation of an epidermoid
Microsurgical operation. Continuation of Fig. 192

A 1 Adjustment of spatula. One sees that Cisterna quadrigemina is free of tumor

2 Posterior and inferior to Corpora quadrigemina, in Fissura horizontalis cerebelli, there are still tumor remnants. (Arrow: approach **b** of Fig. 191 **C**)

3 Preparation of lateral tumor portions at Tentorium edge

B Removal of tumor remnants at Tentorium edge. Vessels and nerves are still sheathed by arachnoidal layer which is to be preserved. Arrows: varying approaches

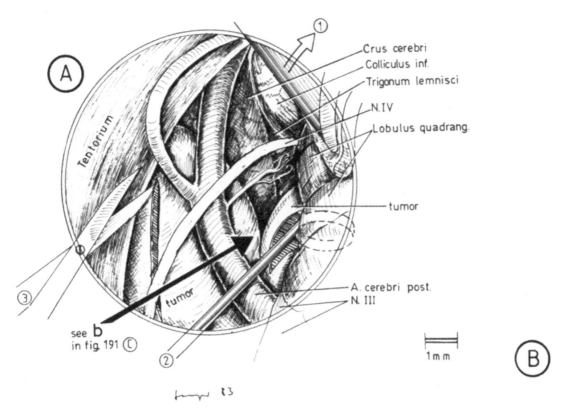

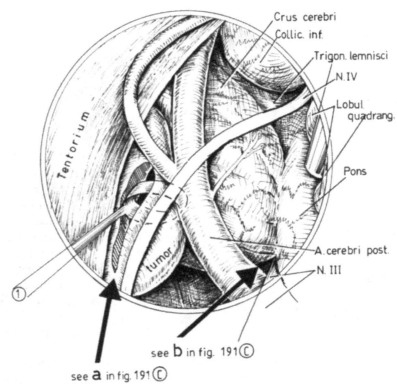

A

Crus cerebri
Colliculus inf.
Trigonum lemnisci
N.IV
Lobulus quadrang.

tumor

Tentorium

tumor

A. cerebri post.
N. III

see b
in fig. 191 ©

1 m m

B

Crus cerebri
Collic. inf.
Trigon. lemnisci
N.IV
Lobul. quadrang.

Tentorium

Pons

tumor

A. cerebri post.
N. III

see b in fig. 191©

see a in fig. 191©

FIG. 194 ⊏⊐ 388

Fig. 194. Basal tumors of posterior Fossa.
Operation of an epidermoid
Microsurgical operation
A 1 Cautious   bipolar   coagulation   close   to
      Trigonum lemnisci with minimal amperage
    2 After pushing N. IV aside, temporo-basal
      tumor portion is removed, which also lies in an
      arachnoidal chamber. Arrow: approach to Cis-
      terna ambiens and temporo-basal region
A' Site after tumor removal. **a, b, c** (arrows):
   approach directions (**a:** to Cisterna ambiens, **b:** to
   Fissura horizontalis cerebelli, **c:** to Cisterna
   ambiens and temporobasal region)
   See also Fig. 191 **C.** Check shows no further
   tumor. Wound closure

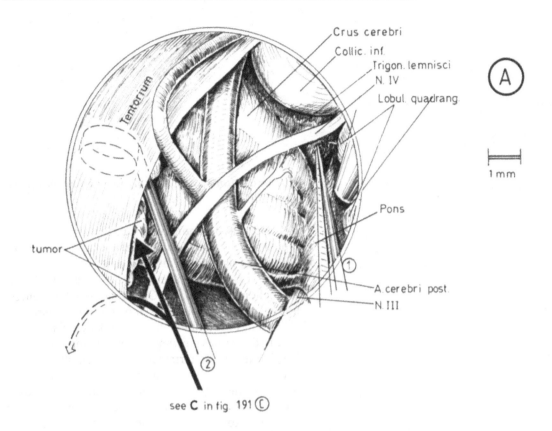

Crus cerebri
Collic. inf.
Trigon. lemnisci
N. IV
Lobul. quadrang.
Tentorium
Pons
tumor
A. cerebri post.
N. III
①
②
1 mm
Ⓐ

see **C** in fig. 191 Ⓒ

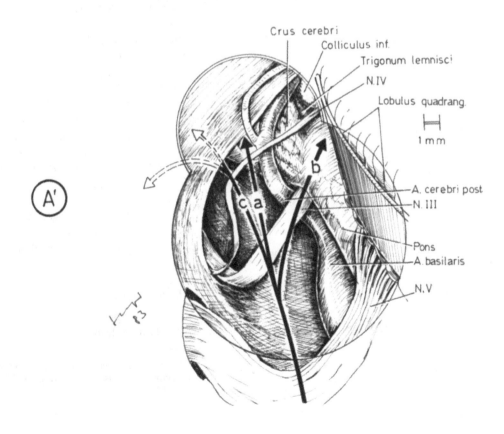

Crus cerebri
Colliculus inf.
Trigonum lemnisci
N. IV
Lobulus quadrang.
1 mm
Ⓐ'
c a
b
A. cerebri post
N. III
Pons
A. basilaris
N. V

FIG. 195 ⊏══⊐ 390

Extradural tumor with shift of Sinus sigmoideus (Figs. 195 to 200)

Fig. 195. Basal tumors of posterior Fossa.
Operation of richly vascularized extradural tumor, with **Sinus sigmoideus displacement**
Clinical example of aneurysmatic bone cyst in left cerebellopontine angle. One year ago hoarseness, noises in left ear, dizziness and vomiting. Neurological findings attributable to left caudal cranial nerves. Due to dangerous bleeding, biopsy attempt by outside hospital had to be terminated. Histological: aneurysmatic bone cyst. Two months later, partial embolization and renewed operative attempt, again terminated due to bleeding. One year later patient refered to our hospital. Additional peripheral VII paresis, postoperatively. After radical tumor removal*, diagnosis was verified
Diagnostic procedures

A	Old trepanation area –t– in preoperative X-ray
B – B"	CT: broad tumor surface connecting to Os petrosum, which shows gross asymmetry as compared to the other side. In addition, tumor reaches skull surface in previous trepanation area –t–
C + C'	Carotis angiogram shows tumor contrast medium uptake from A. carotis externa branches
D	Lateral enlarged detail from C
E	Poor showing of left Sinus sigmoideus in phlebogram, probably indicating medial displacement

Abbreviations:

ao   A. occipitalis
t   Trepanation

---

* N. VII graft reconstruction carried out later on by Prof. Helms, Director, Hals-Nasen-Ohren-Klinik (ENT-Department), University of Mainz.

FIG. 195

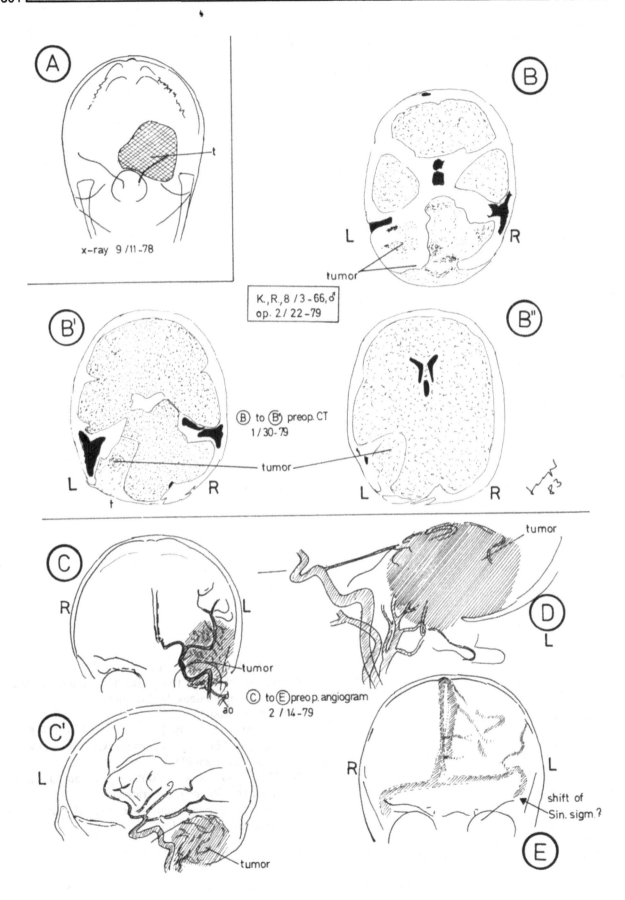

A   x-ray 9/11-78   t

B   tumor

K.,R.,8/3-66,♂
op. 2/22-79

B'   Ⓑ to Ⓑˮ preop. CT
1/30-79
tumor   L   R   †

B"   L   R

C   R   L   tumor   ao

Ⓒ to Ⓔ preop. angiogram
2/14-79

D   tumor   L

C'   L   tumor

E   R   L   shift of Sin. sigm.?

FIG. 196 □==================================□ 392

Fig. 196. Basal tumors of posterior Fossa.
Operation of richly vascularized extradural tumor,
with Sinus sigmoideus displacement
Anatomical sketches

A   Schematic horizontal section based on CT **B'** of
    Fig. 195. Sinus sigmoideus is luxated medially out
    of Sulcus sigmoideus

B   Skull drawing, with Sinus sigmoideus displace-
    ment (projection), superior view.
    Arrows: displacement direction of Sinus sig-
    moideus – broken line –

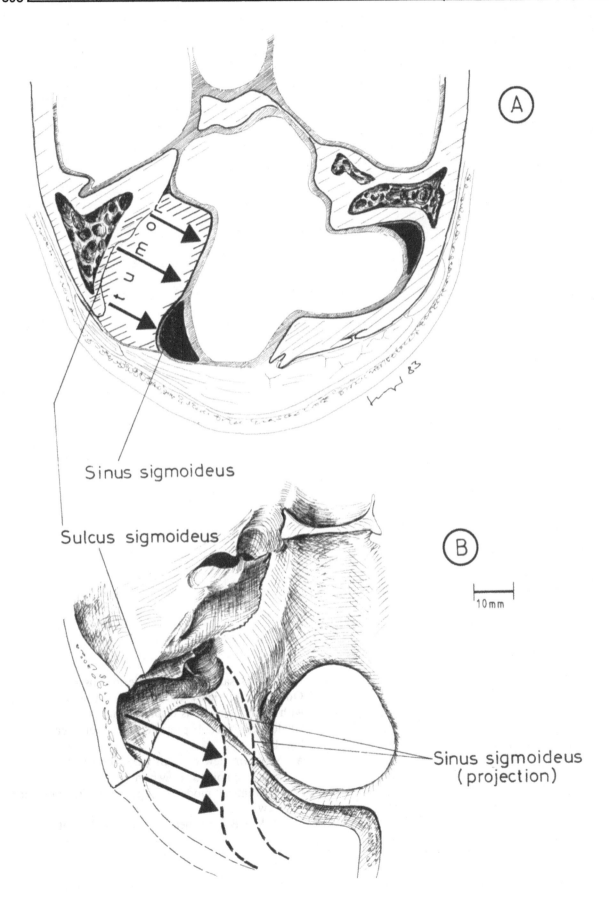

Sinus sigmoideus

Sulcus sigmoideus

Sinus sigmoideus
(projection)

10mm

FIG. 197 394

Fig. 197. Basal tumors of posterior Fossa.
Operation of richly vascularized extradural tumor, with Sinus sigmoideus displacement
Anatomical model presentation. Continuation of Fig. 195
A Superior view of skull base, dura and displaced Sinus sigmoideus drawn in
B Anatomical model of operation site, posterior view
In **A** + **B** dura sheath of N.VII/VIII not shown

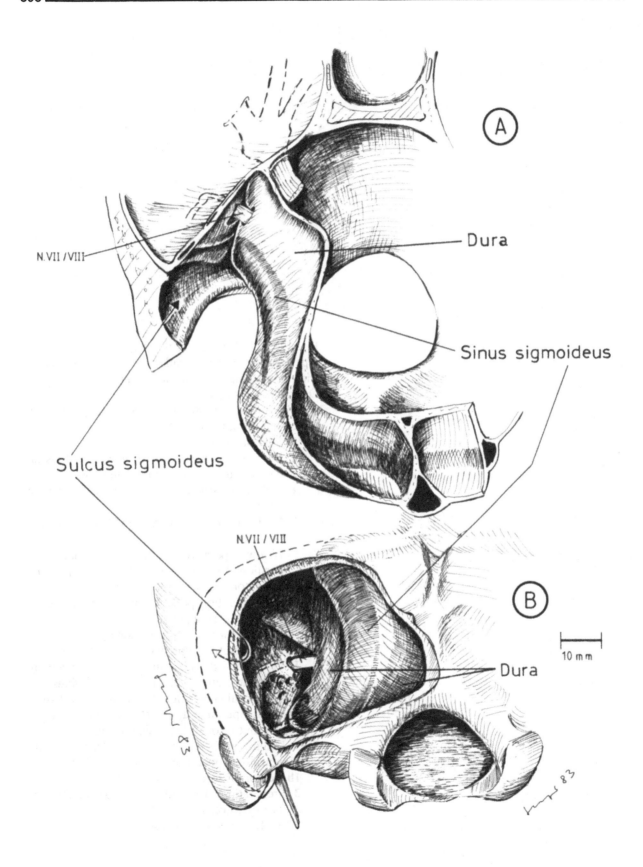

N.VII /VIII

Dura

Sinus sigmoideus

Sulcus sigmoideus

N.VII / VIII

Ⓐ

Ⓑ

10 mm

Dura

FIG. 198 ◻════════════════════════════════════◻ 396

Fig. 198. Basal tumors of posterior Fossa.
Operation of richly vascularized extradural tumor, with Sinus sigmoideus displacement
Operative tumor exposure

A Skin incision, posterior view (correct position on operation table see **B'**)
   1 Skin incision
   2 Monopolar coagulation of subcutis and fascia

B Situation after skin and muscle incision
   1 Incision of scarred periosteum at trepanation edge
   2 Pulling back periosteum, exposure of trepanation edge.
      Arrow: operative approach when patient is positioned on operative table, corresponding to anatomical sketch **B'**

B' During operation patient's head is turned sideways, in this example to the left – the side of tumor – as for acoustic neurinoma operation.
    Arrow: operative approach

C Removal of external tumor capsule scarred by previous operation. At first, relief of Sinus sigmoideus could not be identified within scar tissue. Previous operative approach had been partially carried out through Sinus sigmoideus
   1a Drilling of Os mastoideum, similar to acoustic neurinoma operation
   1b Incision of scarred tumor capsule
   2 Preparation of capsule back from tumor surface by forceps
   3 As **2**, carried out by dissector

FIG. 198

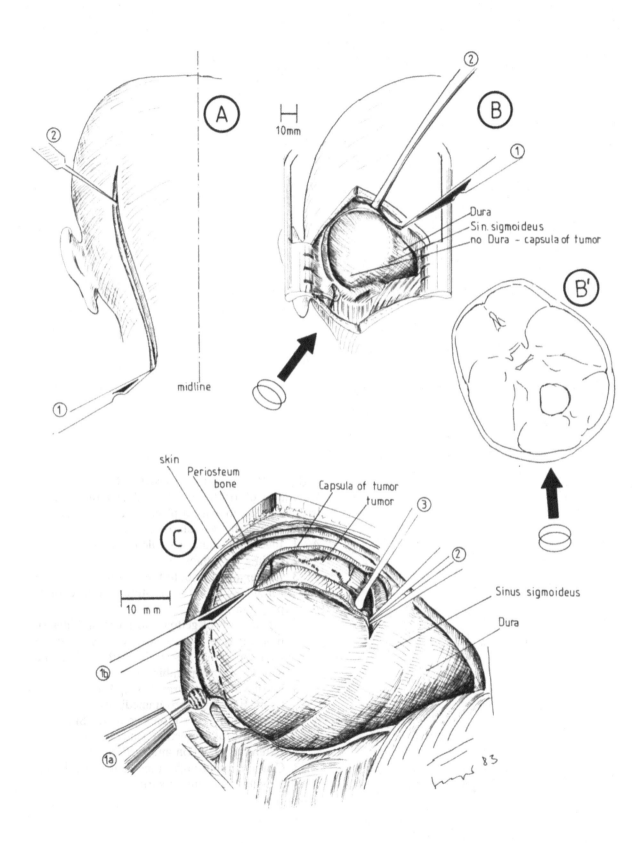

10mm

②

①

Ⓐ

midline

Ⓑ

Dura
Sin. sigmoideus
no Dura – capsula of tumor

Ⓑ′

skin
Periosteum
bone

Capsula of tumor
tumor

③

②

Ⓒ

10 mm

①b

①a

Sinus sigmoideus

Dura

83

Fig. 199. Basal tumors of posterior Fossa.
Operation of richly vascularized extradural tumor, with Sinus sigmoideus displacement
Isolation of richly vascularized tumor

A   1 Incision of tumor capsule portions
      2 Pulling back flaps
      3 Loosening of smooth tumor surface from dura (originally lying on posterior surface of Os petrosum)
      4 Application of gelfoam to bleeding Sinus sigmoideus gaps after removal of scars from previous operative approach. Gelfoam is soaked with Calcium/Thrombin
      5 Fibrinogen concentrate* is squirted under gelfoam. Bleeding stops immediately

B   1 Application of cotton wool to Sinus sigmoideus, for protection against heat
      2 Extensive irrigation and suction
      3 Cautious, thorough, time-consuming bipolar coagulation of tumor surface

---

* Immuno.

FIG. 199

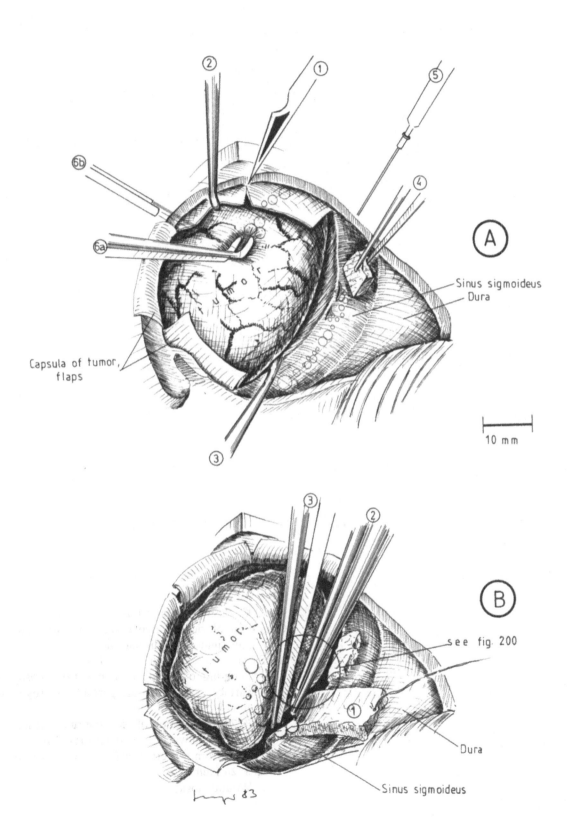

Capsula of tumor, flaps

Sinus sigmoideus
Dura

A

10 mm

B

see fig. 200

Dura

Sinus sigmoideus

FIG. 200 ⊏━━━━━━━━━━━━━━━━━━━━━━━━━━━⊐ 400

Fig. 200. Basal tumors of posterior Fossa.
Operation of richly vascularized extradural tumor, with Sinus sigmoideus displacement
A   Situation after tumor removal
  1 Scraping of tumor remnants from posterior surface of Os petrosum partially destroyed by tumor
  2a + 2b Coagulation of bleeding tumor residuals
B   1a + 1b Removal of tumor-infiltrated bone portions from posterior surface of Os petrosum
     2a + 2b Hemostasis
     Wound closure

FIG. 200

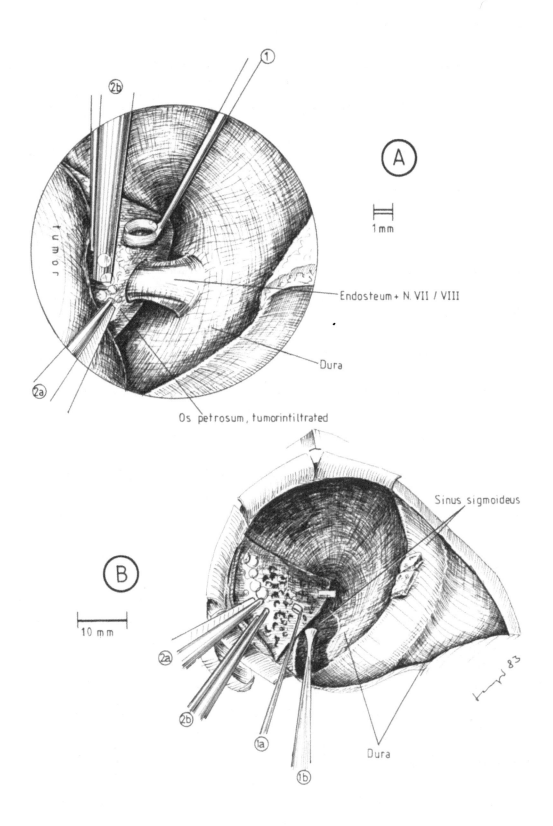

A

1 mm

Endosteum + N. VII / VIII

Dura

Os petrosum, tumorinfiltrated

B

10 mm

Sinus sigmoideus

Dura

References

Chapter 1

Van Alyea, O. E.: Sphenoid sinus. Anatomic study, with consideration of the clinical significance of the structural characteristics of the sphenoid sinus. Arch. Otolaryng. **34**, 225–253 (1941).

Bailey, P.: Tumors of the hypophysis cerebri. In: Cytology and Cellular Pathology of the Nervous System (Penfield, W., ed.), pp. 905–951. New York: Hoeber (1932).

Bailey, P., Cushing, H.: Studies in acromegaly. VII. The microscopical structure of the adenomas in acromegalic dyspituitarism (fugitiative acromegaly). Amer. J. Path. **4**, 545–563 (1928).

Bakay, L.: The results of 300 pituitary adenoma operations. J. Neurosurg. **7**, 240–255 (1950).

Bateman, G. H.: Trans-sphenoidal hypophysectomy. A review of 70 cases treated in the past two years. Trans. Amer. Acad. Ophthal. Otolaryng. **66**, 103–110 (1962).

Benda, C.: Pathologische Anatomie der Hypophysis. In: Handbuch der pathologischen Anatomie des Nervensystems (Flatau, E., Jacobsohn, L., Minor, L., eds.), Bd. 2, pp. 1418–1438. Berlin: S. Karger (1904).

Bergland, R. M., Ray, B. S., Torack, M.: Anatomical variations in the pituitary gland and adjacent structures in 225 human autopsy cases. J. Neurosurg. **28**, 93–99 (1968).

Borchardt, H.: Diskussion zum Vortrag Hochenegg. Verhandl. Ges. Chir. **37**, 85 (1908).

Borchardt, H.: The operative cure of acromegaly by removal of a hypophysial tumor. Ann. Surg. **48**, 783 (1908).

Broeckaert, J.: A contribution to the surgery of the hypophysis. J. Laryngol. **28**, 340–352 (1913).

Broeckaert, J.: Contribution à la chirugie de l'hypophyse. Presse Otolaryngolog. Belge **11**, 297–315 (1912).

Busch, W.: Die Morphologie der Sella turcica und ihre Beziehungen zur Hypophyse. Virchow's Arch. **320**, 437–458 (1951).

Calcaterra, T. C., Rand, R. W.: Current adjuncts for surgery of the sphenoid sinus and pituitary gland. Laryngoscope **86**, 1692–1698 (1976).

Chiari, O.: Ueber eine Modifikation der Schloffer'schen Operation von Tumoren der Hypophyse. Wien. Klin. Wschr. **25**, 5–6 (1912).

Collins, W. F., jr.: Transsphenoidal surgery in pituitary adenomas. In: The Pituitary – a Current Review (Allen, M. B., Mahesh, V. B., eds.), pp. 431–442. New York–San Francisco–London: Academic Press (1977).

Cope, V. Z.: Surgery of the pituitary fossa. Brit. J. Surg. **4**, 107–144 (1916).

Cummings, C. W., Johnson, J.: Transethmoidal approach to the pituitary adenomas. In: Current Techniques in Operative Neurosurgery (Schmidek, H. H., Sweet, W. H., eds.), pp. 173–180. New York: Grune & Stratton (1977).

Cushing, H.: Surgical experiences with pituitary disorders. J. A. M. A. **63**, 1515–1525 (1914).

Cushing, H.: Intracranial tumours. Notes upon a series of two thousand verified cases with surgical-mortality percentages pertaining thereto. Springfield, Ill.: Ch. C Thomas (1932).

Cushing, H.: Dyspituitarism: twenty years later. With special consideration of pituitary adenomas. Arch. Int. Med. **51**, 487–557 (1933).

Denker, A.: Hypophysentumoren. Int. Centralbl. Laryngol. Rhinol. **37**, 225 (1922).

Derome, P. J., Jedynak, C. P., Peillon, F.: Pituitary Adenomas; Biology, Physiopathology and Treatment. Paris: Asclepios (1980).

Dostoiewsky, A.: Ueber den Bau der Vorderlappen des Hirnanhanges. Arch. Mikr. Anat. **26**, 592–598 (1886).

Eiselsberg, A.: The operative cure of acromegaly by removal of a hypophysial tumor. Ann. Surg. **48**, 783–784 (1908).

Eiselsberg, A.: Operations upon the hypophysis. Ann. Surg. **52**, 1–14 (1910).

Eiselsberg, A., Frankl-Hochwart, L.: Über operative Behandlung der Tumoren der Hypophysengegend. Neurol. Zbl. **26**, 994–1001 (1907).

Erdheim, J.: Ueber Hypophysenganggeschwülste und Hirncholesteatome. S. Ber. Akad. Wiss. Wien, Math.-Naturw. Kl. Abt. III, **113**, 537–726 (1904).

Erdheim, J.: Über das eosinophile und basophile Hypophysenadenom. Frankf. Z. Path. **4**, 70–86 (1910).

Escher, F.: Hypophysektomie. Fortschr. Hals-Nasen-Ohrenheilk. **12**, 1–225 (1965).

Fahlbusch, R., Rjosk, H. K., v. Werder, K.: Operative treatment of prolactinproducing adenomas. In: Treatment of Pituitary Adenomas (Fahlbusch, R., Werder, K. v., eds.). Stuttgart: G. Thieme (1978).

Fein, J.: Zur Operation der Hypophyse. Wien. Klin. Wschr. **23**, 1035 (1910).

Ferner, H.: Die Hypophysenzisterne des Menschen und ihre Beziehung zum Entstehungsmechanismus der sekundären Sellaerweiterung. Z. Anat. Entwgesch. **121**, 407–416 (1960).

Fujii, K., Chambers, S. M., Rhoton, A. L.: Neurovascular relationships of the sphenoid sinus. A microsurgical study. J. Neurosurg. **50**, 31–39 (1979).

Guiot, G.: Transsphenoidal approach in surgical treatment of pituitary adenomas: general principles and indications in non-functioning adenomas. In: Diagnosis and Treatment of Pituitary Tumors (Kohler, P. O., Ross, G. T., eds.), pp. 159–178. Amsterdam: Excerpta Medica (1973).

Guiot, G.: Considerations on the surgical treatment of pituitary adenomas. In: Treatment of Pituitary Adenomas (Fahlbusch, R., Werder, K. v., eds.), pp. 202–218. Stuttgart: G. Thieme (1978).

Guiot, G., Derome, P.: Surgical problems of pituitary adenomas. In: Advances and Technical Standards in Neurosurgery (Krayenbühl, H., et al., eds.), Vol. 3, pp. 3–35. Wien–New York: Springer (1976).

Guleke, N.: Die Eingriffe am Gehirnschädel, Gehirn, an der Wirbelsäule und am Rückenmark. In: Allgemeine und spezielle Operationslehre (Guleke, N., Zenker, R., eds.), Vol. 2, 2nd ed., pp. 335–343. Berlin–Göttingen–Heidelberg: Springer (1950).

Halstead, A. E.: Remarks on the operative treatment of tumors of the hypophysis. With the report of two cases operated by an oro-nasal method. Trans. Amer. Surg. Assoc. **28**, 73–93 (1910).

Hamberger, C. A., Hammer, G.: Der transnasale Weg der Hypophysektomie. In: Hals-Nasen-Ohren-Heilkunde (Berendes, J., Link, R., Zöllner, F., eds.), Vol. 1, pp. 795–818. Stuttgart: G. Thieme (1964).

Hamberger, C. A., Hammer, G., Norlén, G., Sjogren, B.: Transantrosphenoidal hypophysectomy. Arch. Otolaryngol. **74**, 22–28 (1961).

Hammer, G., Rådberg, C.: The sphenoidal sinus. – An anatomical and roentgenologic study with reference to transsphenoid hypophysectomy. Acta Radiol. **56**, 401–422 (1961).

Hardy, J.: L'exérèse des adénomas hypophysaires par voie transsphénoidale. Un. Med. Can. **91**, 933–945 (1962).

Hardy, J.: La chirugie de l'hypophyse par voie transsphénoidale ouverte. Etude comparative de deux modalités techniques. Ann. Chir. (Paris) **21**, 1011–1022 (1967).

Hardy, J.: Transsphenoidal microsurgery of the normal and pathological pituitary. Clin. Neurosurg. **16**, 185–216 (1969).

Hardy, J.: Transsphenoidal hypophysectomy. J. Neurosurg. **34**, 582–594 (1971).

Hardy, J.: Transsphenoidal surgery of hypersecreting pituitary tumors. In: Diagnosis and Treatment of Pituitary Tumors (Kohler, P. O., Ross, G. T., eds.), pp. 179–194. Amsterdam: Excerpta Medica (1973).

Hardy, J.: Subnasal trans-sphenoidal approach to the pituitary. In: Microneurosurgery (Rand, R. W., ed.), ed. 2., pp. 105–130. St. Louis: Mosby (1978).

Hardy, J., Townsend, P. R., Gerundulo, D. G.: Forces applied by nasal speculums during transsphenoidal operations. Surg. Neurol. **10**, 361–363 (1978).

Hardy, J., Wigser, S. M.: Transsphenoidal surgery of pituitary fossa tumors with televised radiofluoroscopic control. J. Neurosurg. **23**, 612–620 (1965).

Henderson, W. R.: The pituitary adenomata. A follow-up study of the surgical results in 338 cases (Dr. Harvey Cushing's series). Brit. J. Surg. **26**, 811–921 (1939).

Heimbach, S. B.: Follow-up studies on 105 cases of verified chromophobe and acidophilic pituitary adenomata after treatment by transfrontal operation and x-ray irradiation. Acta Neurochir. (Wien) **7**, 101–155 (1959).

Heuer, G. J.: The surgical approach and the treatment of tumors and other lesions about the optic chiasm. Surg. Gynec. Obstet. **53**, 489–518 (1931).

Hirsch, O.: Eine neue Methode der endonasalen Operation von Hypophysentumoren. Wien. Med. Wschr. **59**, 636–637 (1909).

Hirsch, O.: Zur endonasalen Operation von Hypophysentumoren. Wien. Med. Wschr. **60**, 749–750 (1910).

Hochenegg, J.: Zur Therapie der Hypophysentumoren. Dtsch. Z. Chir. **100**, 317–326 (1909).

Horsley, V.: On the technique of operations on the central nervous system. Brit. Med. J. **2**, 411–423 (1906).

Kahler, O.: Zur Operation der Hypophysentumoren. Z. Ohrenheilk. **75**, 287–308 (1917).

Kanavel, A. B.: The removal of tumors of the pituitary body by an infranasal route. J.A.M.A. **53**, 1704–1707 (1909).

Kanavel, A. B., Grinker, J.: Removal of tumors of the pituitary body. Surg. Gynec. Obstet. **10**, 414–418 (1910).

Karduck, A., Bock, W. J.: Rhinological findings following transantrosphenoidal surgery of the pituitary gland. Acta Otolaryngol. **85**, 449–452 (1978).

Kern, E. B., Laws, E. R., Randall, R., Westwood, W. B.: A transseptal, transsphenoidal approach to the pituitary: An old technique in the managament of pituitary tumors and related disorders. Trans. Amer. Acad. Ophthalmol. Otolaryngol. **84**, 997–1010 (1977).

Killian, G.: Die submucöse Fensterresektion der Nasenscheidewand. Arch. Laryngol. Rhinol. **16**, 362–387 (1904).

Kirchner, J. A., Van Gilder, J. C.: Transethmoidal hypophysectomy: Some surgical landmarks. Trans. Amer. Acad. Ophthalmol. Otolaryngol., sect. Otolaryngol. **80**, 391–196 (1975).

Kocher, T.: Ein Fall von Hypophysis-Tumor mit operativer Heilung. Deutsch. Z. Chir. **100**, 13–37 (1909).

Krogius, A.: Neue Methode, den Nasopharyngealraum für die Operation von Basalfibromen und Hypophysengeschwülsten freizulegen. Zbl. Chir. **36**, 1420 (1909).

Landolt, A. M.: Progress in Pituitary Adenoma Biology. Results of Research and Clinical Applications. In: Advances and Technical Standards in Neurosurgery (Krayenbühl, H., et al., eds.), Vol. **5**, pp. 3–49. Wien–New York: Springer (1978).

Landolt, A. M.: Technique of Transsphenoidal Operation for Pituitary Adenomas. In: Advances and Technical Standards in Neurosurgery (Krayenbühl, H., et al., eds.), Vol. **7**, pp. 119–171. Wien–New York: Springer (1980).

Landolt, A. M., Kistler, G. S.: Morphology of chromophobe adenoma. In: Treatment of Pituitary Adenomas (Fahlbusch, R., Werder, K. v., eds.), pp. 154–171. Stuttgart: G. Thieme (1978).

Landolt, A. M., Siegfried, J.: Zur Behandlung maligner, metastasierender Tumoren mit der stereotaktischen transsphenoidalen Elektrokoagulation der Hypophyse. Schweiz. Med. Wschr. **100**, 1297–1306 (1970).

Landolt, A. M., Wilson, C. B.: Tumors of the sella and the parasellar area in adults. In: Neurological Surgery, 2nd ed. (Youmans, J. R., ed.). Philadelphia: Saunders (1980).

Lang, J.: Klinische Anatomie des Kopfes. Berlin–Heidelberg–New York: Springer (1981).

Lanz, T. von, Wachsmuth, W.: Praktische Anatomie, Vol. 1/1B. Berlin–Heidelberg–New York: Springer (1979).

Lautenschläger, A.: Die prämaxilläre Hypophysenoperation. Chirurg **1**, 30–33 (1929).

Laws, E. R.: Transsphenoidal approach to lesions in and about the sella turcica. In: Current Techniques in Operative Neurosurgery (Schmidek, H. H., Sweet, W. H., eds.), pp. 161–172. New York: Grune & Stratton (1977).

Laws, E. R., Kern, E. B.: Complications of trans-sphenoidal surgery. Clin. Neurosurg. **23**, 401–416 (1976).

Laws, E. R., Trautmann, J. C., Hollenhorst, R. W.: Transsphenoidal decompression of the optic nerve and chiasm. Visual results in 62 patients. J. Neurosurg. **46**, 717–722 (1977).

Loewe, L.: Ueber die Freilegung der Sehnervenkreuzung und der Hypophysis und über die Beteiligung des Siebbeinlabyrinthes am Aufbau der Supraorbitalplatte. Z. Augenheilk. **19**, 456–464 (1908).

Macbeth, R. G.: An approach to the pituitary via a nasal osteoplastic flap. J. Laryngol. Otol. **75**, 70–77 (1961).

Macbeth, R. G.: Hypophysectomy by the nasal route in advanced carcinoma of the breast. J. Roy. Coll. Surg. Edinburgh **6**, 199–205 (1961).

Macbeth, R. G., Hall, M.: Hypophysectomy as a rhinological procedure. Arch. Otolaryngol. **75**, 440–450 (1962).

Montgomery, W. W.: Transethmoidosphenoidal hypophysectomy with septal mucosal flap. Arch. Otolaryngol. **78**, 68–77 (1963).

Moszkowicz, L.: Zur Technik der Operation an der Hypophyse. Wien. Klin. Wschr. **20**, 792–795 (1907).

Mundinger, F., Riechert, T.: Hypophysentumoren – Hypophysektomie. Stuttgart: G. Thieme (1967).

Nager, F. R.: The paranasal approach to intrasellar tumors. J. Laryng. **55**, 361–381 (1940).

Netzer, H. R., McCoy, E. G.: Transseptal transsphenoidal hypophysectomy. A new approach. Arch. Otolaryng. **86**, 252–255 (1967).

Nowikoff, W. N.: Ein neuer Weg für Eingriffe an der Hypophyse. Zbl. Chir. **40**, 1000–1003 (1913).

Nurnberger, J. L., Korey, S. R.: Pituitary chromophobe adenomas. A clinical study of the sella syndrome: Neurology, metabolism, therapy. New York: Springer Publishing Comp. (1953).

Oehlecker, F.: Zur Trepanation des Türkensattels bei Tumoren der Hypophyse und der Gehirnbasis. Langenbeck's Arch. Klin. Chir. **121**, 490–511 (1922).

Olivecrona, H.: The surgical treatment of intracranial tumors. VIII. The pituitary adenomas. In: Handbuch der Neurochirurgie (Olivecrona, H., Tönnis, W., eds.), Vol. 4, part 4, pp. 228–301. Berlin–Heidelberg–New York: Springer (1967).

Palacios, E., Fine, M., Haughton, V. M.: Multiplanar anatomy of the head and neck for computed topography. New York: J. Wiley & Sons (1980).

Parkinson, D.: A surgical approach to the cavernous portion of the carotid artery. Anatomical studies and case report. J. Neurosurg. **23**, 474–483 (1965).

Parkinson, D.: Carotid cavernous fistula: direct repair with preservation of the carotid artery. Technical note. J. Neurosurg. **38**, 99–106 (1973).

Preysing, H.: Beiträge zur Operation der Hypophyse. Verh. Dtsch. Laryng. **20**, 51–66 (1913).

Proust, R.: La chirurgie de l'hypophyse. J. Chir. (Paris) **1**, 665–680 (1980).

Rand, R. W., Heuser, G., Adamas, D. A.: Ten-year experience with stereotaxie cryohypophysectomy. Progr. Neurol. Surg. **6**, 252–271 (1975).

Renn, W. H., Rhoton, A. L.: Microsurgical anatomy of the sellar region. J. Neurosurg. **43**, 288–298 (1975).

Romeis, B.: Hypophyse. In: Handbuch der mikroskopischen Anatomie des Menschen (v. Möllendorf, W., ed.), Vol. 6, part 3. Berlin: J. Springer (1940).

Rhoton, A. L., Jr.: Micro-operative techniques. In: Neurological Surgery (Youman, J. R., ed.), ed. 2., Vol. 1, pp. 1160–1194. Philadelphia: Saunders (1982).

Rhoton, A. L., Jr.: Ring curettes for transsphenoidal pituitary operations. Surg. Neurol. **18**, 28–33 (1982).

Rhoton, A. L., Jr., Hardy, D. G., Chambers, S. M.: Microsurgical anatomy and dissection of the sphenoid bone, cavernous sinus and sellar region. Surg. Neurol. **12**, 63–104 (1979).

Rhoton, A. L., Jr., Merz, W.: Suction tubes for conventional and microscopic neurosurgery. Surg. Neurol. **15**, 120–124 (1981).

Rhoton, A. L., Jr., Yamamoto, I., Peaace, D. A.: Microsurgery of the third ventricle: Part II. Operative approaches. Neurosurgery **8**, 357–377 (1981).

Rubinstein, L. J.: Tumors of the central nervous system. In: Atlas of Tumors Pathology. 2nd series, fascicle 6. Washington, D. C.: Armed Forces Institute of Pathology (1972).

Samii, M., Draf, W.: Course on Surgery of the Skull Base. Hannover, West-Germany (1979).

Samii, M., Draf, W.: Course in the Surgery of the Anterior Skull Base. Hannover, West-Germany (1980).

Samii, M., Jannetta, P. J.: Symposium on Cranial Nerves. Hannover, West-Germany (1980).

Schloffer, H.: Zur Frage der Operation an der Hypophyse. Beitr. Klin. Chir. **50**, 767–817 (1906).

Schloffer, H.: Erfolgreiche Operationen eines Hypophysentumors auf nasalem Wege. Wien. Klin. Wschr. **20**, 621–624 (1907).

Schloffer, H.: Weiterer Bericht über den Fall von operiertem Hypophysentumor. (Plötzlicher Exitus letalis 2½ Monate nach der Operation.) Wien. Klin. Wschr. **20**, 1075–1078 (1907).

Seeger, W.: Atlas of Topographical Anatomy of the Brain and Surrounding Structures. Wien–New York: Springer (1978).

Seeger, W.: Microsurgery of the Spinal Cord and Surrounding Structures. Anatomical and Technical Principles. Wien–New York: Springer (1982).

Smoler, F.: Zur Operation der Hypophysentumoren auf nasalem Wege. Wien. Klin. Wschr. **22**, 1488–1489 (1909).

Svien, H. L., Colby, M. Y.: Treatment for chromophobe adenoma. Springfield, Ill.: Ch. C Thomas (1967).

Tiefenthal: Technik der Hypophysenoperation. Münch. Med. Wschr. **67**, 794 (1920).

Tindall, G. T., Collins, W. F., Kirchner, J. A.: Unilateral septal technique for transsphenoidal microsurgical approach to the sella turcica. J. Neurosurg. **49**, 138–142 (1978).

Tönnis, W., Oberdisse, K., Weber, E.: Bericht über 264 operierte Hypophysenadenome. Acta Neurochir. (Wien) **3**, 113–130 (1953).

Tönnis, W.: Diagnostik der intrakraniellen Geschwülste. In: Handbuch der Neurochirurgie (Olivecrona, H., Tönnis, W., eds.), Vol. 4, part 3, pp. 150–185, Berlin–Heidelberg–New York: Springer (1962).

Trible, W. M., Morse, A. E.: Transpalatal hypophysectomy. Trans. Amer. Laryngol. Rhinol. Otol. Soc. 188–195 (1965).

Vourc'h, G.: L'anesthésie dans les hypophysectomies. In: Adénomes hypophysaires (Guiot, G., ed.), pp. 181–190. Paris: Masson (1958).

West, J. M.: Die Chirurgie der Hypophysis vom Standpunkt des Rhinologen. Arch. Laryngol. Rhinol. 23, 288–295 (1910).

West, J. M.: The surgery of the hypophysis from the standpoint of the rhinologist. J.A.M.A. 54, 1132–1134 (1910).

Wilson, C. B., Dempsey, L. C.: Transsphenoidal microsurgical removal of 250 pituitary adenomas. J. Neurosurg. 48, 13–22 (1978).

Yamamoto, I., Rhoton, Al., Jr., Peace, D. A.: Microsurgery of the third ventricle: Part I. Microsurgical anatomy. Neurosurgery 8, 334–356 (1981).

Zervas, N. T.: Stereotaxic thermal hypophysectomy. Progr. Neurol. Surg. 6, 217–251 (1975).

Chapter 2

Abbie, A. A.: The clinical significance of the anterior choroidal artery. Brain 56, 233–246 (1933).

Agati, D.: Ipertrofie etmoido-sfenoidali a protundenza endocranica. Radiol. Med. 32, 151–154 (1946).

Arnold, F.: Handbuch der Anatomie des Menschen. Vol. 2, pt. 1, p. 465. Freiburg i. Br.: Herder'sche Verlagshandlung (1847) (Cited by Meyer, 1887).

Bacon, T., Duchesneau, P. M., Weinstein, M. A.: Demonstration of the superior ophthalmic vein by high resolution computed tomography. Radiology 124, 129 (1977).

Balèiaux-Wada, D., Mortelmans, L. L., Dupont, M. G., et al.: The use of coronal scans for computed tomography of the orbits. Neuroradiology 14, 89 (1977).

Bedford, M. A.: The "cavernous sinus". Brit. J. Ophthal. 50, 41–46 (1966).

Bendescu, T.: Beiderseitige Optikusatrophie verursacht durch Pneumosinus dilatans der rechten Keilbeinhöhle. Z. Augenheilk. 79, 41–50 (1932).

Bergland, R., Ray, S.: The arterial supply of the human optic chiasm. J. Neurosurg. 31, 327–334 (1969).

Bonnal, J., Thibaut, A., Brotchi, J., et al.: Invading meningiomas of the sphenoid ridge. J. Neurosurg. 53, 587–599 (1980).

Bonnet, P.: La loge caverneuse et les syndromes de la loge caverneuse. Arch. Ophtalmol. (Paris) 15, 357–372 (1955).

Brismar, J., Brismar, G., Davis, K. R.: Superior ophthalmic vein at computed tomography. Acta Radiol. (Stock.) 18, 273 (1977).

Butler, H.: The development of certain human dural venous sinuses. J. Anat. 91, 510–526 (1957).

Cabanis, E. A., Iba-Zizen, M. T., et al.: Tomodensiometric anatomy of the orbital blood vessels. Bull. Soc. Ophthalmol. Fr. 6–7, 511 (1979).

Christensen, J. B., Telford, I. R.: Synopsis of Gross Anatomy with Clinical Correlations, ed. 3, p. 275, New York: Harper and Row (1978).

Clay, C., Vignaut, J., Aubin, M. L., et al.: Phlébographie orbitaire et du sinus caverneux. Gaz. Med. France 80, 2073–2086 (1973).

Crafts, R. D.: A Textbook of Human Anatomy, ed. 2, pp. 503–505. New York: J. Wiley and Sons (1979).

Craig, W. M., Gogela, L. J.: Meningioma of the optic foramen as a cause of slowly progressive blindness. Report of three cases. J. Neurosurg. 7, 44–48 (1950).

van Damme, W., Kosman, P., Wackenheim, A.: A standardized method for computed tomography of the orbits. Neuroradiology 13, 139 (1977).

Dandy, W. E.: Prechiasmal intracranial tumors of the optic nerves. Am. J. Ophthalmol. 5, 169–188 (1922).

Dawson, B. H.: The blood vessels of the human optic chiasm and their relation to those of the hypophysis and hypothalamus. Brain 81, 207–217 (1958).

DiDio, L. J. A.: Synopsis of Anatomy, p. 394. St. Louis: Mosby (1970).

Duke-Elder, S.: Textbook of Ophthalmology, Vol. 1, pp. 102, 182, 184, 188, 401. London: Kimpton (1932).

Dunker, R. O., Harris, A. B.: Surgical anatomy of the proximal anterior cerebral artery. J. Neurosurg. 44, 359–367 (1976).

Gardner, E., Gray, D. J., O'Rahilly, R.: Anatomy. A Regional Study of Human Structure, ed. 4, p. 609. Philadelphia: W. B. Saunders (1975).

Glenn, W. V., Johnson, R. J., et al.: Further investigation and clinical use of advanced CT display capability. Invest. Radiol. 10, 479 (1975).

Goddé-Jolly, D., Cabanis, E. A., et al.: Tomodensiometric anatomy and physiology of the muscle cone. Bull. Soc. Ophthalmol. Fr. 3, 215 (1980).

Grant, J. C. B.: A Method of Anatomy, 6th ed., p. 660. Baltimore: Williams and Wilkins (1958).

Hacker, H.: Venenabflüsse des Gehirns. Deutscher Röntgenkongreß (1967), Part A. Stuttgart: G. Thieme (1968b).

Harris, F. S., Rhoton, A. L., Jr.: Anatomy of the cavernous sinus. A microsurgical study. J. Neurosurg. 45, 169–180 (1976).

Haverling, M., Johanson, H.: Computed sagittal tomography of the orbit. A. J. R. 131, 346 (1978).

Hayreh, S. S., Dass, R.: The ophthalmic artery. Brit. J. Ophthal. 46, 65–97 (1962).

Hollenhorst, R. W., Jr., Hollenhorst, R. W., et al.: Visual prognosis of optic nerve sheath meningiomas producing shunt vessels on the optic disk. Mayo. Clin. Proc. 53, 84–92 (1978).

Hollinshead, W. H.: Anatomy for Surgeons, Vol. 1, p. 156. New York: Hoeber (1954).

Hughes, B.: Blood supply of the optic nerves and chiasma and its clinical significance. Brit. J. Ophthal. 42, 106–125 (1958).

James, B. P., Lawton Smith, J.: Bilateral optic nerve sheath meningiomas presenting as the chiasmal syndrome. Neuro-Ophthalmology Update, pp. 177–183. New York: Masson Publishing USA (1977).

Johnston, T. B., Davies, D. V., Davies, F.: Gray's Anatomy, 32nd ed., p. 757. London: Longmans Green (1958).

Lang, J.: Klinische Anatomie des Kopfes. Berlin–Heidelberg–New York: Springer (1981).

Lanz, T. von, Wachsmuth, W.: Praktische Anatomie, Vol. 1/1 B. Berlin–Heidelberg–New York: Springer (1979).

Lawrence, W., Hirst, M. D., et al.: Sphenoidal pneumosinus dilatans with bilateral optic nerve meningiomas. Case report. J. Neurosurg. **51**, 402–407 (1979).

Leonardi, M., Barbina, V., et al.: Sagittal computed tomography of the orbit. J. Comput. Assist. Tomogr. **1**, 511 (1977).

LeRebellar, M. J., Caillé, J. M., et al.: Tomodensiometric aspects of the normal and pathologic eyeball. Bull. Soc. Ophthalmol. Fr. **80**, 307 (1980).

Liliequist, B.: The subarachnoid cisterns. Anatomic and roentgenologic study. Acta radiol. (Stockh.) Suppl. 185 (1959).

Little, H. L., Chambers, J. W., Walsh, F. B.: Unilateral intracranial optic nerve involvement. Neurosurgical significance. Arch. Ophthalmol. **73**, 331–337 (1965).

Lombardi, G., Passerini, A., Cecchini, A.: Pneumosinus dilatans. Acta Radiol. (Diagn). **7**, 535–542 (1968).

Macialowicz, T.: A case of dilating pneumosinus of the sphenoid sinus and the posterior ethmoid cells. Pol. Rev. Radiolog. Nucl. Med. **33**, 324–330 (1969).

Manelfe, C. L., Pasquini, U., Bank, W. O.: Metrizamide demonstration of the subarachnoid space surrounding the optic nerves. J. Comput. Assist. Tomogr. **2**, 545 (1978).

Manelfe, C., Tremoulet, M., Roulleau, J.: Étude artériographique des branches intracaverneuses de la carotide interne. Neurochirurgie **18**, 581–598 (1972).

Mayer, E. G.: Über Lageanomalien des Planum sphenoidale und ihre diagnostische Bedeutung. Roentgenpraxis **6**, 427–431 (1934).

McGrath, P.: The cavernous sinus; an anatomical survey. Aust. NZ J. Surg. **47**, 601–613 (1977).

Nathan, H., Goldhammer, Y.: The rootlets of the trochlear nerve. Anatomical observations in human brains. Acta Anat. **84**, 590–596 (1973).

Nathan, H., Quaknine, G., Kosary, I. Z.: The abducens nerve. Anatomical variations in its course. J. Neurosurg. **41**, 561–566 (1974).

Palacios, E., Fine, M., Haughton, V. M.: Multiplanar Anatomy of the Head and Neck for Computed Tomography. New York: John Wiley & Sons (1980).

Parkinson, D.: A surgical approach to the cavernous portion of the carotid artery. Anatomical studies and case report. J. Neurosurg. **23**, 474–483 (1965).

Patouillard, P., Vanneuville, G.: Les parois du sinus caverneux. Neurochirurgie **18**, 551–560 (1972).

Paturet, G.: Traité d'Anatomie Humaine, Vol. **IV**, pp. 721–722. Système Nerveux. Paris: Masson (1964).

Perlmutter, D., Rhoton, A. L., Jr.: Microsurgical anatomy of the anterior cerebral-anterior communicating-recurrent artery complex. J. Neurosurg. **45**, 259–271 (1976).

Potter, G. D., Trokel, S. L.: The Optic Canal. In: Radiology of the Skull and Brain: Technical Aspects of Computed Tomography (Newton, T. H., Potts, D. G., eds.), Vol. **5**. St. Louis: Mosby (1981).

Prives, M. G., Lisenkov, N. K., Bushkovich, V. I.: Human Anatomy, ed. **7**, 815 pp. Leningrad: Izdatelstvo "Medisina" (1969).

Quiroz-Gutiérrez, F.: Tratado de Anatomia Humana, Vol. **II**, pp. 146–389. Mexico City: Editorial Porrua (1965).

Rabischong, P., Clay, C., Vignaud, J., et al.: Approche hémodynamique de la signification fonctionnelle du sinus caverneux. Neurochirurgie **18**, 613–622 (1972).

Rhoton, A. L., Jr., Hardy, D. G., Chambers, S. M.: Microsurgical anatomy and dissection of the sphenoid bone, cavernous sinus and sellar region. Surg. Neurol. **12**, 63–104 (1979).

Ridley, H.: The Anatomy of the Brain, p. 39. London: Smith and Walford (1695).

Romanes, G. J.: Cunningham's Textbook of Anatomy, ed. **12**, p. 953. London: Oxford University Press (1981).

Rouvière, H.: Anatomie Humaine. Descriptive et Topographique, ed. **10**, Vol. III, p. 678. Paris: Masson (1970).

Salvolini, U., Cabanis, E. A., et al.: Computed tomography of the optic nerve: Part 1. Normal results. J. Comput. Assist. Tomogr. **2**, 141 (1978).

Samii, M., Draf, W.: Course on Surgery of the Skull Base. Hannover, West Germany (1979).

Samii, M., Draf, W.: Course in the Surgery of the Anterior Skull Base. Hannover, West-Germany (1980).

Samii, M., Draf, W.: Course on the Surgery of the Middle Skull Base. Hannover, West-Germany (1981).

Samii, M., Jannetta, P. J.: Symposium on Cranial Nerves. Hannover, West-Germany (1980).

Schaeffer, J. P.: Morris's Human Anatomy, 11th ed., p. 658. New York: McGray-Hill (1953).

Schott: On some affections of the optic nerve. Arch. Ophthalmol. **6**, 262–283 (1877).

Seeger, W.: Atlas of Topographical Anatomy of the Brain and Surrounding Structures. Wien–New York: Springer (1978).

Seeger, W.: Microsurgery of the Brain. Anatomical and Technical Principles, Vol. 1 + 2. Wien–New York: Springer (1980).

Sinelnikov, P. D.: Atlas of Human Anatomy, Vol. **2**, p. 154. Moscow: Izdatelstvo "Medisina" (1958).

Snell, R. S.: Clinical Anatomy for Students, ed. **2**, Fig. 43. Boston: Little, Brown and Co. (1981).

Sundt, T. M., Jr., Murphey, F.: Clipcrafts for aneurysm and small vessel surgery. Part 3: Clinical experience in intracranial carotid artery aneurysms. J. Neurosurg. **31**, 59–71 (1969).

Sugita, K., Hirota, T., Iguchi, I., et al.: Transient amaurosis under decreased atmospheric pressure with sphenoidal sinus dysplasia. Case report. J. Neurosurg. **46**, 111–114 (1977).

Tadmor, R., New, F. J.: Computed tomography of the orbit with special emphasis on coronal sections: Part 1. Normal anatomy. J. Comput. Assist. Tomogr. **2**, 24 (1978).

Testut, L., Latarjet, A.: Tratado de Anatomia Humana, Vol. II, p. 441. Angiologia-Sistema Nervioso Central. Barcelona: Salvat Editores (1974).

Theron, J.: Les affluents du plexus caverneux. Neurochirurgie **18**, 623–638 (1972).

Thompson, J. S.: Core Textbook of Anatomy, pp. 204–206. Philadelphia: J. B. Lippincott (1977).

Thorek, P.: Anatomy in Surgery, p. 58. Philadelphia: J. B. Lippincott (1951).

Trobe, J. D., Glaser, J. S., Post, J. D., et al.: Bilateral optic canal meningiomas: a case report. Neurosurgery **3**, 68–74 (1978).

Umansky, F., Nathan, H.: The lateral wall of the cavernous sinus. J. Neurosurg. **56**, 228–234 (1982).

Unsöld, R.: Computed Tomography in Ophthalmology, Vol. **22**, No. 4, pp. 45–80. Boston, Massachusetts: Little, Brown and Company (1982).

Unsöld, R.: On the CT diagnosis of optic nerve lesions. Differential diagnostic criteria. Albrecht von Graefes Arch. Klin. Exp. Ophthalmol. **281**, 124 (1982).

Unsöld, R., DeGroot, J., Newton, T. H.: Images of the optic nerve: Anatomic-CT correlation. Am. J. Neuroradiol. **1**, 317 (1980).

Unsöld, R., Newton, T. H., Berninger, W.: The Value and Clinical Application of Multiplanar Computer Reformations in Orbital Diagnosis. In: Diagnostic Radiology 1980. Proceedings of the Annual Postgraduate Course in Diagnostic Radiology, San Francisco, Mar. 3–7, 1980 (Margulis, A. R., Gooding, C. A., eds.). San Francisco: University of California, Department of Radiology (1980).

Unsöld, R., Newton, T. H., DeGroot, J.: CT evaluation of extraocular muscles: Anatomic-CT correlations. Albrecht von Graefes Arch. Klin. Exp. Ophthalmol. **214**, 155 (180).

Unsöld, R., Newton, T. H., Hoyt, W. F.: CT examination technique of the optic nerve. J. Comput. Assist. Tomogr. **4** (4), 560 (1980).

Unsöld, R., Norman, D., Berninger, W.: Multiplanar evaluation of the optic canal from axial transverse CT sections. J. Comput. Assist. Tomogr. **4** (3), 418 (1980).

Vignaud, J., Aubin, M.-L.: Coronal (frontal) sections in computerized tomography of the orbit. J. Neuroradiol. **5**, 161 (1978).

Vignaud, J., Clay, C., Aubin, M. L., et al.: Opacification du sinus caverneux. Intérèt de la tomographie simultanée. J. Radiol. Electrol. Med. Nucl. **53**, 51–53 (1972).

Vignaud, J., Clay, C., Kujas, A., et al.: Phlebo-tomographies simultanées du sinus caverneux. Neurochirurgie **18**, 665–675 (1972).

Vignaud, J., Doyon, D., Aubin, M. L., et al.: Opacification du sinus caverneux par voix postérieure. Neurochirurgie **18**, 649–664 (1972).

Walsh, F. B.: Meningiomas primary within the orbit and the optic canal in Lawton Smith J. (ed.): Neuro-Ophthalmology, Symposium of the University of Miami and the Bascom Palmer Eye Institute, Vol. **V**, pp. 240–266. Hallandale, Florida: Huffman Publishing (1970).

Warwick, R., Williams, P. L. (eds.): Gray's Anatomy, ed. **35**, p. 695. Edinburgh: Longman (1973).

Warwick, R.: In: Anatomy of the Eye and Orbit (Wolff, E., Last, R. J., eds.), 7th ed. London: H. K. Lewis (1976).

Watanabe, T. J., LaMasters, D., et al.: Contrast Enhancement of the Normal Orbit. In International Workshop on Contrast Media in Computed Tomography, Berlin 1981. International Congress Series No. **561**. Amsterdam: Excerpta Medica (1981).

Weinberger, L. M., Adler, F. H., Grant, F. C.: Primary pituitary adenoma and the syndrome of the cavernous sinus. A clinical and anatomic study. Arch. Ophthalmol. **24**, (NS), 1196–1236 (1940).

Weinstein, M. A., Modic, M. T., Risius, B., et al.: Visualization of arteries, veins and nerves of the orbit by sector computed tomography. Radiology **138**, 83 (1981).

Weizenhoffer, A.: Contralateral cavernous sinus thrombosis. NY State J. Med. **32**, 139–142 (1932).

Williams, F. P., Shawker, T. H., Lora, J.: Pneumosinus dilatans of the sphenoid sinus. Bull. Los Angeles Neurol. Soc. **40**, 45–48 (1975).

Winslow, J. B.: Exposition anatomique de la structure du corps humain, Vol. **2**, p. 31. London: Prevost (1732).

Wolff, E.: The Anatomy of the Eye and Orbit, 4th ed., pp. 14, 287, 288, 370. London: Lewis (1954).

Wood Jones, F.: Buchanan's Manual of Anatomy, 8th ed., p. 1175. London: Baillière, Tindall and Cox (1949).

Zozulia, Y. A., Romodanov, S. A., Patsko, Y. V.: Diagnosis and surgical treatment of benign craniobasal tumours involving the cavernous sinus. Acta Neurochir. (Wien) Suppl. **28**, 387–390 (1979).

Chapter 3

Bostroem, A., Spatz, H.: Über die von der Olfactoriusrinne ausgehenden Meningeome und über die Meningeome im allgemeinen. Nervenarzt **2**, 505–521 (1929).

Bradac, G. B.: Some aspects of the venous drainage dynamics with tumors at the bone of the skull in the anterior and middle fossae. Neuroradiology **12**, 115–120 (1976).

Dandy, W. E.: Prechiasmal intracranial tumors of the optic nerve. Amer. J. Ophthal. **5**, 169–188 (1922).

Dietz, H.: Die frontobasale Schädelhirnverletzung. Berlin–Heidelberg–New York: Springer (1970). See there further literature before 1970.

Ehlers, N., Malmros, R.: The suprasellar meningioma. Acta Ophthalmol. (Copenhagen) Suppl. 121 (1973).

Hacker, H.: Venenabflüsse des Gehirns. Deutscher Röntgenkongreß (1967), Part A. Stuttgart: G. Thieme (1968b).

Haensel, G., Seeger, W.: Die mikrochirurgische Behandlung der sogenannten Tuberculum sellae-Meningeome. Acta Neurochir. (Wien) **37**, 111–123 (1977).

Hughes, B.: Blood supply of the optic nerves and chiasma and its clinical significance. Brit. J. Ophthal. **42**, 106–125 (1958).

Kaplan, H. A.: The lateral perforating branches of the anterior and middle cerebral arteries. J. Neurosurg. **23**, 305–310 (1965).

Kaplan, H. A., Browder, J.: Benign tumors of the cerebral dural sinuses. J. Neurosurg. **37**, 576–579 (1972).

Kaplan, H. A., Browder, J.: Atresia of the rostral superior sagittal sinus: substitute parasagittal venous channels. J. Neurosurg. **38**, 602–607 (1973).

Kaplan, H. A., Browder, A., Browder, J.: Nasal venous drainage and the Foramen caecum. Laryngoscope **83**, 327–329 (1973).

Krause, F.: Die spezielle Chirurgie der Gehirnkrankheiten. Bd. 2b u. 3. In: Neue Deutsche Chirurgie, Bd. 49b u. 50. Stuttgart: F. Enke (1941, 1932).

Lang, J.: Klinische Anatomie des Kopfes. Berlin–Heidelberg–New York: Springer (1981).

Lanz, T. von, Wachsmuth, W.: Praktische Anatomie, Vol. 1/1 B. Berlin–Heidelberg–New York: Springer (1979).

Liliequist, B.: The subarachnoid cisterns. Anatomic and roentgenologic study. Acta radiol. (Stockh.) Suppl. 185 (1959).

Logue, V.: Surgery of Meningiomas. In: Operative Surgery Fundamental International Techniques Neurosurgery (Symon, L., ed.), pp. 128–173. London–Boston–Sydney–Wellington–Durban–Toronto: Butterworths (1979).

Love, J. G., Gay, J. R.: Resection of the superior longitudinal sinus. J. Neurosurg. **4**, 182–188 (1947).

McCord, G. M., Goree, J. A., Jimenez, J. P.: Venous drainage to the inferior sagittal sinus. Radiology **105**, 583–589 (1972).

Maltby, G. L.: Resection of longitudinal sinus posterior to the rolandic area for complete removal of a meningioma. Arch. Neurol. Psychiat. **42**, 1135–1139 (1939).

Marc, J. A., Schechter, M. M.: Cortical venous rerouting in parasagittal meningiomas. Radiology **112**, 85–92 (1974).

Okonek, G.: Beitrag zur Erkennung und Behandlung basaler Meningeome. Zbl. Chir. **22**, 1912–1025 (1941).

Olivecrona, H.: The Surgical Treatment of Intracranial Tumors. In: Handbuch der Neurochirurgie 4/IV (Olivecrona, H., Tönnis, W., eds.), pp. 181–184. Berlin–Heidelberg–New York: Springer (1967).

Palacios, E., Fine, M., Haughton, V. M.: Multiplanar Anatomy of the Head and Neck for Computed Tomography. New York: John Wiley & Sons (1980).

Perlmutter, D., Rhoton, A. L., Jr.: Microsurgical anatomy of the anterior cerebral-anterior communicating-recurrent artery complex. J. Neurosurg. **45**, 259–271 (1976).

Pøppen, J. L.: An Atlas of Neurosurgical Techniques. Philadelphia–London: W. B. Saunders Company (1960).

Probst, Ch.: Frontobasale Verletzungen. Pathogenetische, diagnostische und therapeutische Probleme aus neurochirurgischer Sicht. Bern–Stuttgart–Wien: Hans Huber (1971). See there further literature up till 1971.

Samii, M., Draf, W.: Course on Surgery of the Skull Base. Hannover, West Germany (1979).

Samii, M., Draf, W.: Course on the Surgery of the Anterior Skull Base. Hannover, West-Germany (1980).

Samii, M., Jannetta, P. J.: Symposium on Cranial Nerves. Hannover, West-Germany (1980).

Seeger, W.: Atlas of Topographical Anatomy of the Brain and Surrounding Structures. Wien–New York: Springer (1978).

Seeger, W.: Microsurgery of the Brain. Anatomical and Technical Principles, Vol. 1+2. Wien–New York: Springer (1980).

Stephens, R. B., Stilwell, D. L.: Arteries and Veins of the Human Brain. Springfield, Ill.: Ch. C Thomas (1969).

Symon, L.: Olfactory groove and suprasellar meningiomas. In: Advances and Technical Standards in Neurosurgery (Krayenbühl, H., et al., eds.), Vol. **4**, pp. 67–91. Wien–New York: Springer (1977).

Towne, E. B.: Invasion of intracranial venous sinuses by meningioma (dural endothelioma). Ann. Surg. **83**, 321–327 (1926).

Wilson, McClure: The Anatomical Foundation of Neurology of the Brain Subarachnoid Spaces, Chapter 4, pp. 93–103. Boston: Little, Brown (1963 and 1972).

Chapter 4

Ausman, J. I., Diaz, F. G., et al.: Superficial temporal to proximal superior cerebellar artery anastomosis for basilar artery stenosis. Neurosurgery **9**, 56–59 (1981).

Ausman, J. I., Lee, M. C., et al.: Stroke: what's new? Cerebral revascularization. Minn. Med. **59**, 223–227 (1976).

Ausman, J. I., Lindsay, W., et al.: Ipsilateral subclavian to external carotid and STA-MCA bypasses for retinal ischemia. Surg. Neurol. **9**, 5–8 (1978).

Ausman, J. I., Nocoloff, D. M., Chou, S. N.: Posterior fossa revascularization: anastomosis of vertebral artery to PICA with interposed radial artery graft. Surg. Neurol. **9**, 281–286 (1978).

Barner, H. B., Judd, D. R., et al.: Late failure of arterialized in situ saphenous vein. Arch. Surg. **99**, 781–786 (1969).

Barnes, W. T., Jacoby, G. E.: Aneurysm of the common carotid artery due to cystic medial necosis treated by excision and graft. Ann. Surg. **155**, 82–85 (1962).

Baxter, Th. J., O'Brien, B., et al.: The histopathology of small vessels following microvascular repair. Brit. J. Surg. **59**, 617 (1972).

Beall, A. C., Jr., Crawford, E. S., et al.: Extracranial aneurysms of the carotid artery. Report of seven cases. Postgrad. Med. **32**, 93–102 (1962).

Brambilla, G., Paoletti, P., Rodriguez y Baena, R.: Extracranial-intracranial arterial bypass in the treatment of inoperable giant aneurysms of the internal carotid artery. Report of a Case. Acta Neurochir. (Wien) **60**, 63–69 (1982).

Chater, N. L., Popp, J.: Microsurgical vascular bypass for occlusive cerebrovascular disease: Review of 100 cases. Surg. Neurol. **6**, 115–118 (1976).

Chater, N. L., Reichmann, O. H., Tew, J.: Cerebral Revascularization – Scientific Exhibit. American Association of Neurological Surgeons. Los Angeles (1972).

Chater, N. L., Reichmann, O. H., Tew, J.: Cerebral Revascularization for Occlusive Cerebrovascular Disease. Presented at the meeting of the American Association of Neurological Surgeons. Los Angeles, April 8–11 (1973).

Chater, N. L., Spetzler, R.: Anatomical Studies of the Cerebral Cortical Vasculature of Microvascular Surgical Significance. Presented at the international Symposium on Neurosurgery Through the Microscope. Mount Sinai School of Medicine, City University of New York. New York City, June 11–14 (1973).

Chater, N. L., Spetzler, R., Tonnenmacher, K., et al.: Microvascular bypass surgery. Part I: Anatomical studies. J. Neurosurg. **44**, 712–714 (1976).

Chater, N. L., Yaşargil, M. G.: Results of Temporal Artery Bypass Procedures in Treatment of Cerebrovascular Disease. Presented at Congress of Neurological Surgeons. Miami, Florida, October 1971.

DeBakey, M. E.: Concepts underlying surgical treatment of cerebrovascular insufficiency. Clin. Neurosurg. **10**, 310–340 (1964).

De Weese, J. A., Robb, C. G.: Autogenous venous bypass grafts five years later. Ann. Surg. **174**, 346–356 (1971).

Donaghy, R. M. P., Yaşargil, M. G. (eds.): Microvascular Surgery, pp. 75–86. Report of First Conference 1966. St. Louis: Mosby (1967).

Drake, C.: The Intracranial Use of the 'Hunterian' Proximal Ligation in the Treatment of Giant Aneurysm. Presented at American Association of Neurological Surgeons, Toronto, Canada (1977).

Drake, C. G.: Giant intracranial aneurysms: experience with surgical treatment in 174 patients. Clin. Neurosurg. **26**, 12–95 (1979).

Ferguson, G. G., Drake, C. G., Peerless, S. J.: Extracranial-intracranial arterial bypass in the treatment of "giant" intracranial aneurysms. Stroke 8, 11, 1977 (Abstract).

Fields, W. S.: Selection of stroke patient for arterial reconstructive surgery. Am. J. Surg. 125, 527–529 (1973).

Galbraith, J. G., McDowell, H. A.: Stroke and occlusive cerebrovascular disease: review and surgical results in 265 cases. J. Med. Assoc. Alabama 38, 1107–1111 (1969).

Garmella, J. J., Lynch, M. F., et al.: Endarterectomy and thrombectomy for the totally occluded extracranial internal carotid artery: use of Fogarty balloon catheters. Ann. Surg. 164, 325–333 (1966).

Gelber, B. J., Sundt, T. M., Jr.: Treatment of intracavernous and giant carotid aneurysms by combined internal carotid ligation and extra- to intracranial bypass. J. Neurosurg. 52, 1–10 (1980).

Gilsbach, J. M.: Intraoperative Doppler Sonography in Neurosurgery. Wien–New York: Springer (1983).

Gratzl, O., Schmiedek, P., Oeteanu-Nube, V.: Long-term clinical results following extra-intracranial arterial bypass surgery. In: Microsurgery for Stroke (Schmiedek, P., Gratzl, O., Spetzler, R., eds.), pp. 271–275. Berlin–Heidelberg–New York: Springer (1977).

Henschen, C.: XXXVIII. Operative Revaskularisation des zirkulatorisch geschädigten Gehirns durch Auflage gestielter Muskellappen (Encephalo-Myo-Synangiose). Basel, pp. 392–401.

Holbach, K. H., Wassmann, H., Bonatelli, A. P.: A method to identify and treat reversible ischemialterations of brain tissue. In: Microsurgery for Stroke (Schmiedek, P., Gratzl, O., Spetzler, R., eds.), pp. 169–176. Berlin–Heidelberg–New York: Springer (1977).

Hopkins, L. N., Grand, W.: Extracranial-intracranial arterial bypass in the treatment of aneurysms of the carotid and middle cerebral arteries. Neurosurgery 5, 21–31 (1979).

Horváth, M., Pásztor, E., Vajda, J., Nyáry, I.: Posterior fossa revascularization by superficial temporal artery (STA) – superior cerebellar artery (SCA) anastomosis. Acta Neurochir. (Wien) 66, 43–53 (1982).

International Symposium on Microneurosurgical Anastomosis for Cerebral Ischemia. Loma Linda University School of Medicine Loma Linda Calif. June 14–15 (1973).

Jacobson, J. H., Suarez, E.: Microsurgery in anastomosis of small vessels. Surgical Forum 11, 243 (1960).

Khodadad, G.: Occipital artery-posterior inferior cerebellar artery anastomosis. Surg. Neurol. 5, 225–227 (1976).

Khodadad, G.: Short- and long-term results of microvascular anastomosis in the vertebrobasilar system: A critical analysis. Neurol. Res. 3, 33–65 (1981).

Khodadad, G., Singh, R. S., Olinger, C. P.: Possible prevention of brain stem stroke by microvascular anastomosis in the vertebrobasilar system. Stroke 8, 316–321 (1977).

Kletter, G., Koos, W. Th.: Zur Technik der arteriellen experimentellen extra-intra-kraniellen Anastomose. Acta Chir. Austriaca 8, 83 (1975).

Kletter, G., Matras, H., Dinges, H. P.: Zur partiellen Klebung von Mikrogefäßanastomosen im intrakraniellen Bereich. Wien. klin. Wschr. 90, 415–419 (1978).

Kletter, G., Meyermann, R.: Histological Case Control of Microanastomosis. Clinical Microneurosurgery 234. Stuttgart: G. Thieme (1976).

Kletter, G., Meyermann, R.: Histologische Veränderungen nach Mikrogefäßanastomosen. Acta Chirurg. Austriaca 2, 35 (1977).

Kletter, G., Meyermann, R., Koos, W. Th., Schuster, H.: L'importance de la structure histologique de l'artère temporale superficielle pour la fonction de l'anastomose arterielle extra-intracrânienne. Neurochirurgie (Paris) 21, 551 (1975).

Kopaniky, D., Spetzler, R. F.: Severe otorrhagia resulting from a ruptured aneurysm of the extracranial internal carotid artery (in preparation).

Krayenbühl, H.: Comments on the history of external-internal anastomosis for cerebral ischemia. In: Microsurgery for Stroke (Schmiedek, P., Gratzl, O., Spetzler, R., eds.), pp. 3–7. Berlin–Heidelberg–NewYork: Springer (1977).

Lang, J.: Klinische Anatomie des Kopfes. Berlin–Heidelberg–New York: Springer (1981).

Lanz, T. von, Wachsmuth, W.: Praktische Anatomie, Vol. 1/1B. Berlin–Heidelberg–New York: Springer (1979).

Lazar, M. L., Clark, K.: Microsurgical cerebral revascularization: concept and practice. Surg. Neurol. 1, 355–359 (1973).

Lougheed, W. M., Marshall, B. M., et al.: Common carotid to intracranial internal carotid bypass venous graft. J. Neurosurg. 34, 114–118 (1971).

Matras, H., Chiari, F., et al.: Zur Klebung von Mikrogefäßanastomosen. Bericht d. 13. Jtgg. d. Dtsch. Ges. f. plast. und Wiederherstellungschir., 1975, S. 357. Stuttgart: G. Thieme (1977).

Matras, H., Chiari, F., et al.: Neue Wege in der Mikrogefäßchirurgie (eine experimentelle Studie). Bericht d. 17. Tagung der Österr. Ges. f. Chir., Salzburg, 1976. Acta Chir. Austr. Sonder-Supplement S. 458 (1976/77).

Matras, H., Chiari, F., et al.: Zur Klebung kleinster Gefäße im Tierversuch. Dtsch. Z. Mund-Kiefer-Gesichts-Chir. 1, 19 (1977).

Meyermann, R., Kletter, G.: Causes of Stenosis and Embolic Occlusions in Microsurgical Anastomosis. Advances in Neurosurgery 2, 322 (1975).

Miller, C. F. II, Spetzler, R. F., Kopaniky, D. J.: Middle meningeal to middle cerebral arterial bypass for cerebral revascularization. Case report. J. Neurosurg. 50, 802–804 (1979).

Nunn, D. B., Chun, B., et al.: Autogeneous veins as arterial substitutes: A study of their histologic fate with special attention to endothelium. Ann. Surg. 160, 14–22 (1964).

Ohara, I., Utsumi, N., Ouchi, H.: Resection of extracranial internal carotid artery aneurysms with arterial reconstruction. J. Cardiovasc. Surg. 9, 365–373 (1968).

Palacios, E., Fine, M., Haughton, V. M.: Multiplanar Anatomy of the Head and Neck for Computed Tomography. New York: John Wiley & Sons (1980).

Peerless, S. J., Chater, N. L., Ferguson, G. G.: Multiple-vessel occlusions in cerebro-vascular disease – A further follow up of the effects of microvascular bypass on the quality of life and the incidence of stroke. In: Microsurgery for Stroke (Schmiedek, P., Gratzl, O., Spetzler, R., eds.), pp. 251–259. Berlin–Heidelberg–New York: Springer (1977).

Raphael, H. A., Bernatz, P. E., Spittell, J. A., Jr., et al.: Cervical carotid aneurysms: treatment by excision and restoration of arterial continuity. Am. J. Surg. **105,** 771–778 (1963).

Reichmann, O. H.: Experimental lingual-basilar arterial microanastomosis. J. Neurosurg. **34,** 500–505 (1971).

Reichmann, O. H.: Extracranial-intracranial arterial anastomosis. In: Cerebral Vascular Diseases: Ninth Conference (Whisnant, J. P., Sandok, B. A., eds.), pp. 175–185. New York: Grune and Stratton (1975).

Roski, R., Spetzler, R. F., et al.: Reversal of documented seven-year old visual field defect with extracranial-intracranial arteriel anastomosis. Surg. Neurol. **10,** 267–268 (1978).

Roski, R. A., Spetzler, R. F., et al.: Occipital artery to posterior inferior cerebellar artery bypass for vertebrobasilar ischemia. Neurosurgery **10,** No. 1, 44–49 (1982).

Samii, M., Draf, W.: Course on Surgery of the Skull Base. Hannover, West Germany (1979).

Samii, M., Jannetta, P. J.: Symposium on Cranial Nerves. Hannover, West-Germany (1980).

Samson, S., Neuwelt, E. A., et al.: Failure of extracranial-intracranial arterial bypass in acute middle cerebral artery occlusion. Case report. Neurosurgery **6,** 185–188 (1980).

Schmiedek, P., Gratzl, O., et al.: Selection of patients for extracranial arterial bypass surgery based on rCBF measurements. J. Neurosurg. **44,** 303–312 (1976).

Seeger, W.: Atlas of Topographical Anatomy of the Brain and Surrounding Structures. Wien–New York: Springer (1978).

Seeger, W.: Microsurgery of the Brain. Anatomical and Technical Principles, Vol. 1 + 2. Wien–New York: Springer (1980).

Spetzler, R. F.: Extracranial-intracranial arterial anastomosis for cerebrovascular disease. Surg. Neurol. **11,** 157–161 (1979).

Spetzler, R. F., Chater, N. L.: Occipital artery-middle cerebral anastomosis for cerebral artery occlusive disease. Surg. Neurol. **2,** 235–238 (1974).

Spetzler, R., Chater, N.: Microvascular bypass surgery. Part 2: Physiological studies. J. Neurosurg. **45,** 508–513 (1976).

Spetzler, R. F., Chater, N. L.: Microvascular arterial bypass in cerebrovascular occlusive disease. In: Clinical Microneurosurgery (Koos, W. Th., Bock, F. W., Spetzler, R. F., eds.), pp. 242–246. Stuttgart: G. Thieme (1976).

Spetzler, R., Chater, N. L., Mani, J.: The spectrum of intracranial occlusive disease suitable for microvascular bypass. J. Radiol. (submitted).

Spetzler, R. F., Iversen, A. A.: Alleable microsurgical suction device: Technical note. J. Neurosurg. **54,** 704–705 (1981).

Spetzler, R. F., Owen, M. P.: Extracranial-intracranial arterial bypass to a single branch of the middle cerebral artery in the management of a traumatic aneurysm. Neurosurgery **4,** 334–337 (1979).

Spetzler, R. F., Rhodes, R. S., et al.: Subclavian to middle cerebral artery saphenous vein bypass graft. J. Neurosurg. **53,** 465–469 (1980).

Spetzler, R. F., Roski, R. A., et al.: The 'bonnet bypass'. J. Neurosurg. **53,** 707–709 (1980).

Spetzler, R. F., Schuster, H., Roski, R. A.: Elective extracranial-intracranial arterial bypass in the treatment of inoperable giant aneurysms of the internal carotid artery. J. Neurosurg. **53,** 22–27 (1980).

Story, J. L., Brown, W. E., Jr., et al.: Cerebral revascularization: common carotid to distal middle cerebral artery bypass. Neurosurgery **2,** 131–134 (1978).

Story, J. L., Brown, W. E., Jr., et al.: Cerebral revascularization: proximal external carotid to distal middle cerebral artery bypass with a synthetic tube graft. Neurosurgery **3,** 61–65 (1978).

Story, J. L., Brown, W. E., Jr., et al.: Cerebral revascularization: cervical carotid-intracranial arterial long graft bypass. In: Advances in Neurosurgery, Vol. 7 (Marguth, F., Brock M., Kazner, E., et al., eds.), pp. 15–23. Berlin–Heidelberg–New York: Springer (1979).

Sundt, T. M., Piepgras, D. G.: Occipital to posterior inferior cerebellar artery bypass surgery. J. Neurosurg. **48,** 916–928 (1978).

Sundt, T. M., Siekert, R. G., et al.: Bypass surgery for vascular disease of the carotid system. Mayo Clinic Rochester Minn. **51,** 677–692 (1976).

Sundt, T. M., Whisnat, J. P., Piepgras, D. G., et al.: Intracranial bypass grafts for vertebral-basilar ischemia. Mayo Clin. Proc. **53,** 12–18 (1978).

Sundt, T. M., Jr.: Editorial comment to Reference 1. Neurosurgery **9,** 59–60 (1981).

Sundt, T. M., Jr., Campbell, J. K., Houser, O. W.: Transpositions and anastomoses between the posterior cerebral and superior cerebellar arteries. J. Neurosurg. **55,** 967–970 (1981).

Sundt, T. M., Jr., Houser, O. W., et al.: Interposition saphenous vein grafts between the external carotid artery and the proximal posterior cerebral artery for advanced occlusive disease and large aneurysms in the posterior circulation. J. Neurosurg. **56,** 1982 (in press).

Sundt, T. M., Jr., Piepgras, D. G.: Surgical approach to giant intracranial aneurysms. Operative experience with 80 cases. J. Neurosurg. **51,** 731–742 (1979).

Sundt, T. M., Jr., Smith, H. C., et al.: Transluminal angioplasty for basilar artery stenosis. Mayo Clin. Proc. **55,** 673–680 (1980).

Tew, J. M., Jr.: Reconstructive intracranial vascular surgery for prevention of stroke. Clin. Neurosurg. **22,** 264–280 (1975).

Thompson, J. E., Austin, D. J.: Endarterectomy of the totally occluded carotid artery for stroke: Results in 100 operations. Arch. Surg. **95,** 791–801 (1967).

Weinstein, P. R., Chater, N. L., et al.: Extra- to intracranial arterial bypass for occlusive vertebro-basilar cerebrovascular disease. Presented at the meeting of American Association of Neurological Surgeons. Miami, April 1975.

Wilson, J. R., Jordan, P. H., Jr.: Excision of an internal carotid artery aneurysm: restitution of continuity by substitution of external for internal carotid artery. Ann. Surg. **154,** 45–47 (1961).

Yaşargil, M. G., Krayenbühl, H. A., Jacobson, J. H.: Microsurgery Applied to Neurosurgery, 230 pp. Stuttgart: G. Thieme (1969).

Yaşargil, M. G., Krayenbühl, H. A., Jacobson, J. H. II: Microneurosurgical arterial reconstruction. Surgery **67,** 221–233 (1970).

Yaşargil, M. G., Yonekawa, Y.: Results of microsurgical extra-intracranial arterial bypass in the treatment of cerebral ischemia. Neurosurgery **1,** 22–24 (1977).

Chapter 5

Apfelbaum, R. I.: A comparison of percutaneous radiofrequency trigeminal neurolysis and microvascular decompression of the trigeminal nerve for the treatment of tic douloureux. Neurosurgery **1**, 16–21 (1977).

Apfelbaum, R. I.: Surgical management of disorders of lower cranial nerves. In: Current Techniques in Operative Neurosurgery, 2nd ed. (Schmidek, H. H., ed.). New York: Grune/Stratton (1982).

Atkinson, W. J.: The anterior inferior cerebellar artery: Its variations, pontine distributions, and significance in the surgery of cerebello-pontine angle tumors. J. Neurol. Neurosurg. Psychiat. **12**, 137–151 (1949).

Burchiel, K. J., Steege, T. D., Howe, J. F., Loeser, J. D.: Comparison of percutaneous radiofrequency gangliolysis and microvascular decompression for the surgical management of tic douloureux. Neurosurgery **9**, 111–119, (1981).

Campbell, E., Keedy, C.: Hemifacial spasm: A note of the etiology in two cases. J. Neurosurg. **4**, 342–347 (1944).

Cushing, H.: The major trigeminal neuralgias and their surgical treatment based on experiences with 332 gasserian operations; the varieties of facial neuralgia. Am. J. Med. Sci. **160**, 157–184 (1920).

Dandy, W. E.: An operation for the cure of tic douloureux. Partial section of the sensory root at the pons. Arch. Surg. **18**, 687–734 (1929).

Dandy, W. E.: The treatment of trigeminal neuralgia by the cerebellar route. Ann. Surg. **96**, 787–795 (1932).

Dandy, W. E.: Concerning the cause of trigeminal neuralgia. Am. J. Surg. **24**, 447–455 (1934).

Dandy, W. E.: Trigeminal neuralgia and trigeminal tic douloureux. In: Lewis' Practice of Surgery, Vol. 12, pp. 167–187. Hagerstown, Md.: W. F. Prior (1946).

Fisch, U.: The surgical anatomy of the so-called internal auditory artery. In: Disorders of the Skull Base Region; Proceedings: Nobel Symposium, 10th, Stockholm, 1968 (Hamberger, C.-A., Wersäll, J., eds.), pp. 121–130. Stockholm: Almqvist and Wiksell, New York: Wiley (1968).

Gardner, W. J.: The mechanism of tic douloureux. Trans. Am. Neurol. Assoc. **78**, 168–173 (1953).

Gardner, W. J.: Concerning the mechanism of trigeminal neuralgia and hemifacial spasm. J. Neurosurg. **19**, 947–957 (1962).

Gardner, W. J., Miklos, W. V.: Response of trigeminal neuralgia to 'decompression' of sensory route: Discussion of cause of trigeminal neuralgia. JAMA **170**, 1773–1776 (1959).

Gardner, W. J., Sava, G. A.: Hemifacial spasm – A reversible pathophysiologic state. J. Neurosurg. **20**, 240–247 (1962).

German, W. J.: Surgical treatment of spasmodic facial tic. Surgery **11**, 912–914 (1942).

Granit, R., Skoglund, C. R., Leksell, L.: Fibre interaction in injured or compressed region of nerve. Brain **67**, 125–140 (1944).

Haines, S. J., Jannetta, P. J., Zorub, D. S.: Microvascular relations of the trigeminal nerve: An anatomical study with clinical correlation. J. Neurosurg. **52**, 381–386 (1980).

Haines, S. J., Martinez, A. J., Jannetta, P. J.: Arterial cross compression of the trigeminal nerve at the pons in trigeminal neuralgia: Case report with autopsy findings. J. Neurosurg. **50**, 257–259 (1979).

Hanraets, P. R.: Surgical treatment of trigeminal neuralgia following the method of Dandy. Psychiatr. Neurol. Neurochir. **73**, 441–446 (1970).

Hardy, D. G., Rhoton, A. L.: Microsurgical relationships of the superior cerebellar artery and the trigeminal nerve. J. Neurosurg. **49**, 669–678 (1978).

Jannetta, P. J.: Arterial compression of the trigeminal nerve at the pons in patients with trigeminal neuralgia. J. Neurosurg. (Suppl.) **26**, 159–162 (1967).

Jannetta, P. J.: Microsurgical exploration and decompression of the facial nerve in hemifacial spasm. Curr. Topics Surg. Res. **2**, 217–220 (1970).

Jannetta, P. J.: Trigeminal and glossopharyngeal neuralgia. Curr. Diagnosis **3**, 849–850 (1971).

Jannetta, P. J.: Neurovascular compression of the facial nerve in hemifacial spasm. Relief by microsurgical technique. In: Reconstructive Surgery of Brain Arteries (Merei, R. T., ed.), pp. 193–199. Budapest, Hungary: Akademiai Kiado (1974).

Jannetta, P. J.: Neurovascular cross-compression in patients with hyperactive dysfunction symptoms of the eighth cranial nerve. Surg. Forum **26**, 467–469 (1975).

Jannetta, P. J.: Microsurgical approach to the trigeminal nerve for tic douloureux. In: Progress in Neurological Surgery, Vol. 7: Pain – Its Neurosurgical Management (Krayenbühl, H., Maspes, P. S., Sweet, W. H., eds.), pp. 180–200. Basel: S. Karger (1976).

Jannetta, P. J.: Observations on the etiology of trigeminal neuralgia, hemifacial spasm, acoustic nerve dysfunction and glossopharyngeal neuralgia: Definitive microsurgical treatment and results in 117 patients. Neurochirurgia (Stuttg.) **20**, 145–154 (1977).

Jannetta, P. J.: Treatment of trigeminal neuralgia by suboccipital and transtentorial cranial operations. Clin. Neurosurg. **24**, 538–549 (1977).

Jannetta, P. J.: Microsurgery of cranial nerve cross-compression. Clin. Neurosurg. **26**, 607–615, (1979).

Jannetta, P. J.: Treatment of trigeminal neuralgia. Neurosurgery **4**, 93–94 (1979).

Jannetta, P. J., Abbasy, M., Maroon, J. C., Ramos, F. M., Albin, M. S.: Hemifacial spasm: Etiology and definitive microsurgical treatment of hemifacial spasm. Operative techniques and results in 47 patients. J. Neurosurg. **47**, 321–328 (1977).

Jannetta, P. J., Hackett, E., Ruby, J. R.: Electromyographic and electron microscopic correlates in hemifacial spasm treated by microsurgical relief of neurovascular compression. Surg. Forum **21**, 449–451 (1970).

Jannetta, P. J., Rand, R. W.: Microanatomy of the trigeminal nerve. Anat. Rec. 154–362 (1966).

Jannetta, P. J., Rand, R. W.: Transtentorial retro-gasserian rhizotomy in trigeminal neuralgia by microneurosurgical technique. Bull., L. A. Neurol. Soc. **31**, 93–99 (1966).

Lang, J.: Klinische Anatomie des Kopfes. Berlin–Heidelberg–New York: Springer (1981).

Lanz, T. von, Wachsmuth, W.: Praktische Anatomie, Vol. 1/1B. Berlin–Heidelberg–New York: Springer (1979).

Lee, F. C.: Trigeminal neuralgia. J. Med. Assoc. Georgia **26**, 431 (1937).

Lewy, F. H., Grant, F. C.: Physiopathologic and pathoanatomic aspects of major trigeminal neuralgia. Arch. Neurol. Psychiat. **40**, 1126–1134 (1938).

Liliequist, B.: The subarachnoid cisterns. Anatomic and roentgenologic study. Acta radiol. (Stockh.) Suppl. 185, 1959.

Martin, R. G., Grant, J. L., Peace, D., Theiss, C., Rhoton, A. L.: Microsurgical relationships of the anterior inferior cerebellar artery and the facial-vestibulocochlear nerve complex. Neurosurgery **6**, 483–507 (1980).

Matsushima, Y., et al.: A new surgical treatment of moyamoya disease in children: a preliminary report. Surg. Neurol. **15**, 313–320 (1981).

Mazzoni, A.: Internal auditory canal: Arterial relations at the porus acusticus. Ann. Otol. Rhinol. Laryngol. **78**, 797–814 (1969).

Nager, G. T.: Origins and relations of the internal auditory artery and the subarcuate artery. Ann. Otol. Rhinol. Laryngol. **63**, 51–61 (1954).

Naidich, T. P., Kricheff, I. I., George, A. E., Lin, J. P.: The anterior inferior cerebellar artery in mass lesions: Preliminary findings with emphasis on the lateral projection. Radiology **119**, 375–383 (1976).

Nieuwenhuys, R., Voogd, J., van Juijzen, Chr.: The Human Central Nervous System. A Synopsis and Atlas. Berlin–Heidelberg–New York: Springer (1978).

Palacios, E., Fine, M., Haughton, V. M.: Multiplanar Anatomy of the Head and Neck for Computed Tomography. New York: John Wiley & Sons (1980).

Rand, R. W.: Microneurosurgery. 2nd ed. St. Louis: Mosby (1978).

Rand, R. W.: Functional and Anatomic Localization in the Trigeminal Root: in Support of Dandy. In: Current Controversies in Neurosurgery (Morley, T. P., ed.), pp. 533–538. Philadelphia: Saunders (1976).

Rand, R. W.: Microsurgical operations in the treatment of trigeminal neuralgia. J. Microsurg. **1**, 101–107 (1979).

Rand, R. W.: Gardner neurovascular decompression of the trigeminal and facial nerves for tic douloureux and hemifacial spasm. Surg. Neurol. **16**, 329–332 (1981).

Rand, R. W., Jannetta, P. J.: Microneurosurgery: application of the binocular surgical microscope in brain tumors, intracranial aneurysms, spinal cord disease and nerve reconstruction. Clin. Neurosurg. **15**, 319–342 (1967).

Rhoton, A. L.: Microsurgical removal of acoustic neuromas. Surg. Neurol. **6**, 211–219 (1976).

Rhoton, A. L.: Microsurgical neurovascular decompression for trigeminal neuralgia and hemifacial spasm. J. Fla. Med. Assoc. **65**, 425–428 (1978).

Samii, M., Draf, W.: Course on Surgery of the Skull Base. Hannover, West Germany (1979).

Samii, M., Draf, W.: Course on the Surgery of the Posterior Skull Base. Hannover, West-Germany (1982).

Samii, M., Jannetta, P. J.: Symposium on Cranial Nerves. Hannover, West-Germany (1980).

Scoville, W. B.: Partial extracranial section of seventh nerve for hemifacial spasm. J. Neurosurg. **31**, 106–108 (1969).

Seeger, W.: Atlas of Topographical Anatomy of the Brain and Surrounding Structures. Wien–New York: Springer (1978).

Seeger, W.: Microsurgery of the Brain. Anatomical and Technical Principles, Vol. 1 + 2. Wien–New York: Springer (1980).

Spiller, W. G., Frazier, C. H.: Tic douloureux; anatomic and clinical basis for subtotal section of sensory root of trigeminal nerve. Arch. Neurol. Psychiat. **29**, 50–55 (1933).

Sunderland, S.: The arterial relations of the internal auditory meatus. Brain **68**, 23–27 (1945).

Taarnhøj, P.: Decompression of the trigeminal root and the posterior part of the ganglion as treatment in trigeminal neuralgia. Preliminary communication. J. Neurosurg. **9**, 288–290 (1952).

Taarnhøj, P.: Ny operation ved trigeminus neuralgi. Decompression af trigeminusroden og gangliets bageste del. Nord. Med. **47**, 360–361 (1952).

Taarnhøj, P.: Decompression of the trigeminal root. J. Neurosurg. **11**, 299–305 (1954).

Taarnhøj, P.: Trigeminal neuralgia and decompression of the trigeminal root. Surg. Clin. North. Am. **36** (4), 1145–1157 (1956).

Waga, S., Marikawa, A., Kojima, T.: Trigeminal neuralgia: Compression of the trigeminal nerve by an elongated and dilated basilar artery. Surg. Neurol. **11**, 13–16 (1979).

Watt, J. C., McKillip, A. N.: Relation of arteries to roots of nerves in posterior cranial fossa in man. Arch. Surg. **30**, 336–345 (1935).

Willis, T.: The Anatomy of the Brain and Nerves. Tercentenary ed. 1664, Feindel, W. Montreal: McGill University Press. 1965.

Wilson, McClure: The Anatomical Foundation of Neurology of the Brain Subarachnoid Spaces. Chapter 4, pp. 93–103. Boston: Little, Brown. 1963 and 1972.

Wilson, C. B., Torke, C., Prioleau, G.: Microsurgical vascular decompression for trigeminal neuralgia and hemifacial spasm. West. J. Med. **132**, 481–484 (1980).

Wolf, B. S., Huang, Y. P., Newman, C. M.: Lateral anastomotic mesencephalic vein and other variations in drainage of basal cerebral vein. Amer. J. Roentgenol. **89**, 411–422 (1963).

Yaşargil, M. G., Fox, J. L.: The microsurgical approach to acoustic neuromas. Surg. Neurol. **2**, 393–398 (1974).

Chapter 6

Krause, F.: Die spezielle Chirurgie der Gehirnkrankheiten, Bd. 2b u. 3. In: Neue Deutsche Chirurgie, Bd. 49b u. 50. Stuttgart: F. Enke (1941, 1932).

Lang, J.: Klinische Anatomie des Kopfes. Berlin–Heidelberg–New York: Springer (1981).

Lanz, T. von, Wachsmuth, W.: Praktische Anatomie, Vol. 1/1B. Berlin–Heidelberg–New York: Springer (1979).

Liliequist, B.: The subarachnoid cisterns. Anatomic and roentgenologic study. Acta radiol. (Stockh.) Suppl. 185 (1959).

Logue, V.: Surgery of Meningiomas. In: Operative Surgery Fundamental International Techniques Neurosurgery (Symon, L., ed.), pp. 128–173. London, Boston, Sydney, Wellington, Burban, Toronto: Butterworths (1979).

Nieuwenhuys, R., Voogd, J., van Juijzen, Chr.: The Human Central Nervous System. A Synopsis and Atlas. Berlin–Heidelberg–New York: Springer (1978).

Okonek, G.: Beitrag zur Erkennung und Behandlung basaler Meningeome. Zbl. Chir. **22,** 1912–1925 (1941).

Olivecrona, H.: The Surgical Treatment of Intracranial Tumors. In: Handbuch der Neurochirurgie 4/IV (Olivecrona, H., Tönnis, W., eds.), pp. 181–184. Berlin–Heidelberg–New York: Springer (1967).

Palacios, E., Fine, M., Haughton, V. M.: Multiplanar Anatomy of the Head and Neck for Computed Tomography. New York: John Wiley & Sons (1980).

Poppen, J. L.: An Atlas of Neurosurgical Techniques. Philadelphia–London: W. B. Saunders Company (1960).

Samii, M., Draf, W.: Course on Surgery of the Skull Base. Hannover, West-Germany (1979).

Samii, M., Draf, W.: Course on the Surgery of the Posterior Skull Base. Hannover, West-Germany (1982).

Samii, M., Jannetta, P. J.: Symposium on Cranial Nerves. Hannover, West-Germany (1980).

Seeger, W.: Atlas of Topographical Anatomy of the Brain and Surrounding Structures. Wien–New York: Springer (1978).

Seeger, W.: Microsurgery of the Brain. Anatomical and Technical Principles, Vol. 1+2. Wien–New York: Springer (1980).

Seeger, W.: Microsurgery of the Spinal Cord and Surrounding Structures. Anatomical and Technical Principles. Wien–New York: Springer (1982).

Stephens, R. B., Stilwell, D. L.: Arteries and Veins of the Human Brain. Springfield, Ill.: Ch. C Thomas (1969).

Willis, T.: The Anatomy of the Brain and Nerves. Tercentenary ed. 1664, Feindel, W. Montreal: McGill University Press (1965).

Wilson, McClure: The Anatomical Foundation of Neurology of the Brain Subarachnoid Spaces, Chapter 4, pp. 93–103. Boston: Little, Brown (1963 and 1972).

Wolf, B. S., Huang, Y. P., Newman, C. M.: Lateral anastomotic mesencephalic vein and other variations in drainage of basal cerebral vein. Amer. J. Roentgenol. **89,** 411–422 (1963).

Subject Index

Printed by Ferdinand Berger & Söhne Gesellschaft m.b.H., A-3580 Horn

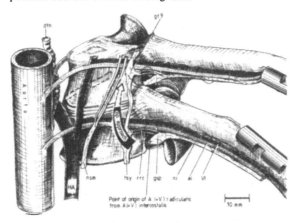

Printed in the United States
By Bookmasters